Gupta and Gelb's Essentials of Neuroanesthesia and Neurointensive Care

Gupta and Gelb's Essentials of Neuroanesthesia and Neurointensive Care

Second Edition

Edited by

Arun Gupta
Cambridge University Hospitals, UK

Adrian Gelb
University of California, San Francisco, USA

Derek Duane
Cambridge University Hospitals, UK

Ram Adapa
Cambridge University Hospitals, UK

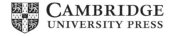

CAMBRIDGE
UNIVERSITY PRESS

University Printing House, Cambridge CB2 8BS, United Kingdom

One Liberty Plaza, 20th Floor, New York, NY 10006, USA

477 Williamstown Road, Port Melbourne, VIC 3207, Australia

314–321, 3rd Floor, Plot 3, Splendor Forum, Jasola District Centre, New Delhi – 110025, India

79 Anson Road, #06–04/06, Singapore 079906

Cambridge University Press is part of the University of Cambridge.

It furthers the University's mission by disseminating knowledge in the pursuit of
education, learning, and research at the highest international levels of excellence.

www.cambridge.org
Information on this title: www.cambridge.org/9781316602522
DOI: 10.1017/9781316556801

© Cambridge University Press 2018

First published 2008 by Elsevier
Second Edition Cambridge University Press 2018

Printed in the United Kingdom by Clays, St Ives plc

A catalogue record for this publication is available from the British Library.

Library of Congress Cataloging-in-Publication Data
Names: Adapa, Ram, 1975– editor. | Gupta, Arun K., editor. | Gelb, Adrian W., editor.
Title: Gupta and Gelb's essentials of neuroanesthesia and neurointensive care / edited by Ram Adapa,
Addenbrooke's Hospital, Cambridge, Derek Duane, Addenbrooke's Hospital, Cambridge, Adrian Gelb,
University of Cambridge San Francisco, Arun Gupta, Addenbrooke's Hospital, Cambridge.
Other titles: Essentials of neuroanesthesia and neurointensive care.
Description: Second edition. | Cambridge, United Kingdom ; New York, NY : Cambridge University Press,
2018. | Revised edition of: Essentials of neuroanesthesia and neurointensive care / [edited by] Arun K.
Gupta, Adrian W. Gelb. Saunders Elsevier, c2008. | Includes bibliographical references and index.
Identifiers: LCCN 2017046824 | ISBN 9781316602522 (paperback)
Subjects: LCSH: Anesthesia in neurology. | Neurological intensive care. | Nervous system – Surgery. | BISAC:
MEDICAL / Anesthesiology.
Classification: LCC RD87.3.N47 E87 2018 | DDC 617.9/6748–dc23
LC record available at https://lccn.loc.gov/2017046824

ISBN 978-1-316-60252-2 Paperback

....

Contents

Section 5 – Neurointensive Care

Contributors

Anthony Absalom
University Medical Center, Groningen, The Netherlands

Ashish Agrawal
University of California, San Francisco, CA, USA

Dr Poppy Aldam
Cambridge University Hospitals, UK

Ricardo Andrade
University of Chicago, Chicago, IL, USA

Shymal Asher
University of Chicago Pritzker School of Medicine, Chicago, IL, USA

Philip E. Bickler
University of California, San Francisco, CA, USA

Anne Booth
Cambridge University Hospitals, UK

Kristine E. W. Breyer
University of California, San Francisco, CA, USA

Erika Brinson
University of California, San Francisco, CA, USA

Nicolas Bruder
Aix Marseille University, Marseille, France

Karol Budohoski
Cambridge University Hospitals, UK

Dr Rowan Burnstein
Cambridge University Hospitals, UK

Eleanor Carter
Cambridge University Hospitals, UK

Joyce Chang
University of California, San Francisco, CA, USA

Xinying Chen
Khoo Teck Puat Hospital, Singapore

Randall Chesnut
University of Washington, USA

Sarah Chetcuti
Cambridge University Hospitals, UK

Jason Chui
Western University, London, Ontario, Canada

Craig D. McClain
Harvard Medical School, Boston, MA, USA

Jonathan P. Coles
University of Cambridge, UK

Rosemary Ann Craen
Western University, London, Canada

Marek Czosnyka
University of Cambridge, Cambridge, UK

Michael McDermott
University of California, San Francisco, CA, USA

Anne L. Donovan
University of California, San Francisco, CA, USA

Ari Ercole
Cambridge University Hospitals, UK

Alana M. Flexman
University of British Columbia,
Vancouver, BC, Canada

Dean Frear
Addenbrooke's Hospital, Cambridge, UK

Tamsin Gregory
Airedale General Hospital, UK

Donald Griesdale
University of British Columbia,
Vancouver, BC, Canada

Shaun E. Gruenbaum
Yale University School of Medicine, New
Haven, CT, USA

Mathew Guilfoyle
Cambridge University Hospitals, UK

Antoine Halwagi
Hôpital Notre-Dame, Montréal,
Canada

Bradley Hay
University of California, San Diego,
CA, USA

Manuel Aliaño Hermoso
Cambridge University Hospitals, UK

Sophia Yi
University of California, San Diego,
CA, USA

Piyush Patel
University of California, San Diego,
CA, USA

Ian Herrick
Western University, London, Ontario,
Canada

Peter Hutchinson
Cambridge University, UK

Kelsey Innes
University of British Columbia,
Vancouver, BC, Canada

Andrea Lavinio
Cambridge University Hospitals, UK

Ronan O' Leary
Cambridge University Hospitals, UK

Chanhuan Z. Lee
University of California, San Francisco,
CA, USA.

Jeremy A. Lieberman
University of California, San Francisco,
CA, USA

Daniel A. Lim
University of California, San Francisco,
CA, USA

Mariska Lont
University Medical Center Groningen UK

Pirjo H. Manninen
University of Toronto, Ontario, Canada

Vaithy Mani
Cambridge University Hospitals, UK

Oana Maties
University of California, San Francisco,
CA, USA

Lingzhong Meng
Yale University School of Medicine, New
Haven, CT, USA

Chris Nixon-Giles
University of British Columbia,
Vancouver, BC, Canada

Hélèe Pellerin
Université Laval, Québec, Canada

Simeone Pierre
Aix Marseille University, Marseille, France

Mark Plummer
Cambridge University Hospitals, UK

Jane E. Risdall
Cambridge University Hospitals, UK

Mark D. Rollins
University of California, San Francisco, CA, USA

Kali Romano
University of British Columbia, Vancouver, BC, Canada

Mark A. Rosen
University of California, San Francisco, CA, USA

Keith J. Ruskin
University of Chicago Pritzker School of Medicine, Chicago, IL, USA

Grant Sanders
Kaiser Permanente, Oakland, CA, USA

Eschtike Schulenburg
Cambridge University Hospitals, UK

Veena Sheshadri
Toronto Western Hospital, Canada

Jane Sturgess
West Suffolk Hospital, Bury St Edmunds, UK

Daniel Scoffings
Cambridge University Hospitals, UK

Mypinder Sekhon
University of British Columbia, Vancouver, BC, Canada

Darreul P. Sewell
University College London Hospitals, London, UK

David Shimabukuro
University of California, San Francisco, CA, USA

Claas Siegmueller
University of California, San Francisco, CA, USA

Sulpicio G. Soriano
Harvard Medical School, Boston, MA, USA

Una Srejic
University of California, San Francisco, CA, USA

Barbara Stanley
Brighton & Sussex University Hospitals, UK

Susan Stevenson
Cambridge University Hospitals, UK

Ivan Timofeev
Cambridge University Hospitals, UK

John H. Turnbull
University of California, San Francisco, CA, USA

Nienke Valens
University Medical Center Groningen, Netherlands

Monica S. Vavilala
University of Washington, Seattle, WA, USA

Lionel Velly
Aix Marseille University, Marseille, France

Joanna L. C. White
Cambridge University Hospitals, UK

Paul Whitney
Brighton & Sussex University Hospitals, UK

Andrew Wormsbecker
University of British Columbia, Vancouver, BC, Canada

Chapter

1

Structure and Function of the Brain and Spinal Cord

Daniel A. Lim and Michael McDermott

Key Points

- The CNS can be organized into five anatomical regions: cerebral hemispheres, diencephalon, brain stem, cerebellum, and spinal cord.
- The anterior two-thirds of the spinal cord are supplied by the anterior spinal artery. This portion of the spinal cord contains lower motor neurons in the ventral horn, descending corticospinal tracts, and ascending spinothalamic tracts.
- The supra-tentorial compartment includes the cerebral hemispheres and the diencephalon. More than 80% of people are left-hemisphere dominant for speech and language function.
- The infra-tentorial compartment contains the brain stem, cerebellum, and cranial nerves 3–12.
- The basal ganglia include caudate, globus pallidus, putamen, and amygdala.

Abbreviations

CNS   Central nervous system
CSF   Cerebrospinal fluid

Contents

- Introduction
- Spinal Cord
- The Supra-Tentorial Compartment

  - The Cerebrum and Neocortices
  - The Diencephalon

- The Infra-Tentorial Compartment

  - The Brain Stem
  - The Cerebellum

- The Extrapyramidal Organs

  - The Basal Ganglia

Introduction

The CNS can be divided grossly into five anatomical regions (Figure 1.1):

(1) spinal cord

(2) cerebral hemispheres

(3) diencephalon

(4) brain stem, consisting of the medulla, pons, and midbrain

(5) cerebellum

For practical purposes, many surgeons divide the intracranial compartment into supra-tentorial and infra-tentorial compartments. The supra-tentorial compartment contains the cerebral hemispheres and the diencephalon, while the infra-tentorial compartment includes the brain stem and cerebellum.

The CNS is bathed in CSF. CSF is created in the ventricles by the choroid plexus at a rate of about 15–20 ml/h in adults (Figure 1.2a) and circulates through the ventricular system to the subarachnoid space. The subarachnoid space is found between the pia mater, which is attached to the brain and spinal cord tissue, and the arachnoid mater, which is a delicate, spiderweb-like connective tissue (Figure 1.2b). Outside the arachnoid is the tough dura mater. Collectively, the pia, arachnoid, and dura mater form the meninges.

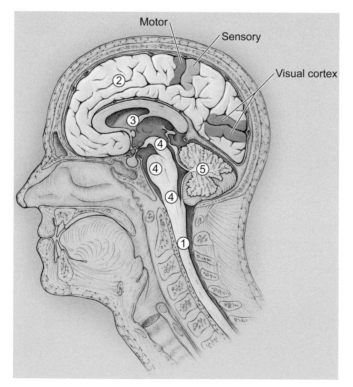

Figure 1.1 Sagittal image showing relationships of (1) spinal cord; (2) cerebral hemispheres; (3) the diencephalon; (4) the brain stem, consisting of the medulla, pons, and midbrain; and (5) the cerebellum.

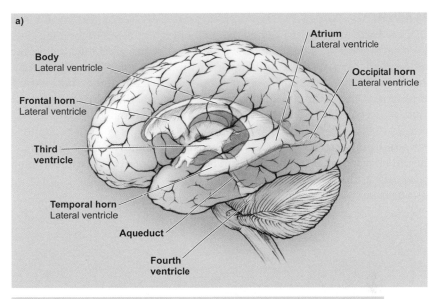

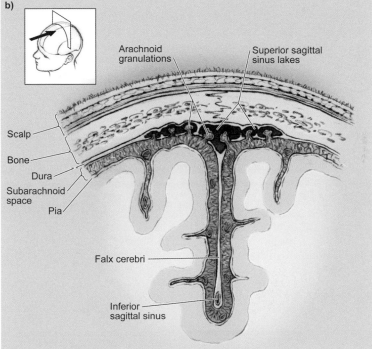

Figure 1.2 (a) Position of the lateral, third and fourth ventricles, and connection pathways. The lateral ventricle is divided into frontal horn, body, atrium, and occipital and temporal horns. Choroid plexus is found in floor of body of ventricle and roof of temporal horn and in the third and fourth ventricles (b) Coronal section showing relationship of arachnoid granulations to superior sagittal sinus.

Spinal Cord

The spinal cord extends from the base of the skull and tapers down to the conus, becoming the filum terminale between T12 and L2 (Figure 1.3). The principal functions of the spinal cord are threefold. First, in its central gray matter lie the cellular circuitry underlying the motor function of most of the body (except for the face, tongue, and mouth), including the anterior horn cells and the indirect pathways which regulate them (reflex loops).

Second, the spinal cord receives sensory input from the peripheral nerves and transmits these to higher structures. The primary ascending tracts are the posterior columns and the lateral spinothalamic tract (Figure 1.4). The posterior columns transmit fine touch, vibration, and proprioception. The lateral spinothalamic tract conveys contralateral pain and temperature. Pain fibers from the dorsal roots ascend or descend one to three segments before synapsing in the spinal cord.

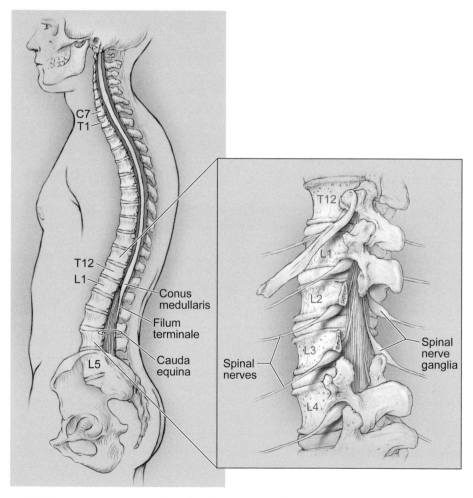

Figure 1.3 Sagittal image of spine and spinal cord with close-up of cauda equina and compound spinal nerves. The spinal cord extends from the base of the skull and tapers down to the conus, becoming the filum terminale between T12 and L2.

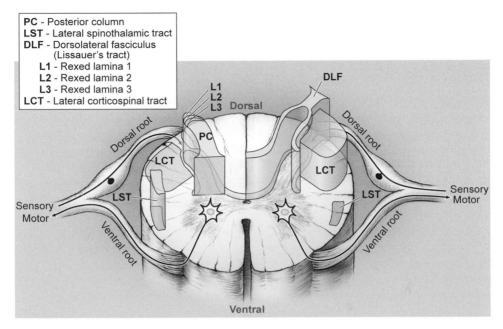

PC - Posterior column
LST - Lateral spinothalamic tract
DLF - Dorsolateral fasciculus
   (Lissauer's tract)
L1 - Rexed lamina 1
L2 - Rexed lamina 2
L3 - Rexed lamina 3
LCT - Lateral corticospinal tract

Figure 1.4 Axial schematic representation of ascending and descending tracts and dorsal horn.

Third, the spinal white matter contains several descending tracts, which are utilized by the higher CNS structures to regulate spinal cord function either by directly stimulating cells or by regulating interneurons that increase or decrease signalling efficiency. The most clinically important of these is the lateral corticospinal tract (Figure 1.4) which conveys voluntary, skilled movement from the contralateral cerebral hemisphere. Many other motor pathways originate from cortical and brainstem structures to control posture and movement. Additionally, there exist descending pathways responsible for the regulation of pain fibers.

The blood supply to the spinal cord comes via paired posterior spinal arteries and a single anterior spinal artery. While the posterior arteries supply the dorsal horns and white matter columns, the anterior spinal artery supplies the anterior two-thirds of the cord. There are six to eight prominent radicular arteries that supply the anterior spinal artery network, most numerous in the cervical region and least in the thoracic. The artery of Adamkiewicz, the main thoraco-lumbar radicular vessel, supplies the spinal cord from T8 to the conus. This artery arises in the T9–L2 region and mostly from the left side of the aorta. Spinal artery perfusion pressure is an important consideration especially in the prone position where intravenous pressures are elevated.

The Supra-Tentorial Compartment

The Cerebrum and Neocortices

The cerebral hemispheres consist of the cerebral cortex, white matter projections, and a few deep structures including the basal ganglia and hippocampus. The cortex is highly

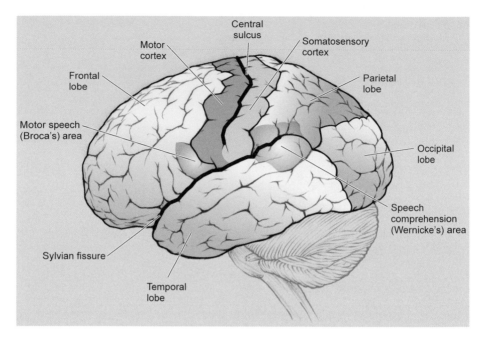

Figure 1.5 The cortex is highly convoluted with infoldings called sulci and bumps or ridges called gyri. Each hemisphere is divided into four major lobes: the frontal, parietal, temporal, and occipital. Motor (Broca's) and receptive (Wernicke's) language areas are shown in the frontal and temporal/parietal lobes, respectively.

convoluted with infoldings called sulci and bumps or ridges called gyri. Each hemisphere is divided into four major lobes: the frontal, parietal, temporal, and occipital (Figure 1.5). The hemispheres are principally defined by the midline interhemispheric fissure, the central sulcus in the posterior frontal lobe, and the large lateral Sylvian fissure.

Not all cortex is created equal, such that some regions can be removed with impunity, while others will cause neurological deficits if injured. Thus, it is essential to understand the location of the so-called eloquent brain regions, as non-eloquent regions are the preferred operative path for most lesions. The eloquent brain regions include the primary motor and sensory cortices, the speech areas (Broca's and Wernicke's areas), the primary visual cortex, the thalamus, the brainstem reticular activating system, the deep cerebellar nuclei, and to some extent the anterior parietal lobes. Many of these lie near or directly adjacent to the Sylvian fissure.

The primary motor cortex and somatosensory cortex straddle the central sulcus. Both the motor and sensory cortex represent the opposite side of the body in a precise topological fashion (Figure 1.6). The visual cortex is in the occipital lobe, primarily on the medial aspect of the hemisphere above and below the calcarine sulcus.

The left hemisphere is dominant for language in nearly all right-handed patients; about 80% of left-handed are still left-hemisphere language dominant with bilateral dominance and right side dominance in about 15% and 5% of patients, respectively. Wernicke's area is behind the primary auditory cortex in the posterior superior temporal lobe. Lesions of Wernicke's area lead to problems with language comprehension, classically causing a fluent aphasia (normal sentence length and intonation, speech devoid of meaning). Broca's area is

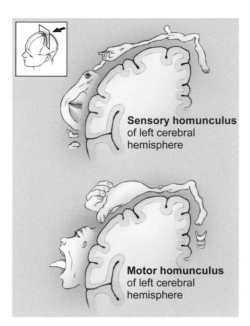

Figure 1.6 Approximate representation of the motor and sensory areas in pre- and post-central sulcus.

located in the frontal lobe premotor cortex and is important for word formation; Broca's area lesions lead to a non-fluent aphasia (faltering, broken speech).

The Diencephalon

The diencephalon sits above the midbrain and consists of the thalamus and hypothalamus. The thalamus is "an information relay station." All sensory modalities except olfaction pass through the thalamus, and there are many reciprocal connections between the thalamus and cerebral cortex as well as with the cerebellum. The thalamus is important for motor control, wakefulness, and sensory information processing. Thalamic lesions thus can produce coma, tremors, and other motor difficulties, as well as sensory problems including pain syndromes.

The hypothalamus, located just inferior to the thalamus, controls endocrine, autonomic, and visceral function. The hypothalamus is connected to the pituitary gland by the infundibulum, which continues as the pituitary stalk (Figure 1.7). The pituitary gland sits within the sella, which is just behind and inferior to the optic chiasm. Hence, tumors of the pituitary can compress the chiasm, producing visual problems (e.g., bitemporal hemianopsia). Hypothalamic releasing and inhibitory factors regulate pituitary hormone release. Vasopressin (or antidiuretic hormone) is made by hypothalamic cells and is transported to the posterior pituitary for release.

The hypothalamus also originates descending fibers which influence the sympathetic and parasympathetic autonomic nervous system. There are discrete nuclei within the hypothalamus which are critical to body homeostasis. Thermoregulation, satiety, and arousal are partially controlled in the hypothalamus. For instance, experimental lesions of the lateral hypothalamus produce anorexia, while medial lesions cause overeating.

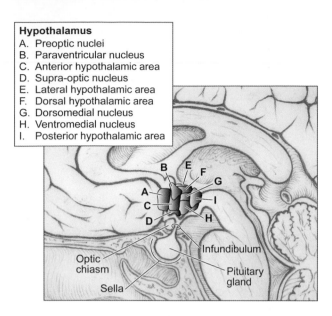

Hypothalamus
A. Preoptic nuclei
B. Paraventricular nucleus
C. Anterior hypothalamic area
D. Supra-optic nucleus
E. Lateral hypothalamic area
F. Dorsal hypothalamic area
G. Dorsomedial nucleus
H. Ventromedial nucleus
I. Posterior hypothalamic area

Figure 1.7 Locations of hypothalamic nuclei in the diencephalon.

The Infra-Tentorial Compartment

The Brain Stem

The medulla, pons, and midbrain comprise the brain stem, a highly complex and clinically critical region of the CNS (Figure 1.1). Unlike any other region of the brain, it is at the same time the anatomic substrate of consciousness, a regulator of autonomic function, the origin and target of numerous different descending regulatory fiber tracts and a few ascending ones, a thoroughfare for tracts having no functional relation to it, the home of 10 of the 12 cranial nerves with their attendant input and output nuclei, and the location of a number of clinically relevant reflexes.

Probably the most clinically important function of the brain stem is its role in maintaining consciousness. Significant injuries to the brain stem lead to stupor and coma, due to injury to the reticular activating system. The brainstem reticular formation consists of a set of interconnected nuclei in the core of the brain stem which mediate the level of alertness.

Equally important are the respiratory control centers located in the medulla and pons. The respiratory control neurons are involved in rhythm generation as well as processing afferent information from central and peripheral chemoreceptors and various lung receptors. Focal medullary injury or edema can lead to life-threatening respiratory arrest.

Many ascending and descending fiber tracts pass through the brain stem. Other tracts, such as the corticobulbar, trigeminothalamic, central tegmental tract, and medial longitudinal fasciculus, have their origin or termination within the brainstem nuclei. For instance, the nuclei for cranial nerves 3 to12 (CNIII–CNXII) are in the brain stem (Table 1.1). Importantly, many of these tracts have close analogues in the spinal cord, and a lack of concordance of deficits between face and body (e.g., a right facial weakness and left hemiparesis) strongly suggests a lesion in the brain stem.

Brainstem function can be grossly tested in comatose patients using the pupillary, corneal, and gag/cough reflexes. The pupillary (light) reflex assesses function at the

Table 1.1 Cranial Nerves and Function

Cranial Nerve	Function	Defined Nucleus Location
I	Smell	Uncus, septal area
II	Vision	Lateral geniculate nucleus
III	Extraocular movement; lid elevation	Midbrain tectum (superior)
IV	Eye movement; down and in	Midbrain tectum (inferior)
V	Sensory to skin of face: Motor to muscles for chewing (V3)	Pons (motor, sensory), medulla, cervical cord (sensory)
VI	Lateral eye movement	Pons (dorsal)
VII	Facial movement; sense of taste (anterior 2/3 tongue)	Pons (ventral)
VIII	Hearing; balance	Pons (dorsal-lateral)
IX	Palate movement/sensation; taste posterior 1/3 tongue	Medulla
X	Vocal cords; parasympathetic supply to viscera	Medulla
XI	Trapezius, sternomastoid supply	Medulla
XII	Muscles of tongue	Medulla

midbrain level, as well as the integrity of the optic and oculomotor nerves. The corneal (blink) reflex assesses brainstem function at the level of the pons. Its afferent limb is the trigeminal nerve and efferent limb is the facial nerve. The gag reflex tests the lower brain stem, or medulla, as well as the glossopharyngeal and vagus nerves.

The vomiting reflex passes through the medulla. Stimulation of certain neurons of the reticular formation leads to impulses descending to lower motor neurons causing contraction of the diaphragm and abdominal muscles.

The Cerebellum

The cerebellum is found in the posterior cranial fossa (Figure 1.1). It is attached to the brain stem by the three cerebellar peduncles at the level of the fourth ventricle. The tentorium, a transverse fold of dura, stretches over the superior part of the cerebellum, separating it from the occipital lobe of the cerebral hemispheres. This intimate relationship between cerebellum and brain stem puts the patient's life in danger in cases of acute cerebellar edema.

The oldest part, the archicerebellum, lies in the antero-inferior flocculonodular lobe, receives input from the vestibular nuclei, and regulates control of eye movements. The paleocerebellum consists of the midline vermis and processes proprioceptive input from the ascending spinocerebellar tracts where it controls axial posture via neocortical projections. The neocerebellum is primarily made up of the lateral hemispheres which receive neocortex input via the middle peduncle and sends processed output back to the neocortex via the thalamus.

Lesions of the cerebellum typically produce deficits ipsilateral to the lesion. This is because the output of the cerebellum is crossed, and it affects primarily the descending motor pathways, which are also crossed. Typical symptoms include ataxia and truncal tremor (titubation), with paleocerebellum (medial) lesions, or limb ataxia or action tremor, with neocerebellum (lateral) lesions.

The Extrapyramidal Organs

The extrapyramidal organs are structures linked not by spatial proximity, but by functional and neuroanatomic similarity. Both structures can be thought of as a form of consultant to the rest of the CNS: receiving and processing input from the neocortex and/or spinal cord, relaying this processed input back to external targets commonly the thalamus, where it modulates motor, emotional, and cognitive function. As a result, damage to the extrapyramidal organs classically causes tremor and incoordination (known as extrapyramidal signs), not paralysis.

The Basal Ganglia

Within the cerebral hemisphere lie the basal ganglia (Figure 1.8). The principal components are the caudate nucleus, putamen, globus pallidus, and amygdala. These organs contain many interconnections as well as reciprocal connections with other brain regions including

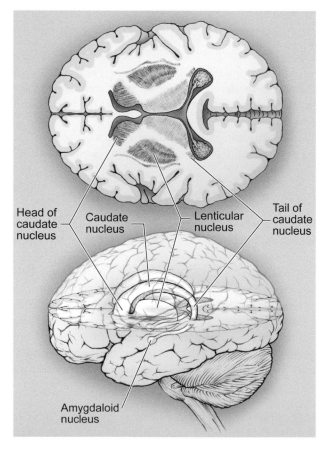

Figure 1.8 Axial and 3D representation of the basal ganglia.

the midbrain, diencephalon, and cerebral cortex. Functionally, these connections can be classified into oculomotor, skeletomotor, limbic, and cognitive circuits, each with different inputs and targets.

Basal ganglia diseases, such as Parkinson's and Huntington's disease, lead to abnormal motor control, alterations of muscular tone, and emergence of irregular, involuntary movements. These diseases can cause emotional and cognitive disturbances, depending on the degree of involvement of the emotional and cognitive circuits.

Further Reading

Gilman, S., Newman, S., Manter, J.T., Gatz, A.J. eds. (2002). *Manter and Gatz's Essentials of Clinical Neuroanatomy and Neurophysiology*, 10th edition, Philadelphia, PA:F.A. Davis.

Kandel, E.R., Schwartz, J.H., Jessell, T.M. eds. (2000). *Principles of Neural Science*, 4th edition, Norwalk, CT: Appleton and Lange.

Cerebral Circulation

2

Barbara Stanley and Paul Whitney

Key Points

- The brain's arterial supply is from the carotid arteries and the vertebrobasilar system.
- The arteries anastomose in the circle of Willis.
- Venous drainage occurs through epithelial lined venous sinuses draining into the internal jugular veins.
- The microcirculation is highly organized, with capillary density correlated with functional activity.
- The blood-brain barrier is formed by highly specialized capillary endothelial cells, astrocytes, pericytes, and the endothelial basement membrane.

Abbreviations

ACA	Anterior cerebral artery
BBB	Blood-brain barrier
CBF	Cerebral blood flow
ICA	Internal carotid artery
ICP	Intracranial pressure
MCA	Middle cerebral artery
PCA	Posterior cerebral artery

Contents

- Introduction
- The Arterial System
- The Venous System
- Cerebral Microcirculation
- Blood-Brain Barrier
- Further Reading

Introduction

The brain is unique among the organs of the body in its ability to maintain its blood flow over a wide range of arterial pressures. The blood flow to the brain is approximately 750 ml/min, i.e., 50 ml/100 g/min or about 14% of resting cardiac output. Regional flow within the brain is also regulated to match regional metabolic demand. Blood flow within the brain is variable with gray matter flow (80–110 ml/100 g/min) almost five times that of white matter (20 ml/100 g/min). Understanding the anatomy and physiology of the cerebral circulation allows prediction of neurological deficits in the event of circulatory compromise.

The Arterial System

The arterial supply is divided into anterior and posterior circulations and comprises two sets of paired arteries. The anterior circulation originates from the ICA. These ascend into the brain through the carotid foramen and give rise to a posterior communicating artery before ending by dividing into the ACA and MCA. The ICA also gives rise to the ophthalmic artery, which supplies the orbital structures including the retina. The ACA and MCA supply the medial side of the frontal lobe and the lateral aspects of the frontal, temporal, and parietal lobes, respectively. The lenticulostriate arteries are penetrating branches of the MCA that arise soon after its origin, and supply the basal ganglia and internal capsule. These branches are end arteries and therefore common sites for embolic and hemorrhagic stroke (Table 2.1 and Figure 2.3).

The posterior circulation originates from the paired vertebral arteries, which ascend through the vertebral foramen and fuse to form the basilar artery at the ponto-medullary junction. The basilar artery subsequently divides into two PCAs. Several important branches arise from the posterior system:

1. spinal arteries (which supply the entire length of the cord)
2. meningeal branches
3. superior cerebellar arteries
4. anterior and posterior inferior cerebellar arteries (supplying the cerebellum)

Table 2.1 Vascular and functional anatomy.

Parent Vessel	Vessel	Structures Supplied/Function
ICA	ACA	Primary motor/somatosensory cortex (leg and foot)
		Medial frontal lobe (motor planning)
ICA	MCA (superior branches)	Primary motor/somatosensory cortex (face and upper limb)
	MCA (inferior branches)	Broca's area (language expression)
		Frontal eye fields (gaze)
		Wernicke's area (language comprehension)
		Primary somatosensory cortex
		Optic radiation (vision)
Basilar	PCA	Occipital lobe (vision)
		Posterior hippocampus (memory)
		Thalamus (subcortical hub for most sensorimotor functions)
Vertebral	Basilar Artery	Posterior fossa (brainstem and cerebellum) along with PCA

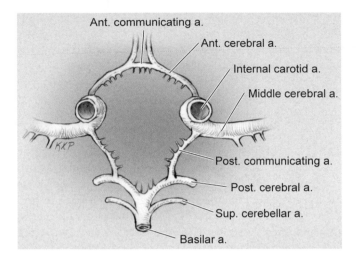

Ant. communicating a.
Ant. cerebral a.
Internal carotid a.
Middle cerebral a.
Post. communicating a.
Post. cerebral a.
Sup. cerebellar a.
Basilar a.

Figure 2.1 Diagrammatic representation of the circle of Willis. This classic polygon is found in less than 50% of brains.

The ICA and ACA form part of the circle of Willis – the anastomotic vascular ring located in the interpeduncular cistern at the level of the tragus of the ear and encircling the pituitary gland, mammillary bodies and optic chiasm. Deep penetrating branches from the circle behave as end arteries and therefore systemic hypotension may result in typical patterns of ischemia at boundary zones (watershed ischemia). These distributions are not always consistent due to the presence of anatomical variations in the circle (Figures 2.1 and 2.2).

The Venous System

Unlike the vascular beds of other organ systems, the cerebral venous drainage does not follow the arterial supply. Instead, small veins combine into pial veins which coalesce into venous sinuses forming superficial and deep drainage systems characterized by limited venous anastomoses (Figure 2.4). Intra- to extracranial anastomoses arise via diploic skull veins. Total intracranial blood volume amounts to approximately 200 ml, of which, most lies within the venous system, which therefore provides the capacitance vessels of the cerebral circulation.

Each hemisphere drains into the nearest dural sinus. These endothelialized, valveless channels lie between folds of dura, are continuous with the endothelial surface of the cerebral veins and are semi-rigid despite lacking a muscular wall. The midline (superior sagittal sinus, inferior sagittal sinus, straight sinus, and occipital sinus) and paramedian sinuses (anterior cerebral veins, basal veins, cavernous sinuses, and transverse sinuses) link up to complete the sinus network which drain into both jugular veins via the sigmoid sinus at the level of the jugular bulbs.

The basal ganglia and other deep structures drain via the internal cerebral and basal veins, forming the great cerebral vein of Galen beneath the splenium of the corpus callosum. The vein of Galen coalesces with the inferior sagittal sinus to form the straight sinus.

Superior cerebral veins, otherwise known as bridging veins, drain the superior and medial surfaces of the cerebral hemispheres and lie beneath the arachnoid on the cortical

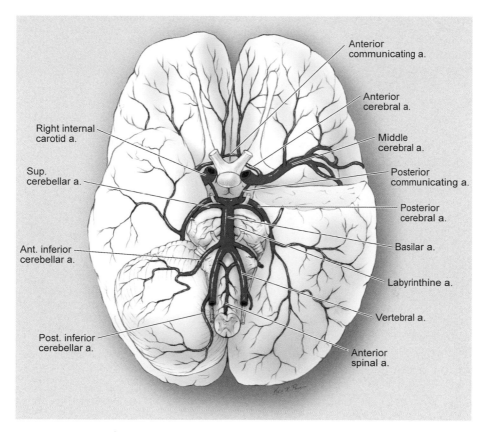

Anterior
communicating a.

Anterior
cerebral a.

Right internal
carotid a.

Middle
cerebral a.

Sup.
cerebellar a.

Posterior
communicating a.

Posterior
cerebral a.

Basilar a.

Ant. inferior
cerebellar a.

Labyrinthine a.

Vertebral a.

Post. inferior
cerebellar a.

Anterior
spinal a.

Figure 2.2 Relationship of the arterial supply to the base of the brain. Note the proximity of the circle of Willis to the optic chiasm and pituitary stalk.

surface, thereby bridging the subdural space. The unique properties of this venous system give rise to multiple clinical implications summarized in Table 2.2.

Cerebral Microcirculation

The cerebral microcirculation consists of highly organized pial surface vessels (<100 μm) branching into arterioles that penetrate the brain perpendicularly. Each arteriole supplies a hexagonal column of tissue, with overlapping boundary zones producing columnar patterns of local blood flow matching the arrangement of neuronal groups and functional units.

Capillaries arise at all laminar levels, the density of which, in adults, relates to the number of synapses and correlates with regional levels of oxidative metabolism. Capillary density at birth is one-third of adult levels, doubling in the first year and reaching adult levels by 4 years. Capillaries are protected from systemic blood pressure surges by the complex branching system and a dual system of twin resistance elements in series: (1) extra-parenchymal vessels under autonomic control and (2) intraparenchymal vessels under intrinsic metabolic and myogenic control which, therefore, react to P_aCO_2 (dual-control hypothesis). At normal physiological P_aCO_2 intraparenchymal tone predominates and

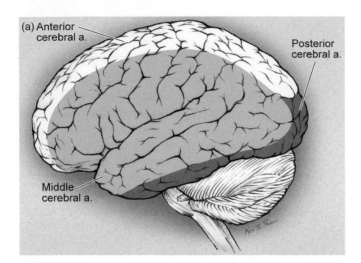

(a) Anterior
cerebral a.

Posterior
cerebral a.

Middle
cerebral a.

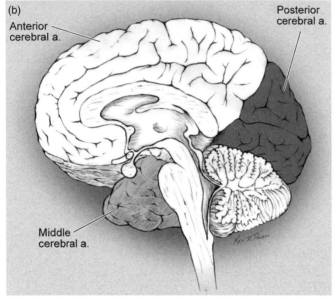

(b)

Posterior
cerebral a.

Anterior
cerebral a.

Middle
cerebral a.

Figure 2.3 A and B, Areas of the brain supplied by the cerebral arteries.

autonomic control has little influence on CBF. However, when intraparenchymal vessels are dilated by hypercapnia, sympathetic stimulation produces a profound reduction in CBF.

Blood-Brain Barrier

The brain parenchyma is supplied by a vast network of microcapillaries, which is separated from brain extracellular fluid by a relatively impermeable anatomical barrier with high electrical resistance, called the blood-brain barrier (BBB). Even small molecules such as mannitol are unable to cross under normal physiological conditions. The BBB is formed by highly specialized capillary endothelial cells, astrocytes and pericytes (the cellular components), and the endothelial basement membrane. The anatomical barrier is sealed by

Table 2.2 Clinical implications of cerebral venous outflow.

Anatomical Property	Clinical Implications
Lack of valves	Head up position improves venous drainage. Outflow obstruction from an internal jugular catheter can theoretically increase risk of raised ICP and surgical bleeding.
Diploic anastomoses	Potential route for cranial spread of organisms from face/paranasal air sinuses.
Intracranial venous drainage Exits the cranium via the jugular bulbs. 70% from ipsilateral hemisphere, 27% contralateral hemisphere, 3% extracranial	Jugular venous oxygenation ($S_{jv}O_2$) can be used as an indication of global cerebral oxygenation.
Semi-rigid Non-muscular walls	High risk of venous air embolus in head up position.
Bridging veins	Increased risk of subdural hemorrhage even from minor head trauma due to traction on bridging veins in atrophic brain or low ICP states (postdural puncture).
Relative lack of anastomoses	Sudden occlusion of large veins or sinuses causes brain swelling or venous infarction due to accumulation of deoxygenated blood in the parenchyma. Dural stenting can be used for treatment of benign intracranial hypertension.

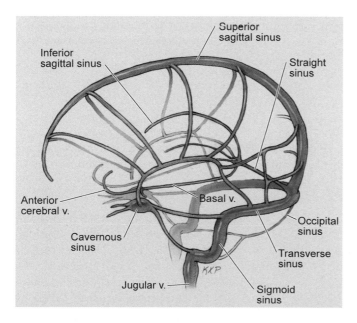

Figure 2.4 Cerebral venous drainage.

interendothelial tight junctions, called zonulae occludentes. The formation of a BBB is unique to the cerebral microenvironment and capillaries from other vascular beds will develop a similar barrier when transplanted into brain tissue. The BBB is not complete throughout the central nervous system. Regions which lie outside the BBB include the posterior pituitary gland, median eminence, area postrema, preoptic recess, paraphysis, pineal gland, and the endothelium of the choroid plexus.

Movement of substances across an intact BBB is a function of lipid solubility, molecular size, and active transport mechanisms. Lipophilic substances traverse relatively easily. Many hydrophilic substances also cross via active transport. There are two potential routes through the barrier: the paracellular route, i.e., in between the tight junctions, and the transcellular route, i.e., through the microvascular endothelial cells, utilizing enzymes and transporters to actively eject or metabolize blood-borne substances. Tight control of the ionic composition of brain extracellular fluid by active processes is energy-intensive and accounts for the high mitochondrial density of capillary endothelial cells.

The combined efforts of passive obstruction (tight junctions), active drug efflux (embedded transporters), and biochemical transformation (metabolism) create an obstacle to drug delivery and very tightly control the biochemistry of the brain environment. Furthermore, it is a dynamic interface capable of reacting to disease and infective or inflammatory states. The barrier is disrupted by disease processes such as ischemia; however, the process takes hours to days. The initial cerebral edema after ischemia is, therefore, cytotoxic rather than vasogenic and mannitol continues to be of use for the reduction of edema in early acute brain injury.

Further Reading

Matta, B.F., Menon, D.K., Smith, S. (2011). *Core Topics in Neuroanaesthesia and Neurointensive Care*. Cambridge: Cambridge University Press.

McCaffrey, G., Davis, T.P.: Physiology and pathophysiology of the blood brain barrier. *J Investig Med* 2012; **60**:1131–1140.

TeachMeAnatomy.info.: Online anatomy resource, March 12, 2016, http://teachmeanatomy.info/neuro/vasculature/arterial-supply-brain/.

TeachMeAnatomy.info.: Online anatomy resource, March 12, 2016, http://teachmeanatomy.info/neuro/vessels/venous-drainage/.

Section 2   Physiology

Chapter

3

Cerebral Blood Flow and Its Control

Susan Stevenson and Ari Ercole

Key Points

- The brain has a high energy and oxygen requirement. Locally, CBF and metabolic demand are coupled by a variety of mechanisms.
- Autoregulation maintains a constant CBF over a range of cerebral perfusion pressures, but this may fail outside this range or after brain injury.
- Failure of CBF may rapidly lead to irreversible neuronal injury.
- Increasing arterial carbon dioxide tension and hypoxemia are both potent cerebral vasodilators.

Abbreviations

ATP	Adenosine triphosphate
BBB	Blood-brain barrier
CBF	Cerebral blood flow
CBV	Cerebral blood volume
CMR	Cerebral metabolic rate
CMR_{glu}	Cerebral metabolic rate for glucose
$CMRO_2$	Cerebral metabolic rate for oxygen
CO	Cardiac output
CO_2	Carbon dioxide
CPP	Cerebral perfusion pressure
CSF	Cerebrospinal fluid
CT	Computed tomography
CT-P	Computed tomography perfusion
CVR	Cerebrovascular resistance
ICP	Intracranial pressure
MAP	Mean arterial pressure
MTT	Mean transit time
$PaCO_2$	Carbon dioxide tension
PaO_2	Arterial oxygen tension
RBC	Red blood cell

SAH	Subarachnoid hemorrhage
SVR	Systemic vascular resistance
TCD	Transcranial doppler

Contents

Introduction

Neuronal function requires a large and continuous supply of oxygen and energy substrate. The brain has the highest metabolic demand of any organ, consuming 20% of the body's resting oxygen consumption (250 ml/min). However, the brain has a limited number of energy substrates with glucose being the main source for production of ATP. Without glucose stores, energy production for neuronal function is completely dependent on CBF. A critical reduction in CBF, i.e., ischemia, is poorly tolerated for all but the briefest of periods with permanent neuronal damage occurring within minutes.

An understanding of the physiology underlying the maintenance of CBF and its relationship with CPP and ICP is paramount to the practice of neuroanesthesia and neurological critical care. Manipulation and optimization of cerebral physiology underpins the management principles of neurological disease. Appropriate treatment aims to reduce and prevent secondary brain injury, and therefore limit the consequences on functional ability.

Determinants of Cerebral Blood Flow

CBF is related to CPP and CVR, as shown by the equation:

$$CBF = CPP/CVR$$

Therefore, factors influencing either CPP or CVR may affect CBF.

Cerebral Perfusion Pressure

Cerebral perfusion pressure is determined by the difference between the upstream MAP and downstream CVP. However, because the cerebral vasculature is enclosed within a rigid non-compliant skull, ICP is substituted for downstream pressure when this exceeds CVP. Therefore:

$$CPP = MAP - ICP.$$

The two dependent variables in this equation can be altered by several other associated factors and thus impact on CPP. MAP is the product of CO and SVR and subject to fluctuations depending on preload, cardiac contractility and vasomotor tone. ICP is determined by the relative volumes of the contents of the skull: the brain parenchyma (85%), blood (5%), and CSF (10%). These volumes are non-compressible, and an increase in one must be compensated by a decrease in another, otherwise ICP increases. For example, under certain circumstances, an increase in CBV through vasodilatation is compensated by displacement of CSF and therefore ICP changes are minimal. However, if this compensation is exhausted then ICP may rise rapidly with only small increases in CBV.

Cerebral Vascular Resistance

CVR is very sensitive to vessel caliber as resistance to flow is inversely proportional to the fourth power of diameter. Arteriolar vasoconstriction or vasodilatation is the predominant method of maintaining CBF in response to changes in CPP and underpins cerebral auto-regulation. Vascular resistance is both locally and globally controlled. Local CMR may vary considerably depending on neuronal activation. Local CBF is adjusted according to local metabolic rate by a mechanism known as flow-metabolism coupling ensuring the necessary demands for function are met.

Autoregulation

Cerebral autoregulation is the process whereby CBF is maintained relatively constant in the face of modest changes of perfusion pressures ensuring consistent delivery of oxygen and metabolic substrate (Figure 3.1). This is frequently erroneously cited as a fixed range of 50–150 mmHg perfusion pressure. The MAP at which CBF begins to drop is approxi-mately 70–90 mmHg with a range of 40–110 mmHg. The upper limit is not well

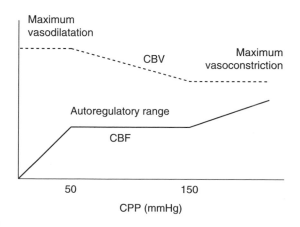

Figure 3.1 Graphic illustration of the independence of CBF on CPP over the autoregulatory range between about 50 and 150 mmHg. Autoregulation is achieved by changes in vascular caliber and is therefore accompanied by a change in CBV. Outside this range, vasodilatation/vasoconstriction is maximal and CBF becomes pressure-passive.

characterized because of ethical issues in deliberately raising blood pressure above a safe threshold. Such autoregulation is achieved through changes in vascular tone with the upper and lower limits of autoregulation representing maximal vasoconstriction and vasodilatation respectively. Consequently, CBV decreases with increasing CPP.

Autoregulation is achieved through multiple mechanisms of varying latencies. A myogenic mechanism, acting in seconds, leads to compensatory vasoconstriction in the face of increased CPP. Conversely, decreases in CPP cause reflex vasodilation. This effect may be modulated by sympathetic activity that shifts the curve to the right. Vasodilation also occurs in response to metabolic products such as hydrogen ions and adenosine and is the basis for metabolic control. Additionally, nitric oxide is released from vascular endothelium during low perfusion states mediating vasodilatation.

Outside the range of autoregulation, CBF becomes dependent on CPP. Below the lower limit, there is the risk of cerebral ischemia. Above the upper limit, hyperemia and hemorrhage may occur. The limits of autoregulation may shift in response to pathological states such as chronic hypertension where the plateau is right-shifted, and such patients are at greater risk of cerebral ischemia during even modest hypotension. There is a wide variation in regional CBF and regional autoregulation may fail in some regions before the global limits of autoregulation are reached.

Physiological Control of Cerebral Blood Flow

$PaCO_2$ is a strong determinant of CBF in both health and disease. CO_2 freely diffuses across the BBB and enters the CSF where the resulting carbonic acid dissociates to hydrogen and bicarbonate ions. Decreasing pH leads to vascular smooth muscle relaxation and an increase in CBF. Indeed, CBF is directly proportional to $PaCO_2$ between about 3 and 10 kPa with an increase of some 25% for each 1 kPa increase in $PaCO_2$ in this range (Figure 3.2).

This strong relationship underlines the importance of meticulous control of alveolar ventilation in neuroanesthesia. In a non-compliant brain, the resultant vasodilatation from even small increases in $PaCO_2$ may cause large increases in ICP. Conversely, hyperventilation reduces CBV and may be effective in reducing ICP (until CSF buffering adapts). However, hyperventilation should be avoided except as a temporary emergency therapy. Even a modest fall in $PaCO_2$ below the normal range may result in substantial regions of cerebral ischemia in brain injured patients.

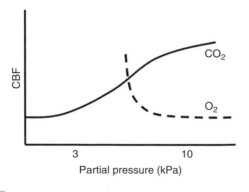

Figure 3.2 Illustration of the influence of $PaCO_2$ and PaO_2 on CBF. CBF shows a strong and approximately linear dependence on $PaCO_2$ over the clinically important range from about 3 to 10 kPa. In contrast, changes in physiological oxygen tensions above 10 kPa have relatively little effect on CBV. However, significant cerebral vasodilatation occurs under hypoxic conditions when PaO_2 falls below 7 kPa.

In addition to $PaCO_2$, low PaO_2 also influences CVR. Hypoxia leads to vasodilation when PaO_2 falls below 7 kPa although this threshold is variable in practice and may be significantly higher in some individuals.

Flow-Metabolism Coupling

Physiological factors affect CBF globally. Regional differences occur with variations in metabolism. CMR is described with reference to the substrates utilized – i.e., oxygen and glucose, $CMRO_2$ and CMR_{glu}, respectively. At rest, the blood flow distribution varies across the microvasculature. During functional activation, flow may be increased by recruitment of capillaries and this closely tracks regional changes in glucose utilization. Flow-metabolism coupling is rapid so that CBF and CMR are matched within seconds. A number of metabolic, endothelial, or neurotransmitter mechanisms have been implicated. While most anesthetic agents reduce CMR in a dose-dependent manner, the degree of flow-metabolism coupling is also changed although this varies with each agent.

Seizure activity may result in massive increases in CMR resulting in a similarly large increase in CBF and CBV. This may increase ICP if intracranial compliance is poor. Temperature is also a potent influence on CMR. Hypothermia decreases CMR and therefore CBF and CBV and is an effective strategy for controlling ICP, albeit without clearly demonstrable benefit in outcome to date. Conversely, pyrexia, which is associated with poor outcomes after acute brain injury, is associated with significant increases in CMR and CBF and possibly worsening ICP control and oxygen supply/demand mismatch.

Neurogenic Control

The neurogenic control of cerebrovascular tone in health is poorly understood. However, both extra- and intracranial cerebral vasculature is richly innervated. Vasoactive mediators include catecholamines, acetylcholine, and nitric oxide as well as 5-hydroxytryptamine, substance P, and neuropeptide Y.

Rheology

Flow and viscosity are inversely related with the main determinant of blood viscosity being hematocrit and RBC mechanical properties. Lower hematocrit results in greater flow, but this benefit is offset by the reduction in oxygen carriage. In addition to effect on cerebral edema, mannitol acts to alter RBC morphology by reducing cell volume, improving deformability, and decreasing blood viscosity and thereby increasing CBF.

Measurement of Cerebral Blood Flow

Measuring CBF can aid clinicians in the diagnosis of acute neurological conditions and subsequent development of complications. The ideal measurement of CBF would be performed at the bedside, avoid radiation or contrast exposure, be operator independent, and produce continuous real-time measurements of regional CBF. Numerous techniques for measuring CBF have been described although all suffer from limitations. However, two technologies – TCD ultrasonography and CT-P imaging – are clinically important.

Transcranial Doppler Ultrasonography

TCD directly measures the Doppler shift in frequency of ultrasound scattered from moving RBCs. Depending on available bone windows, the middle, anterior, or posterior cerebral arteries as well the vertebral, basilar, and carotid arteries may be insonated. It should be noted that the Doppler shift is a measure of blood velocity rather than flow and the technique records the pulsatile waveform of velocity against time. This is related to CBF under the assumption of constant cross-section, which is only approximately true. Furthermore, the technique is not sensitive to local changes in CBF.

Despite these limitations, TCD is straightforward, safe, and provides results in real time. TCD is particularly useful in carotid endarterectomy surgery during ipsilateral carotid clamping to determine if sufficient contralateral supply exists to avoid the need for shunting. It is also used during this surgery for the detection of micro-emboli. TCD may also be helpful in the detection and monitoring of vasospasm that may complicate aneurysmal subarachnoid hemorrhage (aSAH) where blood velocity may be increased through the narrowed vessels.

Computed Tomography-Perfusion Scanning

CT-P scanning generates a temporal map of the passage of iodinated contrast through the cerebral circulation. After the intravenous injection of contrast, serial CT scans are triggered after the appearance of contrast in the arterial blood. The degree of attenuation is directly related to the concentration of contrast within each voxel. Since the rate at which contrast arrives at a particular voxel depends on local CBF, a spatial map of CBF can be inferred. Furthermore, from the MTT of the contrast, a measure of local CBV can also be derived using the central volume principle which states that CBF = CBV/MTT. Other temporal parameters may also be obtained from the technique.

CT-P provides detailed information on tissue ischemia where CBF is reduced (Figure 3.3). Furthermore, regions of infarction can be further distinguished by a matching area of decreased CBV. As a result of the spatial sensitivity, CT-P is invaluable in the diagnosis of acute ischemic stroke and delayed neurological deficits after aSAH. CT-P is able not only to detect regions of ischemia but also to identify the extent of potentially salvageable brain. The

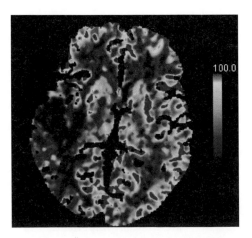

100.0

Figure 3.3 CT-P showing CBF in a patient with aneurysmal subarachnoid hemorrhage. As in health, blood flow is unevenly distributed – being higher near the gray matter of the cortex. Additionally, there is a region of critically low CBF in the territory of the right parieto-temporal middle cerebral artery corresponding to ischemia, in this case caused by vasospasm (white arrow).

huge amount of information from CT-P must, however, be balanced against a significant exposure of the patient to both contrast and radiation.

Further Reading

Aaslid, R., Lindegaard, K.F., Sorteberg, W., et al: Cerebral autoregulation dynamics in humans. *Stroke* 1989; **20**(1):45–52.

Coles, J., Minhas, P., Fryer, T., et al: Effect of hyperventilation on cerebral blood flow in traumatic head injury: Clinical relevance and monitoring correlates. *Crit Care Med 2002;* **30**(9):1950–1959.

Johnston, A.J., Steiner, L.A., Gupta, A.K., et al: Cerebral oxygen vasoreactivity and cerebral tissue oxygen reactivity. *Br J Anaesth* 2003; **90**(6):774–786.

Ter Laan, M., van Dijk, J.M.C., Elting, J.W., et al: Sympathetic regulation of cerebral blood flow in humans: A review. *Br J Anaesth* 2013; **111**(3):361–367.

Chapter

4

Cerebral Metabolism

Sarah Chetcuti and Jonathan P. Coles

Key Points

- The brain has the highest metabolic requirements of any organ in the body.
- Brain function is dependent on a continuous delivery of oxygenated blood and energy substrates.
- Oxidation of glucose fuels the majority of energy requirements.
- Cerebral blood flow varies regionally to match differing metabolic needs across the brain.

Abbreviations

ATP	Adenosine triphosphate
CBF	Cerebral blood flow
CMR	Cerebral metabolic rate
CMRglu	Cerebral metabolic rate of glucose
$CMRO_2$	Cerebral metabolic rate of oxygen
NADH	Nicotinamide adenine dinucleotide
NADPH	Nicotinamide adenine dinucleotide phosphate
OEF	Oxygen extraction fraction
OER	Oxygen extraction ratio
TCA	Tricarboxylic acid

Contents

Introduction

The human brain accounts for only 2% to3% of total body weight but receives about 15% of resting cardiac output (750 ml/min) and consumes about 20% (150 µmol/100 g/min) of the oxygen and 25% (30 µmol/100 g/min) of the glucose required by the body at rest. Up to 60% of this high-energy expenditure is required for the maintenance of transmembrane electro-chemical gradients, while 40% is dedicated to preserving the structural integrity of the membrane along with the synthesis and release of neurotransmitters. CMR is defined as the rate at which the brain utilizes metabolic substrates, e.g., oxygen ($CMRO_2$) or glucose (CMRglu), or generates by-products, e.g., lactate. Even though the brain has the highest metabolic requirements of any organ in the body, it has a very small reserve of metabolic substrates. Therefore, normal functioning of the central nervous system is highly dependent on adequate and continuous provision of energy substrates and removal of the waste products of metabolism.

Mechanisms of Cellular Metabolism (Neuro-energetics)

Although the human brain has the capacity to metabolize ketones, lactate, fatty acids, glycerol, and a variety of amino acids, the conventional view is that glucose oxidation fuels most of the energy requirements. Indeed, the brain is a major consumer of glucose, and more than 90% of all glucose taken up by cerebral tissue is oxidized to CO_2 and water. The rest is metabolized through the pentose phosphate pathway to the reduced form of NADPH, glycogen, galactose, glycoprotein, or to lactate and pyruvate through glycolysis. The glycogen stores of the brain are very small and do not provide a useful reservoir of glucose. In fact, at the normal rate of ATP production, the available stores of glycogen would be exhausted in less than 3 minutes.

Glucose

The body is well designed to ensure delivery of glucose to the brain without a fall in blood glucose levels. At rest, the brain extracts about 10% of the glucose delivered within blood, but this can be increased if blood flow is decreased. In response to a decrease in blood glucose below about 4 mmol/L (72 mg/dl), regulatory mechanisms (glycogenolysis and gluconeogenesis) are initiated that act to restore blood glucose levels. However, if these initial mechanisms fail and blood glucose levels fall further, brain function may likely deteriorate.

The rate-limiting step in glucose metabolism is transport of glucose into the cell. Glucose is transported via facilitated diffusion from the blood to the brain by membrane-based carrier systems. Once intracellular, glucose is phosphorylated to form glucose-6-phosphate, which traps the molecule within the cell, and maintains a concentration gradient that helps draw more glucose into the cell. Glucose is subsequently metabolized through the processes of glycolysis, the TCA cycle and the electron transport chain (Figure 4.1).

Glycolysis is the first stage of brain energy metabolism and the term given to a series of chemical reactions in the cell cytoplasm that convert glucose into two molecules of pyruvate. This reaction results in a net gain of two molecules of ATP.

In the absence of oxygen, pyruvate is reduced to lactate, which may remain within the cell to be later metabolized, or be transported back into the bloodstream. Under aerobic conditions, pyruvate enters the mitochondria, where it passes through a series

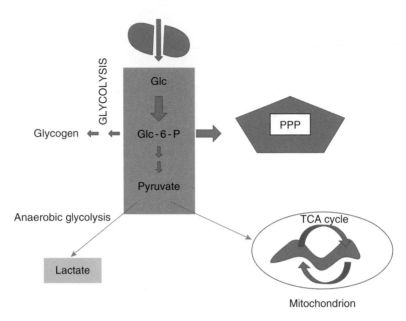

Figure 4.1 Glucose metabolism. Glucose (Glc) is transported into the cell via GLUT transporters and is phosphorylated to form Glucose-6-phosphate (Glc-6-P). Glc-6-P is metabolized via the glycolytic pathway to pyruvate. Pyruvate is transported into the mitochondria and enters the TCA cycle or, in the absence of oxygen, is converted to lactate. Glu-6-P is also the substrate for the pentose phosphate shunt pathway (PPP) which results in synthesis of nucleic acid precursors.

of cyclic reactions and is oxidized to form carbon dioxide and water. This is called the TCA cycle and results in the generation of reduced coenzymes (NADH and flavin adenine dinucleotide), which contain stored energy, and guanosine triphosphate. The reduced coenzymes are subsequently oxidized by the transfer of electrons within the electron transport chain, and this generates 34 molecules of ATP. Therefore, 38 molecules of ATP can be generated from the aerobic metabolism of each molecule of glucose:

$$C_6H_{12}O_6 + 6O_2 + 38ADP + 38Pi \rightarrow 6CO_2 + 6H_2O + 38ATP$$

This contrasts with the two molecules of ATP that can be generated under anaerobic conditions. It is clear from this summary that the energy requirements of the brain cannot be met from anaerobic metabolism alone. A Pasteur effect (enhanced rate of glycolysis when oxygen is limited as a compensation for the decline in ATP generation by oxidative metabolism) also occurs in brain tissue, but even at its maximal rate, anaerobic glycolysis is unable to provide sufficient energy.

This high metabolic requirement for oxygen (40–70 ml O_2/min) must be met by delivery, which depends on the oxygen content of the blood (typically, 20 ml/ 100 ml blood) and CBF (typically, 50 ml/100 g brain/min). Therefore, under normal circumstances, delivery (150 ml/min) is much greater than demand (40–70 ml/min), and around 40% of the

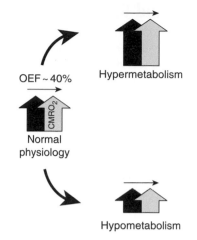

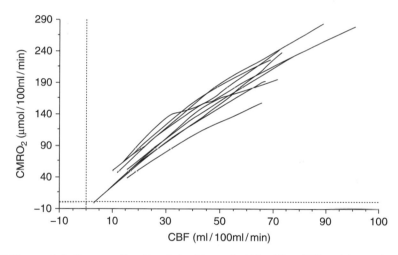

Figure 4.2 Flow-metabolism coupling. Top: In health, cerebral blood flow (CBF) and the cerebral metabolic rate of oxygen ($CMRO_2$) are tightly coupled such that the amount of oxygen extracted from blood is similar across the brain despite differing levels of regional metabolism. This local matching of flow to metabolic demand results in a normal oxygen extraction fraction (OEF) of approximately 40%. **Bottom:** Summary data from a group of 10 healthy controls who underwent physiologic imaging of CBF and $CMRO_2$ via [15]O positron emission tomography. The data demonstrate the close coupling between CBF and $CMRO_2$ across the healthy human brain.
Data obtained by the author within the Wolfson Brain Imaging Centre, Department of Clinical Neurosciences, University of Cambridge, UK.

oxygen delivered in blood is extracted. This so-called OER or OEF can be increased for short periods when either delivery is reduced or demand is increased (Figure 4.2). However, if the supply of oxygen remains insufficient, the energy-requiring processes that sustain normal cellular function and integrity will fail.

Ketone Bodies, Amino, and Organic Acids

Preservation of cerebral function after prolonged fasting suggests that the brain can use alternative substrates for metabolism, particularly after a period of adaptation. In states of prolonged starvation and in the developing brain, ketone bodies (acetoacetate and β-hydroxybutyrate) can become important metabolic substrates within the brain. In addition, some amino and organic acids can be taken up and metabolized within the brain. Overall, these are minor energy substrates except during periods of metabolic stress, such as during acute hypoglycemia and ischemia.

Lactate

The brain can consume lactate as a substrate, particularly during periods of hypoglycemia or elevated blood lactate, e.g., strenuous exercise. Traditionally, it was believed that pyruvate conversion to lactate only occurred in cases of oxygen deficit. However, there is evidence that lactate production can also occur in fully oxygenated circumstances, termed aerobic glycolysis. Lactate shuttling theories suggest that lactate produced by astrocytes is transferred and used by active neurons in health, and that lactate can serve as a fuel following brain injury. These hypotheses are still debated and currently the subject of further scientific review. Thus, although there is evidence that neurons can use lactate under certain conditions, the conventional view is that glucose is the major fuel for oxidative metabolism within active neurons.

Flow-Metabolism Coupling

Cerebral activity varies across the brain and is reflected in changes in cerebral metabolism that determine the requirement for CBF. There are numerous physiological mechanisms to ensure that CBF is maintained and matched to local functional activity. The process of matching oxygen and glucose delivery to metabolic requirements is termed flow-metabolism coupling. Indeed, close matching of flow to metabolism normally results in remarkably little variation in OEF across the brain despite wide regional variations in CBF and $CMRO_2$ (Figure 4.2).

When cerebral function is depressed after coma, energy requirements are reduced and CBF, $CMRO_2$, and glucose use are decreased. Conversely, epileptiform activity or hypermetabolism associated with excitotoxicity may increase energy requirements and necessitate an increase in CBF. Anesthesia and hypothermia suppress brain metabolism and lead to coupled reductions in blood flow.

Further Reading

Mergenthaler, P., Lindauer, U., Gerald, A.D., et al: Sugar for the brain: The role of glucose in physiological and pathological brain function. *Trends Neurosci* 2013; **36**(10):587–597.

Taher, M., Leen, W.G., Wevers, R.A., Willemsen, M.A.: Lactate and its many faces. *Eur J Paediatr Neurol* 2016 January; **20**(1):3–10.

Intracranial Compartment and Intracranial Pressure

Karol P. Budohoski

Key Points

- ICP is a dynamic measurement and reflects the ability of intracranial buffering mechanisms to accommodate extra volume.
- CSF and venous blood provide the majority of the buffering capacity.
- Pressure is related to volume in an exponential fashion and once buffering mechanisms are exhausted small increases in volume can lead to substantial increases in pressure.
- Causes of increased ICP include mass lesions such as neoplasms, intra- and extra-axial hematomas, cerebral edema, and obstruction of CSF flow.
- Intracranial hypertension can present with non-specific and varied symptoms which can rapidly progress to fatality. In patients presenting with altered consciousness, headaches, and papilledema, intracranial hypertension should be included in the differential diagnosis.
- Computed tomography can be used to assess the presence and degree of intracranial pressure but direct measurement remains the gold standard.

Abbreviations

BBB	Blood-brain barrier
CBV	Cerebral blood volume
CPP	Cerebral perfusion pressure
CSF	Cerebrospinal fluid
CT	Computed tomography
CVP	Central venous pressure
GCS	Glasgow Coma Scale
ICP	Intracranial pressure
MAP	Mean arterial pressure
PEEP	Positive end expiratory pressure

Contents

- Pathophysiology of Intracranial Hypertension
  - Brain Parenchyma
  - Cerebral blood volume
  - Cerebrospinal fluid
  - Additional Non-Physiological Volumes
- Clinical Features of Raised Intracranial Pressure
  - Acute Presentation
    - Altered Level of Consciousness
    - Brain Herniation
  - Subacute and Chronic Presentation
    - Headache
    - Vomiting
    - Papilledema
    - Abducens Nerve Palsy
- Radiological Features of Raised Intracranial Pressure

Introduction

ICP refers to the pressure within the intracranial compartment referenced to atmospheric pressure. It represents the dynamic relationship between changes in cranio-spinal volume and the buffering capacity of the system.

Normal ICP ranges from 5 to 15 mmHg but transient physiological elevations occur, for example, during a change of head position, valsalva maneuvers, and coughing. In cases of deranged physiology, such as after traumatic brain injury, it is generally accepted that a sustained ICP greater than 20 mmHg is harmful.

The gold standard technique for measuring ICP is by direct measurement of CSF pressure in the ventricular system of the brain. The origin of this technique dates back to Quincke who first performed a lumbar puncture in 1891 and Lundberg who pioneered direct ventricular catheterization. More recently, intraparenchymal probes have gained in popularity due to their ease of use and relative safety.

Measuring ICP allows for the calculation of CPP which represents the difference between the pressure in the cerebral arterial system and the pressure of blood in the outflow tracts, i.e., CVP. Because the brain is housed in a rigid skull, ICP in most circumstances remains higher than CVP, and hence is a more accurate determinant of CPP which is usually calculated as the MAP minus the ICP value, i.e., CPP = MAP – ICP.

There is abundant data demonstrating an association between raised ICP (greater than 20 mmHg), decreased CPP (CPP less than 50 mmHg), and poor neurological outcomes. Therapies directed and maintaining specific targets of ICP and CPP form the basis of most modern neurointensive therapy protocols for intracranial hypertension and are endorsed by the Brain Trauma Foundation.

Pressure-Volume Relationship

The cranial vault can be considered to comprise three compartments. The first of these, the brain parenchyma, occupies approximately 1400 ml while the CBV and CSF volume

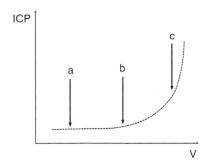

Figure 5.1 Diagram illustrating the intracranial pressure-volume relationship: **(a)** initially with working buffering mechanisms ICP remains unchanged despite changes in volume; **(b)** point at which ICP starts to increase is termed the point of decompensation; and **(c)** further increases of volume following exhaustion of buffering mechanisms results in substantial increases in ICP. Compliance (C) $= \frac{\Delta V}{\Delta ICP}$; Elastance $= \frac{1}{C}$; ICP = intracranial pressure; V = volume.

account for almost 150 ml each of the second and third compartments. The relationship between different intracranial volumes and pressure is described by the Monroe-Kellie doctrine. This states that an increase in the volume of one intracranial compartment will lead to a rise in ICP unless it is matched by an equal reduction in the volume of another compartment.

The buffering compartments are the CSF and CBV as the brain parenchyma is relatively incompressible. Any additional volume is therefore accommodated by displacing CSF through the foramina of Luschka and Magendie into the subarachnoid space and venous blood through the jugular and emissary veins outside of cranium. Only in infants with open fontanelles can expansion of total intracranial volume be observed. The amount of additional volume that can be accommodated is relatively small and in the acute situation, a reduction in arterial blood inflow (ischemia) as well as brain shifting and herniation usually represent exhaustion of the compensatory mechanisms resulting in critically elevated ICP.

The intracranial pressure-volume relationship is demonstrated in Figure 5.1. Initially, additional volume can be effectively buffered resulting in a minimal change in ICP. However, with exhaustion of compensatory reserve, further increases in volume result in large increases in ICP. This relationship at any given point on the curve can be calculated as intracranial *compliance* (C) which is equal to the change in volume (ΔV) divided by the change in pressure (ΔP). However, it is the reciprocal, i.e., elastance, which is clinically important as that is the change in pressure for a change in volume. This can be measured directly using invasive pressure monitors while injecting or withdrawing a known volume of CSF.

Pathophysiology of Intracranial Hypertension

The mechanisms of intracranial hypertension can be classified depending on the compartment where additional volume is present.

Brain Parenchyma

An increase in the volume of the brain parenchyma can result from additional water content causing brain edema. Depending on whether water accumulates in the extracellular or intracellular spaces we describe different types of cerebral edema (Table 5.1). In the majority of pathological states, all three types will be present and the importance of this classification and recognition of the prevailing type is related to the treatment response to steroids and hyperosmotic medications.

Table 5.1 Types of Cerebral Edema

Characteristic	Vasogenic Edema	Cytotoxic Edema	Interstitial Edema
Intra- vs extracellular	Extracellular	Intracellular	Extracellular
Pathophysiology	Increased capillary permeability/ disruption of BBB	Impaired ion transport/ metabolic failure	Direct effect of hydrostatic pressure
White vs gray matter	White matter	Gray and white matter	White matter
Cause	Neoplasms/ infection/late stage infarction	Trauma/early stage infarction	Hydrocephalus
Effect of steroids	Effective	Not effective	Not effective
Effect of osmotherapy	Effective	Effective	Not effective

Cerebral Blood Volume

Mismatch between inflow of arterial blood and outflow of venous blood leads to changes of total CBV. Venous obstruction which reduces venous outflow can be caused by a sinus thrombosis, tight cervical collar, right heart strain, a pulmonary embolus and high PEEP. An increase in arterial inflow may result from causes such as loss of autoregulation, hypoxia, cortical spreading depolarizations and seizures.

Cerebrospinal Fluid

Reduced absorption of CSF in the arachnoid villi or obstruction of CSF flow through the ventricles and subarachnoid spaces leads to the development of hydrocephalus and increased ICP. Common causes of obstructive hydrocephalus include; vascular malformations, intraventricular hemorrhage and tumors causing direct pressure on the ventricular system. Communicating hydrocephalus usually results from infections, subarachnoid hemorrhage, and traumatic brain injury.

Additional Non-physiological Volumes

Space occupying lesions, whether intra- or extra-axial, provide additional volume to the intracranial compartment and lead to the development of intracranial hypertension.

Clinical Features of Raised Intracranial Pressure

Depending on the acuteness and extent of the pathophysiological process, intracranial hypertension can manifest with relatively mild symptoms such as headaches to coma and death. In acute conditions, relatively small additional intracranial volumes can lead to a rapid rise in ICP and subsequent coma. In chronic conditions, such as communicating

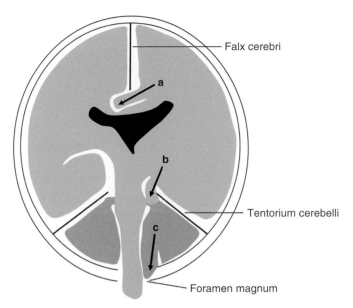

Figure 5.2 Types of brain herniation: **(a)** subfalcine herniation; **(b)** transtentorial herniation; and **(c)** tonsilar herniation.

Falx cerebri

Tentorium cerebelli

Foramen magnum

hydrocephalus or slow-growing neoplasms, large additional volumes can be accommodated with relatively mild symptomatology.

Acute Presentation

Altered Level of Consciousness

This is caused by compression of the supramedullary reticular activating system or bithalamic and/or bicortical damage.

Brain Herniation

Brain herniation is a clinical sign of exhausted compensatory reserve and results from the displacement of brain tissue through natural passages within the cranial cavity. It is a poor prognostic sign and should always be considered a neurosurgical emergency (Figure 5.2).

Transtentorial herniation is caused by a downward and medial shift of the temporal lobe or lobes through the tentorial incisura, leading to compression of the oculomotor nerve, rostral brainstem with its supramedullary reticular activating system, and the cerebral peduncle. Clinically this manifests as an ipsilateral dilated and unreactive pupil, contralateral hemiparesis, and decreasing level of consciousness. The clinical pattern is known as a "localizing sign" and can be used to direct surgical intervention in the absence of imaging. However, occasionally, compressive forces cause the contralateral occulomotor nerve and cerebral peduncle of the midbrain to impinge on the contralateral edge of the tentorium cerebelli, forming an indentation in the crus known as Kernohan's notch. This produces a "false localizing sign" resulting in the opposite clinical presentation.

Tonsilar herniation, on the other hand, is a manifestation of expansion of the posterior fossa, where the tonsils of the cerebellum herniate through the foramen magnum compressing the medulla. Tonsilar herniation often manifests as cardiorespiratory collapse and may produce a Cushing's reflex which consists of a triad of bradycardia, hypertension, and respiratory irregularity. It is a vasopressor response, probably related to increased sympathetic activation as a salvage mechanism due to direct injury to the brainstem. It can be seen in one third of patients with refractory intracranial hypertension.

Subacute and Chronic Presentation

Headache

This is often due to stretching and compression of the dura and cerebral blood vessels on the brain surface. Typically, it is generalized and worsened with recumbency, hypoventilation and straining. It is more often seen with focal lesions rather than generalized edema due to greater distortion of the dura.

Vomiting

Caused by irritation of the vagus nucleus and brainstem and in the context of intracranial hypertension, it is not frequently associated with nausea.

Papilledema

CSF pressure is directly transmitted through the optic nerve sheath to the optic disc. Increased pressure may lead to swelling of the optic disc, which in turn results in ischemic changes to the optic nerve and visual deterioration. It requires up to 24 hours to develop, so the absence of papilledema cannot be used to definitively rule out intracranial hypertension. If it results from high ICP it should be present bilaterally and may lead to permanent visual loss.

Abducens Nerve Palsy

The abducens nerve is susceptible to compression due to its long intracranial course before exiting the skull. Abducens palsy is thought to occur as a result of compression at the level of petroclival ligament, i.e., the level of upper clivus.

Neurological Deficits

These are related to compression of eloquent areas by mass lesions. They typically present as a result of focal lesions caused by neoplasms and hemorrhages.

Radiological Features of Raised Intracranial Pressure

Radiological imaging can reveal space occupying lesions such as neoplasms, hemorrhages, and infections; however, it may not always reveal signs of intracranial hypertension when mass lesions are not present. Previous studies have confirmed that it is impossible to predict ICP on the basis of the CT scan in situations of acute trauma. Nevertheless, certain of the following radiological features may indicate raised ICP (Figure 5.3):

- Effacement of cerebral sulci
- Loss of gray-white differentiation

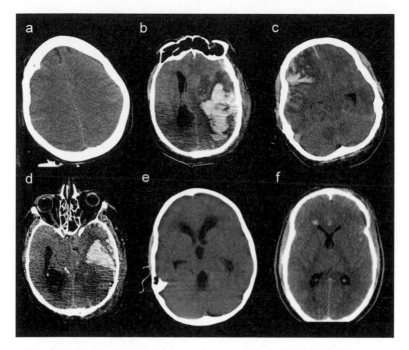

Figure 5.3 Images depicting the radiological features of intracranial hypertension: **(a)** diffuse swelling with loss of gray-white differentiation in ischemic/hypoxic injury; **(b)** large left-sided intraparenchymal hematoma with mass effect manifested as effacement of lateral ventricle, subfalcine herniation and midline shift; **(c)** right fronto-temporal contusions and obliteration of basal cisterns; **(d)** left temporal hematoma causing transtentorial herniation with clear compression of the temporal lobe on the midbrain, the temporal horn in visible medial to the tentorial edge; **(e)** acute hydrocephalus with dilated temporal horns and periventricular lucency best seen around the frontal horns of the lateral ventricles; and **(f)** imaging in keeping with diffuse axonal injury with scattered petechial hemorrhages in a patient with poor GCS. No clear radiological signs of intracranial hypertension; however, ICP in this patient was consistently >25 mmHg. This example demonstrates that it is frequently difficult to judge ICP on basis of CT imaging. CT, computed tomography; GCS, Glasgow Coma Scale; ICP, intracranial pressure.

- Compression of cerebral ventricles
- Midline shift (subfalcine herniation)
- Compression of basal cisterns
- Transtentorial or tonsilar herniation
- Acute hydrocephalus with periventricular lucency (hypodensity around ventricles representing transudated-type fluid originating from the ventricles due to high hydrostatic pressure)

Further Reading

Bratton, S.L., Chestnut, R.M., Ghajar, J., et al: Guidelines for the management of severe traumatic brain injury. VI. Indications for intracranial pressure monitoring. *J Neurotrauma* 2007; **24**(Suppl 1):S37–S44.

Chesnut, R.M., Temkin, N., Carney, N., et al: A trial of intracranial-pressure monitoring in traumatic brain injury. *N Engl J Med* 2012; **367** (26):2471–2481. doi:10.1056/NEJMoa1207363.

Hiler, M., Czosnyka, M., Hutchinson, P., et al: Predictive value of initial computerized tomography scan, intracranial pressure, and state of autoregulation in patients with traumatic brain injury. *J Neurosurg* 2006; **104**(5):731–737. doi:10.3171/jns.2006.104.5.731.

Morton, R., Ellenbogen, R. Intracranial hypertension. In: Ellenbogen, R., Abdulrauf, S., Sekhar, L., (Eds.). *Principles of Neurological Surgery*. 3rd ed. Philadelphia, PA: Elsevier;2012.

Chapter

6

Cerebral Ischemia

Bradley Hay, Sophia Yi, and Piyush Patel

Key Points

- Electroencephalographic evidence of cerebral ischemia occurs at a blood flow of approximately 20 ml/100 g/min.
- Brain infarction is characterized by a central area of severe ischemia, called the ischemic core, and a surrounding area of moderate ischemia called the penumbra.
- Global cerebral ischemia produced by cessation of blood flow results in selective neuronal necrosis in the hippocampus, cortex, cerebellum, and striatum.
- Cytotoxic edema occurs early during ischemia. At later stages, breakdown of the blood-brain barrier results in the development of vasogenic edema.
- BBB disruption occurs in acute and late stages of cerebral ischemia.
- Excitotoxicity is the excessive release of glutamate which activates postsynaptic receptors leading to a massive increase in intracellular calcium concentration and activation of other unregulated processes that cause neuronal death.
- Apoptosis contributes to delayed neuronal death which occurs for a long period after ischemia.
- The influx of inflammatory cells, activation of astrocytes and microglia, together with the release of cytokines into the ischemic territory results in substantial collateral damage.
- Healing of the brain, together with restoration of cerebrovascular carbon dioxide reactivity and cerebral autoregulation, occur over a period of 4 to 6 weeks.

Abbreviations

AMPA	α-amino-3-hydroxy-5-methyl-4-isoxazolepro-pionate
ATP	Adenosine triphosphate
BBB	Blood-brain barrier
CBF	Cerebral blood flow
CNS	Central nervous system
CPP	Cerebral perfusion pressure
EEG	Electroencephalograph
eNOS	Endothelial nitric oxide synthase
IL-1	Interleukin-1
IL-6	Interleukin-6

iNOS	Inducible nitric oxide synthase
MAP	Mean arterial pressure
NMDA	N-methyl-D-aspartate
nNOS	Neuronal nitric oxide synthase
NO	Nitric oxide
NOS	Nitric oxide synthase
TNF	Tumor necrosis factor

Contents

- Introduction
- Cerebral Blood Flow and Ischemia
- Pathophysiological Mechanisms
  - Excitotoxicity
  - Blood-Brain Barrier Disruption
  - Tissue Acidosis
  - Apoptosis and Necrosis
  - Nitric Oxide
  - Inflammation
- Time Course of Injury and Repair
- The Neurovascular Unit
- Summary
- Further Reading

Introduction

The CNS, despite having a relatively high metabolic rate, does not have substantial reserves of oxygen and energy substrates. The CNS is therefore intolerant of a reduction in CBF for all but brief periods. The pathophysiology of cerebral ischemia is complex; a wide variety of cellular processes, initiated by ischemia, have been shown to be integral to neuronal injury. Emphasis will be placed on CBF thresholds that result in specific patterns of injury, and a summary of the processes thought to play a major role in CNS injury is provided.

Cerebral Blood Flow and Ischemia

When MAP decreases below the lower limit of autoregulation, CPP becomes pressure dependent. When average CBF is reduced to about 20 ml/100 g/min, the EEG shows signs of slowing, and below this threshold it is suppressed (Figure 6.1). At 10 ml/100 g/min, energy failure characterized by K^+ efflux and Ca^{2+} influx occurs. Once the membrane depolarizes, neurons undergo death within a short time unless CBF is restored.

Cerebral ischemia is generally categorized into global and focal ischemia. The former is characterized by a widespread reduction in CBF (e.g., during cardiac arrest). Lack of oxygen and glucose leads to a dramatic reduction in cellular ATP levels within a few minutes, resulting in neuronal injury or death. Neurons in the hippocampus, layer 3 of the cerebral cortex, the striatum, and the Purkinje cells of the cerebellum are more vulnerable to ischemia.

Focal ischemia (e.g., stroke) is characterized by blood flow reduction in a major vessel in the brain. Within the ischemic territory, the region supplied by end-arteries undergoes

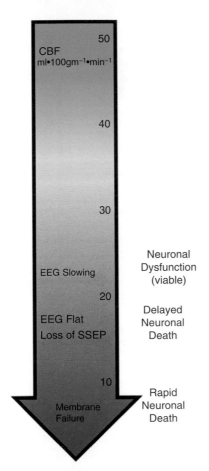

Figure 6.1 Flow thresholds for electrophysiologic dysfunction and cell death in the brain.

rapid cell death and is referred to as the ischemic core. Surrounding the core is a potentially viable area of the brain called the penumbra. The penumbra is rendered sufficiently ischemic to be electrically silent but has not yet undergone ischemic depolarization. It is viable for several hours and can be salvaged by restoration of flow. Within the penumbra, cerebral autoregulation and cerebral reactivity to carbon dioxide are attenuated or abolished making it exquisitely sensitive to changes in CPP and CO_2 tension. Secondary insults in the form of hypoxia and hypotension occurring over the next few hours to days may gradually recruit the penumbra into the core. Once the infarction has fully evolved, the necrotic tissue is gradually resorbed over a period of weeks and the resulting cystic cavity is lined by a glial scar. In the region surrounding the infarction, autoregulation and CO_2 reactivity are re-established in most situations in about 4 to 6 weeks.

Pathophysiological Mechanisms

Excitotoxicity

Energy failure is the central event in the pathophysiology of ischemia. Maintenance of normal ionic gradients across the cell membrane is an active process that requires ATP.

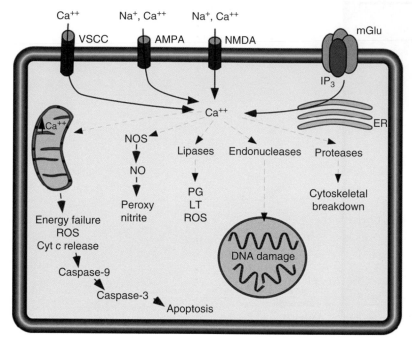

Figure 6.2 Excitotoxicity. Excessive release of glutamate leads to glutamate receptor activation, neuronal depolarization, influx of calcium, release of calcium from the endoplasmic reticulum, and unregulated enzyme activation. See text for details.

When ATP levels are critically low, ionic homeostasis is no longer maintained and rapid influx of Na^+, efflux of K^+, and depolarization of the membrane takes place (Figure 6.2). Simultaneously, depolarization of presynaptic terminals leads to massive release of the excitatory neurotransmitter, glutamate. Excessive glutamate-mediated injury is referred to as excitotoxicity. Glutamate activates NMDA and AMPA receptors, resulting in membrane depolarization and influx of Ca^{2+} and Na^+. This massive increase in intracellular Ca^{2+} is toxic to the cell and activates a variety of cellular processes that contribute to injury. These include activation of proteases, lipases, and DNases which gradually damage cellular constituents. The excess Ca^{2+} that is buffered by the mitochondria, results in their damage from free radical formation and oxidative injury. Membrane depolarization leads to mitochondrial permeability transition, when cytochrome c, an integral component of the electron transport system, is released into the cytoplasm and leads to the activation of caspases resulting in cell apoptosis.

Activation of platelets within cerebral microvessels, as well as the influx of white blood cells into damaged areas, aggravates ischemic injury by occluding the vasculature. Furthermore, the influx of Na^+ and Ca^{2+} into neurons leads to uptake of water from the extracellular space causing cytotoxic edema. Depending on the severity of the injury, BBB breakdown occurs about 2 to 3 days after injury permitting entry of plasma proteins into the brain substance further increasing cerebral swelling (vasogenic edema). The development of post-ischemic edema can be significant enough to result in substantial increases in intracranial pressure and further ischemia.

Blood-Brain Barrier Disruption

After stroke, BBB compromise occurs in two phases; an early immediate phase that is apparent upon restoration of flow, followed by, a delayed opening 2 to 3 days after the stroke. BBB damage results in vasogenic edema and is a major contributor to secondary injury as well as intracerebral hemorrhage. The extent of BBB injury is dependent upon size of the stroke, degree of vascular occlusion, and the extent of reperfusion. The disruption of tight junction proteins and opening of the barrier junctions due to oxidative stress induced by free radical generation after ischemia, initiates the BBB dysfunction (see Chapter 2).

Tissue Acidosis

In the absence of oxygen, anaerobic metabolism supervenes resulting in low ATP synthesis and the generation of lactate. With hyperglycemia, a greater amount of substrate is available for anaerobic metabolism and therefore the reduction in tissue pH is greater than might occur with normoglycemia.

Apoptosis and Necrosis

Cell death is conventionally classified as apoptotic or necrotic. Programmed cell death, or apoptosis, is the result of a coordinated production and activation of a variety of proteases, called caspases, which lead to the breakdown of key cellular constituents. The neuron is fragmented in the later stages of the process and then resorbed with minimal damage and disruption to its neighboring cell. In contrast, necrosis of neurons is caused primarily by energy failure. This results in inhibition of protein synthesis, cellular swelling, rupture of cell membrane, and intense inflammation capable of injuring adjacent cells. During ischemia, those neurons that survive necrosis may undergo delayed cell death by apoptosis and thus contribute to the ongoing neuronal loss for several weeks after the initial ischemia.

Nitric Oxide

Ischemia can cause the formation of iNOS and activate nNOS, (Figure 6.3) to produce NO. The combination of NO and superoxide anion results in the production of peroxynitrite which can damage cellular proteins, membranes, and DNA. By contrast, the NO produced by eNOS is a vasodilator, has anti-inflammatory and antithrombotic effects and in the setting of ischemia, maintains CBF and reduces neuronal injury. Therefore, NO has a dual role in the pathophysiology of cerebral ischemia.

Inflammation

Ischemia induces inflammation early in the process. Expression of adhesion molecules such as intercellular adhesion molecule (ICAM), vascular cell adhesion molecule (VCAM), and selectins on endothelial cells and the expression of integrins on leukocytes lead to the recruitment and adhesion of leukocytes in the microcirculation of the ischemic territory. In addition to occlusion of the microcirculation, leukocytes release proteolytic enzymes and free radicals, thereby augmenting injury. Efforts to block adhesion molecules reduce the influx of leukocytes into the brain and reduce injury. Leukocytes, neurons and glial cells also elaborate a variety of proinflammatory cytokines. These cytokines, which

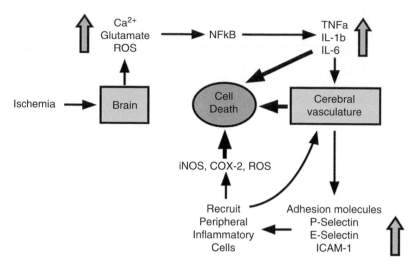

Figure 6.3 Inflammation in the ischemic brain. Activation of the transcription factor NfkB leads to the synthesis and subsequent release of inflammatory cytokines. Expression of adhesion molecules in cerebral vessels results in recruitment of inflammatory cells into the brain. These inflammatory cells contribute to neuronal injury.

include IL-1, IL-6, and TNF-α, mediate the inflammatory response and also serve to recruit more inflammatory cells (Figure 6.3). Cytokine receptor antagonists reduce cerebral infarction, at least in the acute phase. However, long-term suppression of these cytokines actually enhances injury. This suggests that proinflammatory cytokines, though deleterious in the acute phase of ischemia, are nonetheless necessary for long-term neuronal survival.

Neurogenic inflammation arises from the local release of specific neuropeptides such as Substance P (SP) and calcitonin gene-related peptide (CGRP) from primary sensory neurons which surround blood vessels in abundance. These neuropeptides then act directly on vascular endothelial and smooth muscle cells causing vasodilation and increased permeability resulting in plasma extravasation and edema, and, along with other mediators, attract and activate both innate immune cells (mast cells, dendritic cells), and adaptive immune cells (T-lymphocytes). Neurogenic inflammation is an important driver of cerebral edema and resultant neurological deficits.

Time Course of Injury and Repair

With the onset of ischemia, excitotoxicity predominates during the first minutes to hours. Inflammatory mechanisms are subsequently activated and they peak several days later. Of importance is the observation that microglial activation can be observed for as long as 6 months after ischemia. This long-term inflammation in the brain has led some to characterize ischemic injury not as an acute process only but also as a chronic encephalopathic process. The disruption of the BBB occurs at about 2 to 3 days post ischemia. The brain responds to the ischemic injury by initiating several processes in an attempt to limit the extent of injury and to facilitate repair and regeneration (Figure 6.4).

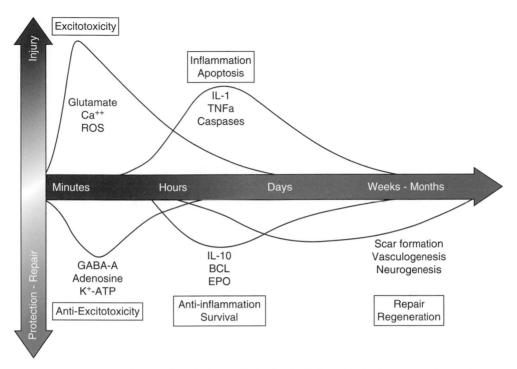

Figure 6.4 Time course of neuronal death after cerebral ischemia. Excitotoxicity leads to neuronal necrosis rapidly. Inflammation and neuronal apoptosis contribute to ongoing cell death for a period that extends from several days to weeks.

The Neurovascular Unit

Much of the investigation into the pathophysiology of ischemic injury has focused on neurons. It is now clear that stroke leads to injury of neurons, astrocytes, oligodendrocytes, and vascular endothelium. The simultaneous activation of the immune cells, including microglia and the influx of inflammatory cells into the brain, contribute to the extent of injury. Increasingly, therapeutic interventions are now being focused on the protection and restoration of the entire neurovascular unit. The tissue components that are injured during ischemia are diagrammatically presented in Figure 6.5.

Summary

A multitude of processes contribute to neuronal injury after ischemia, but not all them produce injury at the same time. Whereas necrosis occurs early in response to excitotoxicity, ongoing neuronal loss from BBB disruption, apoptosis, necrosis, and inflammation can continue well after the initial ischemic insult. It is therefore not surprising that attempts to reduce injury by interventions that target a single pathway have not met with success in humans. Combination therapies, each targeting a specific mechanism that is operative at specific times in the pathophysiology of stroke are more likely to be effective. Finally, the demonstration of inflammation in the CNS as late as 6 to 8 months after ischemia in experimental models indicates that neuronal loss (and

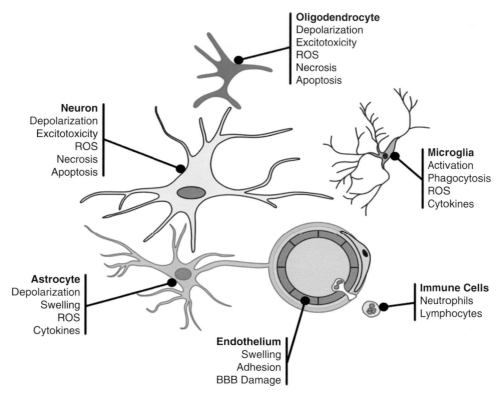

Figure 6.5 The neurovascular unit, comprised of neurons, astrocytes, microglia, and microvessels, is shown in the figure. Ischemia leads to injury to each components of the unit. The type of injurious process that is triggered is shown in the figure.

perhaps neuronal replacement through neurogenesis) is not limited to the acute phase of ischemia. As such, ischemic cerebral injury maybe regarded as a chronic encephalopathic disease.

Further Reading

Astrup, J., Siesjo, B.K., Symon, L.: Thresholds in cerebral ischemia: The ischemic penumbra. *Stroke* 1981; **12**:723–725.

Back, T., Kohno, K., Hossmann, K.A.: Cortical negative DC deflections following middle cerebral artery oc- clusion and KCl-induced spreading depression: Effect on blood flow, tissue oxygenation, and electroen cephalogram. *J Cereb Blood Flow Metab* 1994; **14**:12–19.

Dirnagl, U.: The pathobiology of injury after stroke: The neurovascular unit and beyond. *Ann NY Acad* 2012; **1268**:21–25.

Endres, M., Laufs, U., Liao, J.K., Moskowitz, M.A.: Targeting eNOS for stroke protection. *Trends Neurosci* 2004; **90**:281–289.

Hossmann, K.A.: Ischemia-mediated neuronal injury. *Resuscitation* 1993; **26**:225–235.

Knowland, D., Arac, A., Sekiguchi, K.J., et al: Stepwise recruitment of transcellular and paracellular pathways underlies blood-brain barrier breakdown in stroke. *Neuron* 2014; **82**:603–617.

Polster, B.M., Fiskum, G.: Mitochondrial mechanisms of neural cell apoptosis. *J Neurochem* 2004; **90**:1281–1289.

Prakash, R., Carmichael, S.T.: Blood-brain barrier breakdown and neovascularization processes after stroke and traumatic brain injury. *Curr Opin Neurol* 2015; **28**:556–564.

Rosenberg, G.A.: Ischemic brain edema. *Prog Cardiovasc Dis* 1999; **42**:209–216.

Siesjo, B.K.: Pathophysiology and treatment of focal cerebral ischemia. Part I: Pathophysiology. *J Neurosurg* 1992; **77**:169–184.

Zheng, Z., Yenari, M.A.: Post-ischemic inflammation: Molecular mechanisms and therapeutic implications. *Neurol Res* 2004; **26**:884–892.

Brain Protection

Bradley Hay, Sophia Yi, and Piyush Patel

Key Points

- There does not appear to be any difference among intravenous or volatile anesthetic agents with respect to their neuroprotective efficacy.
- Most anesthetic agents reduce the vulnerability of the brain to ischemic injury.
- Maintenance of cerebral perfusion pressure within the normal range for a patient who is at risk for cerebral ischemic injury is essential.
- Arterial carbon dioxide levels should be maintained in the normal range unless hyperventilation is used for short-term brain relaxation.
- Hyperglycemia can exacerbate ischemic injury and treatment with insulin should be considered.
- The use of mild hypothermia for the management of low-grade aneurysm clipping or traumatic brain injury may not be of benefit. Hyperthermia should always be treated.
- Seizures can augment cerebral injury and should be treated urgently.
- At present, brain protection relies on maintenance of physiologic homeostasis rather than pharmacological agents.

Abbreviations

AMPAR	α-amino-3-hydroxy-5-methyl-4-isoxazolepropionic acid receptor
ATP	Adenosine triphosphate
CMR	Cerebral metabolic rate
CBF	Cerebral blood flow
CBV	Cerebral blood volume
$CMRO_2$	Cerebral metabolic rate for oxygen consumption
CNS	Central nervous system
CPP	Cerebral perfusion pressure
DBP	Diastolic blood pressure
EEG	Electroencephalography
GABA	Gamma-aminobutyric acid
ICP	Intracranial pressure
MAP	Mean arterial pressure

NMDA	N-methyl-D-aspartate
NMDAR	N-methyl-D-aspartate receptor
SAH	Subarachnoid hemorrhage
SBP	Systolic blood pressure
TBI	Traumatic brain injury

Contents

Introduction

The risk of ischemic cerebral injury which can occur during neurosurgical, cardiac, and carotid artery surgery has led to considerable interest in identifying approaches that reduce the vulnerability of the brain to ischemia. This chapter briefly reviews the available information about the neuroprotective efficacy of anesthetic agents and the physiologic management of a brain at risk of ischemic injury.

Influence of Anesthetic Agents on Ischemic Brain

The approach to the problem of cerebral ischemia was initially focused on reducing the brain's requirement for ATP, assuming the brain would be able to tolerate ischemia for a longer time. Given that anesthetic agents suppress CMR and in some circumstances, increase CBF, it is not surprising that they have been extensively investigated as potential neuroprotective agents. Unfortunately, nearly all the evidence comes from animal studies, and very few human trials are available for guidance.

Barbiturates

Barbiturate drugs can produce burst suppression on the EEG but in global ischemia they have not been shown to reduce ischemic injury. By contrast, barbiturates can reduce the extent of focal cerebral injury. In humans, thiopental loading has been demonstrated in a single study to reduce post–cardiopulmonary bypass neurological deficits. More recent animal studies, in which brain temperature was tightly controlled, have confirmed only a modest protective effect of barbiturates. In addition, lower doses that produce burst suppression may yield a reduction in injury that is of similar magnitude to that achieved with much larger doses. Long-term neuroprotection with barbiturates has not yet been demonstrated.

Volatile Anesthetics

A large number of animal investigations have shown that the volatile agents halothane, isoflurane, sevoflurane, and desflurane can reduce cerebral injury in focal ischemia. However, there does not appear to be a substantial difference among the agents but the protective efficacy is as large as that of barbiturates.

In most experimental studies, injury was evaluated a few days after the ischemic insult. Therapeutic strategies that are neuroprotective in the short-term may not produce long-lasting benefit because of the continuous loss of neurons in the post-ischemic period. Volatile anesthetics can produce neuroprotection for short periods but it is not sustained beyond two weeks which suggests that these agents delay but do not prevent neuronal death. In models of very mild focal ischemia, sustained neuroprotection with sevoflurane has been shown suggesting that volatile agents can produce long-term neuroprotection provided the severity of injury is very mild. Once neuronal injury occurs, infarct expansion may preclude long-term neuroprotection.

Propofol

Propofol can also produce burst suppression, reducing $CMRO_2$ by up to 50%. Experimental studies with this agent have shown a substantial reduction of ischemic injury produced by stroke with similar efficacy to that of barbiturates and volatile anesthetics. With mild cerebral ischemic insults, sustained neuroprotection has been demonstrated but this is not the case with moderate to severe injury.

Ketamine

Ketamine is a potent NMDA receptor antagonist. In models of focal ischemia, substantial neuroprotection has been demonstrated but the adverse neuropsychiatric side effects have restricted its clinical use for this purpose. NMDA receptor antagonists have been employed for the treatment of acute stroke in humans but none of the clinical trials have shown neuroprotective efficacy.

Etomidate

Etomidate can reduce $CMRO_2$ by up to 50% by producing EEG burst suppression. Unlike barbiturates, etomidate is cleared rapidly and does not cause myocardial depression or hypotension. However, in human investigations of focal ischemia, etomidate leads to a greater degree of tissue acidosis and hypoxia than desflurane anesthesia. The detrimental effects of etomidate have been confirmed in experimental studies which have shown that brain injury increases after its administration.

Pharmacological Agents

A wide variety of agents have shown considerable efficacy in reducing cerebral infarction in experimental models of stroke. These include (1) NMDAR and AMPAR antagonists, (2) GABA agonists, (3) calcium channel blockers, and (4) trophic factors. With the sole exception of nimodipine (and nicardipine) in subarachnoid hemorrhage, no other agent has demonstrated neuroprotection in clinical trials.

Influence of Physiologic Parameters on Ischemic Brain

Physiologic parameters such as MAP, $PaCO_2$, blood glucose, and body temperature have a significant influence on outcome after cerebral ischemia.

Temperature

Experimental studies have shown that a reduction in temperature of only a few degrees ($\approx$33°C–34°C) can dramatically reduce the brain's vulnerability to ischemic injury. However, in a large multicenter trial mild hypothermia did not result in either short- or long-term improvement in neurological outcome after cerebral aneurysm surgery with similar findings in a trial of hypothermia in head-injured patients. These important outcome studies have forced re-evaluation of the use of mild hypothermia in the operating room.

In contrast, increases in brain temperature, often as small as 1°C, during and after ischemia can aggravate cerebral injury. Ischemia that normally results in scattered neuronal necrosis produces cerebral infarction when body temperature is elevated. It therefore seems prudent to avoid hyperthermia in patients who are at risk of cerebral ischemia or have suffered an ischemic insult.

Cerebral Perfusion Pressure

Cerebral autoregulation maintains a relatively stable CBF over a range of blood pressures. However, because of a lack of clinical trial data, absolute guidelines regarding blood pressure targets cannot be recommended. The selection of these targets is dependent on the patient's pre-existing blood pressure, co-morbid medical conditions, and the nature and extent of CNS injury. Where feasible, it is preferable to titrate blood pressure management to the patient's baseline measurements. About a third of patients with severe TBI have a disruption in cerebral autoregulation and a rise in MAP can lead to elevated ICP due to increased CBV and hyperemia. Therefore, a CPP of 60–70 mmHg is usually adequate in head-injured patients (see Chapter 34).

In patients with an acute ischemic stroke, intravenous thrombolytic therapy administered within 4.5 hours after symptom onset is the most widely proven reperfusion intervention. Recent clinical trials have also demonstrated efficacy of mechanical endovascular therapy (with the intention of clot retrieval and removal) within 6 hours of symptom onset in patients eligible for thrombolytic therapy. Prior to lytic therapy most recommendations suggest a SBP ≤185 mmHg and DBP ≤110 mmHg. Patients that are not eligible for thrombolytic therapy should not have their hypertension treated unless it is severe (SBP > 220 mmHg or DBP > 120 mmHg) and when treatment is indicated, MAP should not be decreased >15% over the first 24 hours after ischemic stroke.

For reasons that are not yet clear, retrospective data indicates that neurologic outcome may be worse in patients who have undergone endovascular therapy under general anesthesia with SBP less than 140 mmHg. It is therefore reasonable to maintain blood pressure in the normal range for these patients or a SBP greater than 140 mmHg if general anesthesia is chosen.

In patients with SAH, regional CBF reductions have been repeatedly observed. While an increase in blood pressure can improve CBF and reduce neurologic deficits, the risk of aneurysmal rupture with induced hypertension must be taken into consideration. Current European Stroke Organization guidelines call for the treatment of systolic hypertension in excess of 180 mmHg and if anti-hypertensive therapy is initiated, the mean arterial pressure should be maintained at or above 90 mmHg.

Hypotension has been shown to be quite deleterious to an injured (ischemic or traumatic) brain. Hypotension can increase cerebral infarct volumes significantly and should be avoided in patients who have suffered a stroke. Similarly, hypotension has been demonstrated to be one of the most important contributors to a poor outcome in patients who have sustained head injury. Maintenance of adequate MAP and CPP is therefore critical. Elevation of MAP by α-agonists is reasonable while maintaining adequate intravascular volume.

Blood Glucose

In a normal brain that is adequately perfused, glucose is metabolized aerobically but when the brain is rendered ischemic, glucose is then metabolized anaerobically and the end products of this pathway are lactic acid and ATP. During hyperglycemia, the supply of glucose to the ischemic brain is increased and the amount of lactic acid produced is considerable and cerebral pH decreases. This acidosis contributes significantly to neuronal necrosis. Acute hyperglycemia is associated with reduced salvage of penumbral tissue and greater final infarct size. Hyperglycemia is associated with a higher incidence of intracerebral hemorrhage, reduced benefit from recanalization after thrombolytic therapy and overall increased neurological injury.

Treatment of hyperglycemia with insulin has been shown to reduce neurological injury. Consequently, it has been suggested that hyperglycemia is treated in patients at risk for cerebral ischemia and in those who have suffered an ischemic insult. What is not certain is the glucose level at which treatment is indicated. In patients with acute stroke, TBI, and SAH, aggressive reduction in blood glucose has not been shown to be of benefit which may relate to episodes of hypoglycemia which in itself can be detrimental. Based on the available data, it is reasonable to treat hyperglycemia in the setting of acute stroke or TBI when glucose levels are in excess of 180 mg/dl and avoid hypoglycemia with frequent measurement of blood glucose levels.

Arterial Carbon Dioxide Tension

Manipulation of arterial carbon dioxide tension is a potent means of altering CBF and CBV. Hypocapnia in patients with ischemic or traumatic CNS injury can be detrimental. Prophylactic hyperventilation has not been shown to be of any benefit in patients with stroke. In fact, laboratory data have shown that hypocapnia can significantly decrease CBF in an ischemic brain and in head injured patients hypocapnia is associated with worse outcomes.

Seizure Prophylaxis

Seizure activity is associated with increased neuronal activity, increased CBF and CBV (and consequently increased ICP), and cerebral acidosis. Untreated seizures can produce neuronal necrosis even with normal cerebral perfusion. Prevention plus rapid treatment of seizures is therefore an important goal (see Chapter 42).

Summary

At present, our ability to pharmacologically protect the brain and make it less vulnerable to ischemic injury is limited. The available data indicate that it is the anesthetized state per se rather than the choice of specific anesthetics that reduces the vulnerability of the brain to ischemic injury. While volatile agents, barbiturates, and propofol have been shown to reduce cerebral injury in experimental models of ischemia, the durability of this protection is limited. In human studies, anesthetics have not shown protective efficacy in comparison to a sedated state. Even if anesthetics provide some degree of protection, this protection is easily obviated by even small degrees of anesthesia-induced blood pressure reduction. Consequently, for purposes of reducing ischemic cerebral injury, the emphasis should be placed on physiologic homeostasis.

Further Reading

Berkhemer, O.A., Fransen, P.S., Beumer, D., et al: A randomized trial of intraarterial treatment for acute ischemic stroke. *N Engl J Med* 2015; **372**:11–20.

Connolly, E.S. Jr, Rabinstein, A.A., Carhuapoma, J.R., et al: Guidelines for the management of aneurysmal subarachnoid hemorrhage. *Stroke* 2012; **43**:1711–1737.

Davis, M.J., Menon, B.K., Baghirzada, L.B., et al: Anesthetic management and outcome in patients during endovascular therapy for acute stroke. *Anesthesiology* 2012; **116**(2):396–405.

Jinadasa, S., Boone, D.: Controversies in the management of traumatic brain injury. *Anesthesiol Clin* 2016; **34**:557–575.

Kawaguchi, M., Furuya, H., Patel, P.M.: Neuroprotective effects of anesthetic agents. *J Anesth* 2005; **19**:150–156.

Powers, W.J., Derdeyn, C.P., Biller, J., et al: 2015 American Heart Association/American Stroke Association focused update of the 2013 guidelines for the early management of patients with acute ischemic stroke regarding endovascular treatment. *Stroke* 2015; **46**:3024–3039.

Quillinan, N., Herson, P.S., Traystman, R.J.: Neuropathophysiology of brain injury. *Anesthesiol Clin* 2016; **34**:453–464.

Steiner, T., Juvela, S., Unterberg, A., et al: European Stroke Organization guidelines for the management of intracranial aneurysms and subarachnoid haemorrhage. *Cerebrovasc Dis* 2013; **35**:93–112.

Todd, M.M., Hindman, B.J., Clarke, W.R., Torner, J.C.: Mild intraoperative hypothermia during surgery for intracranial aneurysm. *N Engl J Med* 2005; **352**:135–145.

The Brain Trauma Foundation: The American Association of Neurological Surgeons. The Joint Section on Neurotrauma and Critical Care. Hyperventilation. *J Neurotrauma* 2000; **17**:513–520.

Chapter

8

Intravenous Anesthetic Agents

Nienke Valens and Anthony Absalom

Key Points

- Propofol, thiopentone, and etomidate have similar effects on overall cerebral hemodynamics and metabolism.
- All three above agents reduce $CMRO_2$ consumption and maintain responsiveness to CO_2 and autoregulation.
- Ketamine may be associated with an increase in CBF and ICP.
- Benzodiazepines have a small effect on blood flow and metabolism.
- Propofol and remifentanil are ideal agents for continuous infusion for maintenance of anesthesia. They allow rapid return of consciousness and assessment of neurological status, even after prolonged infusion.

Abbreviations

BZ	Benzodiazepine
CBF	Cerebral blood flow
CBV	Cerebral blood volume
$CMRO_2$	Cerebral metabolic rate of oxygen
CO_2	Carbon dioxide
CPP	Cerebral perfusion pressure
EEG	Electroencephalogram
fMRI	Functional magnetic resonance imaging
GABA	Gamma-aminobutyric acid
ICP	Intracranial pressure
NMDA	N-methyl-D-aspartate
PET	Positron-emission tomography
TCI	Target controlled infusion

Contents

- Introduction
- Propofol
- Thiopental

- Etomidate
- Dexmedetomidine
- Ketamine
- Benzodiazepines
- Total Intravenous Anesthesia
- Further Reading

Introduction

The mechanisms of action of anesthetic agents remain an area of intense investigation. With the exception of ketamine, which acts via antagonism of the NMDA receptor, most intravenous anesthetic agents (such as propofol, thiopentone, and etomidate) probably act by an agonist effect at the $GABA_A$ receptor, causing an increase in the duration of opening of $GABA_A$-dependent chloride channels. The increased time of opening permits increased passage of chloride ions which serves to cause membrane hyperpolarization and therefore inhibition of neuronal transmission. It is likely that each agent binds to a separate site on the $GABA_A$ receptor and that the different effects of each drug (such as amnesia, sedation, and hypnosis) are mediated by distinct sub-units of the receptor. Although current evidence favors involvement of the $GABA_A$ receptor, it is likely that intravenous anesthetic agents also have significant effects on other receptors and ion channels.

BZs have sedative rather than hypnotic effects. They also act at the $GABA_A$ receptor by binding to the α-subunit of the activated receptor. Two subtypes of BZ receptors have so far been identified. BZ_1 is responsible for anxiolysis and the receptors are located mainly in the cerebellum and spinal cord. BZ_2 receptors facilitate the anticonvulsant and sedative effects of BZs. They are located in the cerebral cortex, hippocampus, and spinal cord.

Functional imaging studies, using techniques such PET and fMRI show that although the intravenous anesthetic agents can have similar clinical effects, they cause distinct (and very different) effects on regional blood flow and metabolism. Despite this, except for ketamine, they all cause global reductions in CBF and metabolism.

Although the intravenous anesthetic agents cause slowing of the surface EEG, the only exception being ketamine, there are agent-specific differences which are discernible to an expert or expert system. In general, the agents other than ketamine cause a dose-dependent progressive shift of power from the higher to the lower frequencies. At deep levels of anesthesia, a burst suppression pattern occurs. With increasing levels of suppression, fewer bursts occur and finally at excessively deep levels of anesthesia or overdose an isoelectric pattern will be found.

An "ideal" intravenous anesthetic agent for use in neuroanesthesia and neurocritical care should possess certain properties. Such an agent would:

- Allow rapid recovery of consciousness
- Permit early assessment of neurological status
- Be rapidly titratable
- Have minimal effects on other organ systems
- Provide analgesia
- Have anti-epileptic properties (or at least be non-epileptogenic)
- Have advantageous effects on cerebral hemodynamics, in particular:
  - Maintenance of cerebrovascular autoregulation

- Maintenance of vasoreactivity to CO_2
- Reduction of $CMRO_2$ coupled with a decrease in CBF
- Reduction of CBV
- Reduction or no alteration of ICP

No agent currently available fulfills all the above criteria. The agents most commonly used for induction of anesthesia for neurosurgery are propofol, thiopental, and etomidate. Although all three agents can induce anesthesia, they have distinct advantages and disadvantages, particularly during neurosurgery which are discussed below.

Propofol

Propofol is now the most widely used agent for intravenous induction and intravenous maintenance of anesthesia during neurosurgical procedures. It has also recently been used successfully for providing conscious sedation during awake craniotomy surgery.

It provides smooth induction of anesthesia with minimal excitatory effects and a rapid, clear-headed recovery. Although there have been case reports of convulsions, these are believed to be "pseudoseizures", as they have not been found to be associated with abnormal EEG activity. Propofol is generally regarded as having anti-convulsive effects (and is sometimes used as a treatment of refractory status epilepticus). It causes a dose-dependent reduction in arterial blood pressure which may in turn compromise CPP.

With regard to neuroanesthesia, propofol can have the following effects:

- Produce a progressive reduction in CBF
- Produce a reduction in $CMRO_2$ of up to 60%
- Produce a reduction in ICP, particularly when elevated from baseline
- Maintain cerebral autoregulation
- Maintain flow-metabolism coupling
- Maintain vasoreactivity to CO_2
- Demonstrate free radical scavenging properties
- Block calcium channels and antagonize glutamate receptors (in vitro)

Thiopental

Thiopental use is diminishing as a first-choice induction agent. Other than occasional use for rapid sequence induction, the clinical use of thiopental is mostly limited to neurocritical care for deep barbiturate coma to reduce ICP in patients with refractory intracranial hypertension. Thiopental has a very large volume of distribution such that after repeated bolus doses or prolonged infusion, significant accumulation and delayed recovery can occur.

Thiopental can have the following effects and uses:

- Produces a reduction in CBF coupled to a decrease in $CMRO_2$
- Causes a decrease in CBV and ICP
- Provides protection against focal ischemia in animals.
- Possesses free radical-scavenging properties
- Reduces calcium influx
- May cause blockade of sodium channels
- Can be used to treat status epilepticus

Etomidate

Etomidate remains a drug of interest due to its cardiovascular stability on induction of anesthesia, which may be relevant when maintenance of CPP is vital. It has similar effects on CBF, $CMRO_2$, and autoregulation as thiopental and propofol. However, it is a potent suppressant of corticosteroid synthesis, an effect that may occur after a single dose in critically ill patients. For this reason, the widespread use of etomidate has declined.

Etomidate causes epileptiform EEG changes and in susceptible patients, even low doses may induce seizures. It has therefore been used to unmask seizure foci during intra-operative EEG mapping for epilepsy surgery.

Dexmedetomidine

Dexmedetomidine is an α_2-adrenergic agonist. It has dose-dependent clinical effects which include anxiolysis, analgesia, and sedation. These are thought to be mediated via effects on α_2 receptors located in the brainstem (locus coeruleus). The nature of the sedation resembles natural sleep in terms of EEG features and clinical effects (patients remain rousable). Adverse effects include bradycardia and biphasic effects on arterial blood pressure. At lower doses, sympatholysis can cause hypotension, whereas at higher doses direct stimulation of α_2 receptors present on vascular smooth muscle can increase peripheral resistance causing hypertension and a decline in cardiac output.

With regard to anesthesia for neurosurgery, dexmedetomidine has been shown to:

- Induce rousable sedation
- Cause matched reductions in $CMRO_2$ and CBF in healthy volunteers
- Have minimal effects on respiratory drive
- Preserve vasoreactivity to CO_2
- Have minimal or no effects on evoked potentials
- Have little effect on epileptiform activity in the EEG
- Have no clear anti-convulsant effect in humans

Ketamine

Ketamine is an NMDA antagonist with sympathomimetic activity. The use of ketamine in neuroanesthesia has been limited due to the perception that it raises ICP and has unwanted side effects including emergence reactions, vivid dreaming, out of body experiences and delusions.

In the United Kingdom, ketamine is available as a racemic mixture of (R–) and (S+) Stereoisomers. S (+) ketamine is twice as potent as (R–) ketamine and may be associated with fewer side effects. It has a larger elimination clearance and a larger volume of distribution.

Ketamine is known to have the following effects:

- Increased $CMRO_2$ and CBF (but usually not when used in low doses as an adjunct to other anesthetic agents)
- Increase ICP when used alone for maintenance of anesthesia
- Demonstrates cerebral protection via NMDA antagonism in animals

- Has minimal respiratory depressant effects
- Preserves vasoreactivity to CO_2

Benzodiazepines

BZs may be associated with prolonged sedation which limits their use as induction agents for neuroanesthesia but at lower doses may be prescribed for premedication. These agents are useful for sedation on the intensive care unit in traumatic brain-injured patients undergoing hypothermia treatment when propofol metabolism is impaired allowing lipid accumulation.

BZs can have the following effects:

- Cause a modest reduction in CBF
- Cause a modest reduction in $CMRO_2$
- Cause a modest reduction in ICP
- Preserve vasoreactivity to CO_2
- Preserve cerebral autoregulation
- Increase seizure threshold

However, a plateau effect occurs, whereby increasing doses do not produce greater reductions in these variables. All effects are reversed by flumazenil, a competitive BZ antagonist but its use may precipitate seizures.

Total Intravenous Anesthesia

The use of intravenous agents for the maintenance of anesthesia is popular. Propofol is the agent most suited to prolonged infusion since its context-sensitive half time does not increase appreciably with time. Therefore, following prolonged infusion, there is a rapid return of consciousness facilitating assessment of neurological status.

Remifentanil is a pure mu (μ) receptor agonist. It possesses ester linkages which are degraded by non-specific tissue and plasma esterases. It has a constant context-sensitive half time making it ideal for use in addition to propofol for maintenance of anesthesia. This agent allows good analgesia and muscle relaxation during surgery but minimizes post-operative sedation, nausea, and vomiting that may occur with longer-acting opiates. Provision of alternative drugs to ensure adequate postoperative analgesia is essential after painful surgical interventions.

Both propofol and remifentanil can be used by simple infusions for maintenance of anesthesia. The usual dose ranges for propofol are 3–12 mg/kg/h and for remifentanil 0.05–0.5 mcg/kg/min. With the development of commercially available microprocessor-controlled infusion pumps, propofol and remifentanil can now be given for both induction and maintenance of anesthesia using TCI systems based on three compartment model algorithms. The pumps require the patient's weight and age to be entered in order to calculate the appropriate infusion rate based on an estimated plasma concentration. The usual target propofol levels are 4–6 µg/ml and 2–4 µg/ml for induction and maintenance respectively. Typical target concentrations for remifentanil are 4–8 ng/ml. The use of TCI systems has been shown to result in improved hemodynamic stability during induction of anesthesia which is particularly beneficial for neurosurgical cases.

	Target Receptor	ICP	CMRO2	Respiratory Depression	Cardiovascular Depression	Indication
Propofol	GABA	↓↓	↓↓	++	++	Induction & maintenance of anesthesia
Thiopental	GABA	↓↓	↓↓	++	+	Induction of anesthesia; Deep barbiturate coma
Etomidate	GABA	↓↓	↓↓	++	–/+	Induction of anesthesia (cardiovascularly unstable patients)
Ketamine	NMDA	↑/↓	↑	–	–	Hypovolemic trauma patient
Dexmedetomidine	α_2-adrenoceptor	↓	↓	–	Concentration dependent	Functional neurosurgery
Benzodiazepine	GABA	↓	↓	+	+	ICU sedation Sedative premedication;

Summary (qualitative) of the pharmacodynamic effects of intravenous anesthetic agents.

Further Reading

Absalom, A.R., Struys, M.R. (2005) *An Overview of TCI and TIVA*. Belgium: Academia Press.

Hemmings, H.C. Jr., Akabas, M.H., Goldstein, P. A., et al: Emerging molecular mechanisms of general anesthetic action. *Trends Pharmacol Sci* 2005; **26**(10):503–510.

Rozet, I., Metzner, J., Brown, M., et al: Dexmedetomidine does not affect evoked potentials during spine surgery. *Anesth Analg* 2015; **121**:492–501.

Souter, J., Rozet, I., Ojemann, J., et al: Dexmedetomidine sedation during awake craniotomy for seizure resection: Effects on electrocorticography. *J Neurosurg Anesthiol* 2007; **19**:38–44.

Chapter

9 Volatile Anesthetic Agents

Una Srejic

Key Points

- All inhaled vapors decrease cerebral metabolism except nitrous oxide.
- All inhaled vapors are cerebral vasodilators at higher concentrations, with desflurane and isoflurane causing more vasodilation than sevoflurane.
- Vasodilation causes an increase in cerebral blood flow, cerebral blood volume, and intracranial pressure, and progressively impairs cerebral autoregulation. Hyperventilation producing hypocapnia can offset the cerebral vasodilation.
- No human randomized studies validate neuro-protection or preconditioning by anesthetic vapors.
- Manipulation of cardiac output, mean arterial pressure, and arterial carbon dioxide tension can minimize some of the adverse effects of inhaled agents on intracranial pressure.

Abbreviations

AR	Autoregulation
CBF	Cerebral blood flow
CBV	Cerebral blood volume
$CMRO_2$	Cerebral metabolic rate for oxygen
CO	Cardiac output
CPP	Cerebral perfusion pressure
CSF	cerebrospinal fluid
ICP	Intracranial pressure
MAP	Mean arterial pressure

Contents

- Introduction
- Physiology: Cerebral Blood Flow, Metabolism, and Autoregulation
- Nitrous Oxide
- Isoflurane

- Sevoflurane
- Desflurane
- Xenon
- Further Reading

Introduction

Knowledge of the pharmacological effects of inhaled anesthetics on $CMRO_2$, AR, and vascular reactivity is essential when administering a neurosurgical anesthetic. Manipulation of these physiologic parameters with inhaled agents can have beneficial or detrimental effects on ICP and neuronal survival post injury.

Physiology: Cerebral Blood Flow, Metabolism, and Autoregulation

Under normal conditions, population averaged CBF is relatively constant at MAP of 60–150 mmHg. CBF is influenced by vascular tone and local environmental chemicals (neuronal nitric oxide, vasoactive intestinal peptide (VIP), potassium, metabolites, prostaglandins, glutamate, and calcium), and is maintained at about 50 ml/100 g/min. CBF can be affected by many factors including MAP < 60 mmHg > 150 mmHg, low PaO_2, $PaCO_2$, vascular spasm, seizures and cardiac output (CO) (see Chapter 3).

The inhaled anesthetics (isoflurane, desflurane, and sevoflurane) have in common a twofold effect on CBF. $CMRO_2$ decreases with the administration of these vapors. Up to a minimum alveolar concentration (MAC) of approximately 0.6, there is a coupled slight vasoconstriction of the cerebral vessels, resulting in a decrease in CBF. Beyond 0.6 MAC of isoflurane and desflurane there is progressive separation of CBF and $CMRO_2$ whereby CBF increases despite continue reduction in $CMRO_2$. This is often referred to as "uncoupled" although there is still coupling but at a different slope of the CBF-$CMRO_2$ relationship. With sevoflurane, this does not occur until above 1–1.5 MAC. This progressive cerebral vasodilation, impairs AR resulting in pressure dependent blood flow. When AR is impaired, ischemia or luxury perfusion with resulting edema or hemorrhage can occur. Xenon and nitrous oxide (N_2O) do not affect the brain in this manner.

The brain responds differently to inhaled anesthetics under normal and pathological conditions. In the presence of hypoxia, acidosis, edema, and inflammation, cerebral AR can be lost regionally ("vasoparalysis"). This can result in unpredictable physiologic changes in these areas.

In the normal brain, vascular changes in response to $PaCO_2$ are preserved. Hyperventilation and hypocapnia can override the vasodilation induced by inhaled agents at >0.6 MAC. Because excessive hypocapnia can result in reduced blood flow and potentially ischemia, common clinical practice is to target the $PaCO_2$ between 32 and 35 mmHg if using a vapor anesthetic. Excessive vasodilation with hypercapnia can cause an increase in ICP by increasing intracranial blood volume. Isoflurane, desflurane, and sevoflurane all increase ICP as the concentration increases, with sevoflurane having the least effect. By virtue of their systemic vasodilating properties, they also decrease MAP, CPP, and CBF (Chapter 3).

Inhaled anesthetics decrease $CMRO_2$ by decreasing the electrical activity of the brain until the point of isoelectricity ("flat line" EEG). At this point, $CMRO_2$ is decreased by 60%

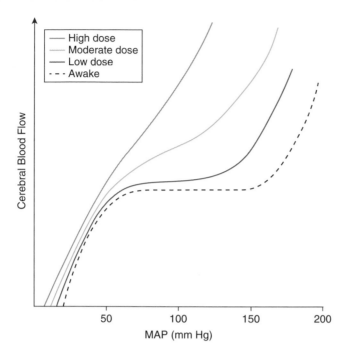

Figure 9.1 Inhaled anesthetic agents and cerebral autoregulation Schematic representation of the effect of increasing concentrations of a typical volatile anesthetic drug on autoregulation of cerebral blood flow. Dose-dependent cerebral vasodilation results in attenuation of autoregulatory capacity. Both the upper and lower thresholds are shifted to the left.
MAP, Mean arterial pressure.
(With permission from Miller's Anesthesia, published 2015, Chapter 17, Figure 17–10)

and cannot be decreased further by anesthetics except with the addition of hypothermia (Chapter 4).

Neuromonitoring of the somatosensory evoked potential (SSEP), motor evoked potential (MEP), brainstem auditory evoked potential (BAEP), and visual evoked potential (VEP) show progressively increased latency and decreased amplitude of the waveforms with increasing dose of inhaled agents. MEP and VEP waves are the most sensitive to inhaled agents and SSEP/BAEP, the least (Chapter 49).

Although neuroprotective and pre-conditioning properties of inhaled agents are observed in rodents, there are still no prospective or randomized human clinical trials to support this in the clinical arena (Figure 9.1).

Nitrous Oxide

N_2O is an N-methyl-D-aspartate (NMDA) receptor blocker (like ketamine and xenon), therefore, it does not share the same mechanism of action as the other inhaled agents. N_2O does not affect AR and cerebral vascular tone. When given alone, N_2O can stimulate the sympathetic nervous system and increase CBF, CBV, $CMRO_2$, and subsequently ICP. As N_2O is rarely given as a sole neurosurgical anesthetic, it is of not great clinical significance. However, in patients with critically increased ICP, N_2O combined with inhaled agents is not recommended as part of the anesthetic regimen.

Conversely, in elective neurosurgical cases, N_2O can be safely combined with IV anesthetics (propofol, narcotics, and benzodiazepines) and mild-moderate hyperventilation to offset some of its natural properties. N_2O enlarges airspaces and may lead to pneumocephalus. Although a controversial subject, N_2O can increase the incidence of postoperative nausea and vomiting.

Isoflurane

Below 0.6 MAC, isoflurane decreases $CMRO_2$ and has minimal effect on CBF. Over 1.1 MAC, isoflurane can increase CBF by 20% and impair AR. This dose dependent vasodilation can increase ICP. The EEG can be made isoelectric at 2 MAC. Thus, in patients with severely increased ICP, TIVA (total intravenous anesthesia) may be a better choice than an inhalational/opioid anesthetic.

Sevoflurane

Similar to isoflurane, sevoflurane decreases CBF and $CMRO_2$ below 0.6 MAC and increases them above 1 MAC. Being the least vasoactive, sevoflurane can preserve CBF best up to 1–1.5 MAC and maintains AR. Thus, increases in ICP over 1 MAC are greatest with desflurane than with isoflurane and least with sevoflurane.

Sevoflurane is the least pungent of the inhaled agents so is ideal for inhaled inductions in children. Because of its low blood/gas solubility, it also dissipates very quickly and promotes a faster emergence.

Sevoflurane can be associated with seizure-like activity on the EEG, in seizure-prone patients, those taking anti-convulsants, patients with a history of febrile seizures, or those receiving a high-dose inhalation induction. Usually, sevoflurane-induced spiking does not have any sequelae. In these patients, hyperventilation and using a MAC greater than 1.5 are best avoided.

Approximately 40% of preschool children may get emergence agitation after sevoflurane anesthesia. This can be minimized with small doses of clonidine, dexmedetomidine, or propofol on emergence.

Desflurane

At 1 MAC, desflurane causes the most vasodilation, followed by isoflurane and then sevoflurane. AR is lost at >1 MAC. Desflurane is the only currently used inhaled anesthetic known to increase CSF production and alter CSF dynamics. This property may contribute to increased ICP. Like sevoflurane, desflurane has a low blood/gas partition coefficient and can be easily and quickly exhaled for a rapid emergence. Its sympathetic stimulating properties can increase the heart rate, CO, and CBF.

Xenon

Xenon, an inhaled noble gas, has anesthetic properties of hemodynamic stability, cardio-protection, and experimental neuro-protection. A non-competitive NMDA receptor blocker, xenon facilitates rapid induction and emergence with no teratogenicity. However, it is very expensive and not widely used clinically in the United States (used in Europe). Like other inhaled agents, xenon decreases $CMRO_2$ causing a decrease in CBF in gray matter (increases CBF in white matter), and decreased ICP. It also has a very low blood/gas partition coefficient of 0.115. Currently, it is being studied for use in ASA III-IV patients as a possible replacement for N_2O (Table 9.1).

Table 9.1 Summary of the Effects of Inhalational Anesthetics on CBF, CMRO$_2$, and ICP

	CBF	CMRO$_2$	ICP
N$_2$O	↑↑	↑ or →	↑↑
Xenon	↓ (Gray) ↑ (White)	↓	↑ or →
Isoflurane	↑ or →	↓↓	→ or ↗ or ↑
Sevoflurane	↓ or → or ↗	↓ or ↓↓	→ or ↗ or ↑
Desflurane	↓ or ↑	↓↓	↑ or →

Arrows indicate semi-quantitative changes.
↗: slight increase, ↑:increase, ↑↑:marked increase, →:unchanged ↓:decrease, ↓↓:marked decrease (with permission from: Adapted from Cottrell and Young's *Neuroanesthesia* 5th Ed. Chapter 5. Table 5-1.
CBF, cerebral blood flow; CMRO$_2$, cerebral metabolic rate of oxygen consumption; ICP, intracranial pressure

Further Reading

Cottrell, J.E., Young W. (2010). *Neuroanesthesia*. Philadelphia, PA: Mosby Elsevier, Chapter 5, Table 5-1, pp. 78–95.

Holmstrom, A., Akeson, J.: Desflurane increases intracranial pressure more and sevoflurane less than isoflurane in pigs subjected to intracranial hypertension. *J Neurosurg Anesth* 2004; **16**:136–143.

Jovic, M., Unic-Stojanovic, D., Isenovic, E., et al: Anesthetics and cerebral protection in patients undergoing carotid endarterectomy. *J Cardiothorac Vasc Anesth* 2015; **29**(1):178–184.

Lieberman, J.A., Feiner, J., Lyon, R., Rollins, M. D.: Effect of hemorrhage and hypotension on transcranial motor-evoked potentials in swine. *Anesthesiology* 2013; **119**:1109–1119.

Meng, L.Z., Gelb, A., Regulation of cerebral autoregulation by carbon dioxide. *Anesthesiology* 2015; **122**:196–205.

Meng, L.Z., Hou, W., Chui, J., Han, R., Gelb, A. W.: Cardiac output and cerebral blood flow, *Anesthesiology* 2015; **123**:1198–1208.

Maze, M.: Preclinical neuroprotective actions of xenon and possible implications for human therapeutics: A narrative review. *Can J Anesth* October 27, 2015 (epub ahead of print) PMID 26507536.

Miller, R., et al: (2015), *Miller's Anesthesia*, 8th ed. Chapter 17, Figure 17-10, Philadelphia, PA: Elsevier Saunders.

Petersen, K.D., Landsfeldt, U., Cold, G.E., et al: Intracranial pressure and cerebral hemodynamics in patients with cerebral tumors. A randomized prospective study of patients subjected to craniotomy in propofol-fentanyl, isoflurane-fentanyl or sevoflurane-fentanyl anesthesia. *Anesthesiology* 2003; **98**:329–336.

Stocchetti, N., Maas, A.I., Chieregato, A., van der Plas, A.A.: Hyperventilation in head injury: A Review. *Chest* 2005; **127**:1812–1827.

Chapter 10

Opioids and Adjuvant Drugs

Mariska Lont and Anthony Absalom

Key Points

- Opioids have minimal effects on cerebral blood flow, metabolism, and intracranial pressure provided normocapnia and normotension are maintained.
- Pain after craniotomy can be significant and perioperative use of modest doses of morphine does not increase the incidence of sedation, nausea, or depressed airway reflexes.
- Naloxone is best avoided in neurosurgical patients as abrupt opioid reversal can have detrimental effects on cerebral hemodynamics
- Succinylcholine causes a mild temporary elevation in ICP and is not contraindicated when rapid airway control is required. With the availability of sugammadex, rocuronium is a safe and reliable alternative.
- For control of perioperative hypertension, adrenoreceptor antagonists, and calcium channel blockers are preferred to vasodilators as they reduce blood pressure without increasing cerebral blood volume and ICP.

Abbreviations

5-HT	5-hydroxytryptamine
BBB	Blood brain barrier
CBF	Cerebral blood flow
CMR	Cerebral metabolic rate
EEG	Electroencephalographic
HS	Hypertonic saline
ICP	Intracranial pressure
ICU	Intensive care unit
NMBA	Neuromuscular blocking agent

Contents

- – Electrical Activity
- – Postoperative Analgesia
- – Other Effects
- Naloxone
- α_2-Adrenergic Agonists
- Neuromuscular Blocking Drugs
- Antihypertensive Agents
  - – Direct acting Vasodilators
  - – Adrenoreceptor Antagonists
  - – Calcium Channel Blockers
- Miscellaneous Agents
  - – Glucocorticoids
  - – Osmotic Agents

Opioids

Opioid analgesics are an important adjunct to the sedative and hypnotic anesthetic agents. In addition to providing analgesia, limiting hypertensive responses to painful stimuli, opioids also have a hypnotic-sparing effect that can help provide improved intraoperative hemodynamic stability and more rapid emergence. The opioid analgesics commonly used in neuroanesthesia include morphine, fentanyl, sufentanil, remifentanil, and alfentanil. Sufentanil is a highly selective opioid agonist used in North America and Europe, but not in the United Kingdom. It is 10–15 times more potent than fentanyl with a shorter elimination half-life. Remifentanil has unique pharmacokinetic characteristics resulting in a more rapid onset and offset of action. This results from susceptibility of its ester linkages to non-specific esterases widely present in blood and tissues. Therefore, it has a context-insensitive duration of action following an infusion (i.e., its duration of effect is independent of duration of administration).

Cardiovascular Effects

Opioids are sympatholytic yet they increase parasympathetic tone. In large doses, all opioids are associated with bradycardia but any resulting hypotension usually responds to atropine or glycopyrrolate. Opioids greatly potentiate the effects of hypnotic agents. Moderate doses of remifentanil can significantly reduce propofol requirements needed to prevent the effects of noxious stimuli. Hypotension may also occur if the dose of hypnotic agent is not reduced accordingly when moderate or large doses of opioids are used.

Respiratory Effects

There is profound synergism between the depressant respiratory effects of opioids and hypnotics. Opioids are known to attenuate airway reflexes and can prevent coughing in response to the presence of an endotracheal tube. The pharmacokinetic profile of remifentanil makes it an ideal agent for use in combination with other sedative drugs during operations where neuromuscular paralysis is not used to facilitate electrophysiological monitoring.

Cerebral Hemodynamics

High opioid doses may cause modest reductions in CBF and $CMRO_2$ if normocapnia is maintained. The effects are probably minimal in the clinical dose range under normal circumstances. Some studies have shown an increase in ICP after the administration of opioids. This may be secondary to autoregulatory vasodilation after a reduction in mean arterial and cerebral perfusion pressures. However, the effect was not demonstrated when mean arterial pressure was maintained with vasopressors. Opioids are useful for attenuating the adverse effects on cerebral hemodynamics during stimulating procedures such as intubation, suctioning, and skull pin application.

Cerebral Electrical Activity

EEG changes are dose-dependent and small doses of fentanyl and sufentanil produce minimal EEG changes. However, very high doses of fentanyl, 30–70 μg/kg, can result in delta wave activity (high voltage, slow waves). There may be a ceiling effect for the EEG changes produced during sufentanil infusion. Even though higher dose of opioids may alter the latency and amplitude of sensory evoked potentials, this does not preclude their use for monitoring spinal cord function. In general, opioids have minimal effects on auditory and motor evoked potentials.

Postoperative Analgesia

The moderate to severe pain from craniotomy can lead to sympathetic stimulation and hypertension which is a risk factor for post-craniotomy hematoma. Opioids have been underused in the perioperative period for fear of sedation, pupillary changes, nausea, and suppression of airway reflexes. However, there are many studies showing that the use of morphine does not significantly increase the incidence of these adverse effects. Commonly used opioids for postoperative analgesia include morphine, piritramide, fentanyl, oxycodone, and tramadol. Use of codeine is dwindling because it is ineffective in up to 30% of patients who lack the enzyme to convert it to morphine.

Other Effects

Opioids have the potential to cause nausea and vomiting by stimulation of serotonin $(5\text{-}HT_3)$ and dopamine receptors in the chemoreceptor trigger zone. Prolonged infusions or repeated doses of longer-acting agents can cause impaired gastric emptying, ileus, constipation, pupillary constriction, pruritus, and blurred vision. Postoperative nausea and vomiting are less common after propofol and remifentanil anesthesia possibly because of the antiemetic effect of propofol combined with the rapid clearance of remifentanil. Large intraoperative doses of opioids other than remifentanil, may result in delayed emergence from anesthesia.

Naloxone

Naloxone is a potent competitive antagonist at the μ opioid receptor but has a weaker affinity for the κ and δ receptors. The drug has minimal effects on CBF and oxygen metabolism. Although it can be used to reverse opioid-induced sedation and respiratory depression, it will also antagonize the analgesic effects. Abrupt opioid reversal with naloxone can result in pain, hypertension, arrhythmias, myocardial ischemia, and intracranial hemorrhage. It should be used cautiously in doses of approximately 1.5 µg/kg titrated to clinical effect. The effects of a bolus of naloxone last only 20–30 minutes and thus the patient may return to a narcotized state if a longer-acting opioid had been used.

α_2-Adrenergic Agonists

These agents cause sedation, analgesia, and anxiolysis. Clonidine and dexmedetomidine are the two commonly used drugs. Dexmedetomidine is more selective with a 1600-fold greater sensitivity for α_2 than α_1 receptors. They produce their sedative effects by an agonist action on α_2 receptors in the locus ceruleus consequently reducing neural activity in ascending projections. Reduced sympathetic activity and associated reduced catecholamine levels make them promising neuroprotective agents.

Dexmedetomidine reduces CBF as a result of activity inhibition in ascending arousal projections and probably not via direct cerebrovascular effects. However, it can cause *systemic* vasoconstriction via activation of vascular smooth muscle α_2 receptors. Limited animal studies have shown that $CMRO_2$ is unaffected, despite reduced CBF causing concerns about cerebral oxygen delivery and a possible increase in oxygen extraction. Human studies, however, suggest that flow-metabolism coupling is maintained, and that matched reductions in CBF and $CMRO_2$ occur. As yet, there is no clear evidence on the safety of dexmedetomidine use in patients with injured brains.

Dexmedetomidine is now available in Europe although it is currently licensed only for sedation in ICUs. In the operating room, it is a useful adjuvant providing potential benefit when used for sedation during conscious functional procedures such as deep-brain electrode implantation, awake craniotomy, and epilepsy surgery.

Neuromuscular Blocking Agents

Succinylcholine has the potential to increase ICP but the rise is minimal and transient. The clinical significance of this increase is unknown and these concerns should not preclude its use in situations where rapid control of the airway is required. The rise in ICP can be minimized by pre-treatment with nondepolarizing neuromuscular blockers. Rapid intubation conditions can also be obtained by administration of rocuronium 1.2 mg/kg. Deep neuromuscular blockade induced by rocuronium can be rapidly antagonized by sugammadex, a selective neuromuscular blocker binding agent. This can be useful where neuromonitoring or diagnostic procedures are required soon after endotracheal intubation.

It is important to recognize that the metabolism of some NMBAs can be accelerated by certain anticonvulsant medication such as phenytoin or carbamazepine. For example, carbamazepine almost doubles the clearance of vecuronium. On the other hand, intraoperative magnesium sulphate administration can prolong the neuromuscular blockade induced by non-depolarizing agents.

Antihypertensive Agents

Perioperative hypertensive episodes can result in increased ICP and may cause intracranial hemorrhage in patients with disturbed cerebral autoregulation. Dangerous levels of hypertension may occur during laryngoscopy, at incision or during extubation and can be treated with either direct-acting vasodilators, adrenoreceptor antagonists or calcium channel blockers.

Direct Acting Vasodilators

Direct acting vasodilators such as sodium nitroprusside, glyceryltrinitrate, and hydralazine reduce blood pressure by relaxing vascular smooth muscle and decreasing vascular resistance. They must be used with caution because the cerebral vasodilatation can result in increased cerebral blood volume and ICP with a reduction in cerebral perfusion. Moreover, if the blood vessels in the abnormal regions of the brain are selectively sensitive to vasodilators, a steal-phenomenon and worsening of ischemic injury could result. To reduce the risk of rebound hypertension, these drugs must be withdrawn slowly.

Adrenoreceptor Antagonists

Labetalol is one of the more commonly used adrenoreceptor blockers. It has both α- and non-cardioselective β-adrenergic blocking actions. The ratio of α to β-blocking effects is 1:7. Unlike the direct-acting vasodilators, it reduces the mean arterial pressure without a concomitant increase in ICP. Labetalol improves cerebral perfusion pressure when compared to sodium nitroprusside in postoperative neurosurgical patients with refractory hypertension. Esmolol, an ultrashort-acting β-adrenoceptor antagonist metabolized by plasma esterases, is commonly used to control perioperative surges in blood pressure. Urapidil is a systemic postsynaptic α_1-antagonist capable of inhibiting catecholamine induced vasoconstriction. Its use in the context of neuroanesthesia has seen a recent increase.

Calcium Channel Blockers

Nicardipine blocks the influx of calcium ions into cardiac and smooth muscle. This results in a decrease in systemic vascular resistance with little or no negative inotropic effect and no effect on ICP. A favorable pharmacokinetic profile makes it easy to titrate. During hypertensive emergencies, nicardipine has clear benefits over longer-acting calcium channel antagonists which may cause cerebral vasodilatation. The use of nimodipine in subarachnoid hemorrhage is discussed in Chapter 35.

Miscellaneous Agents

Glucocorticoids

Glucocorticoids stabilize the BBB and increase absorption of cerebrospinal fluid. They are beneficial in reducing vasogenic edema in primary and metastatic brain tumors improving generalized symptoms such as headache and altered mental status more than focal deficits. In traumatic brain injury, glucocorticoids have been associated with an increased risk of death. The use of steroids in acute spinal cord injury has not been shown to improve long-term motor function. A disadvantage of glucocorticoid use is the associated hyperglycemia which may be associated with a worse postoperative neurologic outcome and an increased risk of postoperative infections.

Osmotic Agents

Mannitol and HS are osmotic agents that are commonly used to treat acute increases in ICP. By creating an osmotic gradient, they draw water out of tissues into the vascular compartment reducing blood viscosity. The resultant increase in CBF induces autoregulatory vasoconstriction that may reduce ICP. Mannitol (0.25–0.5 g/kg) has free radical scavenging properties and is dependent on an intact BBB to be most effective. It can accumulate in injured tissues leading to rebound effects and should not be used if the serum osmolality exceeds 320 mosmol/kg.

HS is administered both as an intermittent bolus or as a continuous infusion with varying volumes and tonicity (3%–23.4%). It is increasingly being used for intraoperative brain relaxation and according to the limited evidence available, HS significantly reduces the risk of brain swelling during craniotomy. However, further studies investigating long-term outcome parameters are currently in progress.

Further Reading

Haldar, R., Kaushal, A., Gupta, D., Srivastava, S., Singh, P.K.: Pain following craniotomy: Reassessment of the available options. *Biomed ResInt* 2015; **2015**:509164.

Ortega Gutiérrez, S., Thomas, J., Reccius, A., et al: Effectiveness and safety of nicardipine and labetalol infusion for blood pressure management in patients with intracerebral and subarachnoid haemorrhage. *Neurocritical Care* 2013; **18**:13–19.

Prabhakar, H., Singh, G.P., Anand, V., Kalaivani, M.: Mannitol versus hypertonic saline for brain relaxation in patients undergoing craniotomy (Review). *Cochrane Database Syst Rev* 2014; **7**: CD010026.

Chapter

11

Preoperative Assessment

Eleanor Carter and Amit Prakash

Key Points

- Preoperative assessment of neurosurgical patients is central to planning safe and effective perioperative care.
- It encompasses a standard assessment that is applicable to all patients and specific elements relevant to particular procedures and groups of patients.
- Comorbid conditions including medications required for their treatment need to be reviewed and optimized prior to neurosurgical interventions.
- Communication of information relating to morbidity and mortality risk estimation is an important part of a patient's assessment.

Abbreviations

AED	Antiepileptic drug
ASA	American Society of Anesthesiologists
CNS	Central nervous system
GCS	Glasgow Coma Scale
ICP	Intracranial pressure
INR	International normalized ratio
LMWH	Low molecular weight heparin

Contents

- Introduction
- The Preoperative Assessment Clinic
- Generic Preoperative Assessment
    - Routine History and Examination
    - Neurological Assessment
- Medication Management
    - Anticoagulant and Antiplatelet Agents
    - Corticosteroids

- – Antiepileptic Drugs
- – Antiparkinson Drugs
- Investigations
- Procedure Specific Preoperative Assessment
  - – Tumor Surgery
  - – Vascular Surgery
  - – Functional Neurosurgery
  - – Surgery for Traumatic Brain Injury
  - – Spinal Surgery
- Preoperative Risk Assessment
- Consent
- Postoperative Planning
- Further Reading

Introduction

Preoperative assessment is central to planning safe and effective perioperative care in neurosurgery. This process focuses on collating patient- and procedure-specific information, optimizing management of comorbid conditions, and estimating surgical risks for each patient. The objective is to communicate collaboratively and inform patients prior to surgery while formulating individualized evidence-based perioperative care plans.

The Preoperative Assessment Clinic

Preoperative assessment is typically performed in a dedicated outpatient clinic, ideally, 4–6 weeks prior to elective surgery. Depending upon patient access and urgency, appointments should be made available for "walk-in-patients" needing expedited neurosurgical procedures. The clinic should be anesthetist-led with multidisciplinary input from surgeons, physicians, specialist nurses, pharmacists, and occupational therapists. This form of integrated preoperative assessment approach has been shown to decrease day of surgery cancellations, improve the patient's experience, and reduce complication rates and perioperative mortality.

Generic Preoperative Assessment

Neurosurgery encompasses a wide range of procedures, but common elements of preoperative assessment exist. The overarching goal is to determine the patient's baseline health and functional status and from this, identify and minimize risks. Preoperative information can be gathered from multiple sources including the patient, family members, and medical notes.

Routine History and Examination

Pertinent information should be sought from the patient regarding: (1) current and past medical diseases, (2) previous surgery and anesthetic complications, (3) prescribed and non-prescribed medications, (4) relevant family medical conditions, and (5) functional status of organ systems and social history (current employment, driving status and home support). This level of detail is required as certain medical conditions are directly associated

Table 11.1 Medical Conditions Directly Associated with Neurosurgical Pathology

Intracranial aneurysm	Hypertension Cigarette smoking, recreational drug use, especially cocaine Adult polycystic kidney disease, Ehlers-Danlos syndrome, Marfan's syndrome
Arteriovenous malformation	Neurofibromatosis type 1 (NF1), Sturge-Weber, Osler-Weber-Rendu, von Hippel-Lindau (VHL) syndromes
Carotid artery stenosis	Atherosclerosis, hypertension, diabetes mellitus Cigarette smoking
Brain tumors	Primary cancer elsewhere in body NF1, tuberous sclerosis, VHL, Li-Fraumeni, Turner, Turcot, Gorlin syndromes, human immunodeficiency virus
Pituitary lesions	Hypo- or hyperpituitarism, multiple endocrine neoplasia 1
Acoustic neuroma	Neurofibromatosis type 2
Cerebral or spinal infections	Infective focus elsewhere in body, immunocompromize
Spinal deformities	Cerebral palsy, spina bifida, muscular dystrophy Ankylosing spondylitis, rheumatoid arthritis Restrictive lung disease

with neurosurgical pathology (Table 11.1) and many of the interventions required can impact on the patient's ability to live independently.

A preliminary examination includes a cardiopulmonary and airway assessment. Neurosurgical patients, especially those with cervical spine disease, have higher rates of difficult ventilation and intubation, which if unanticipated can lead to life-threatening complications.

Neurological Assessment

A preoperative neurological assessment establishes the patient's baseline status which is used as a comparator if new neurological deficits are detected postoperatively. The history should include details about symptoms, diagnoses, current neurological deficits, and response to treatment. Any signs or symptoms consistent with raised ICP including headaches, nausea, vomiting, blurred vision, or confusion are particularly important and can guide perioperative neuro-protection strategies. In patients with epilepsy, the frequency and type of seizures, any premonitory features, and treatment responsiveness should be ascertained. A focused neurological examination includes assessment of a patient's GCS, pupil size, reactivity and establishing laterality, and extent of cranial or peripheral nerve deficits. The ability of the patient to communicate appropriately and fluently should be assessed as it has implications for awake procedures and other types of functional or ablative neurosurgery.

Medication Management

In addition to routine medications, attention should be paid to perioperative management of corticosteroids (used for control of cerebral edema) anti-epileptics, anticoagulants and antiplatelet agents. Drug allergies and reactions to dyes and contrast agents should be established.

Anticoagulant and Antiplatelet Agents

The majority of anticoagulant and antiplatelet drugs are withheld prior to neurosurgery due to the risk of bleeding and its devastating consequences. However, interventional procedures (aneurysm coiling, cerebral stenting procedures) carry a high risk of thrombosis and hence require antiplatelet agents perioperatively.

Typically, aspirin and clopidogrel are withheld for ten days preoperatively to ensure normal platelet function at the time of surgery. Warfarin is stopped for 5 to 7 days preoperatively to aim for an INR of less than 1.2. Bridging therapy with LMWH may be warranted in certain patients at very high risk of thromboembolism. The management of newer direct acting oral anticoagulants such as rivaroxaban, dabigatran, and apixaban, often require specialist hematology advice.

Corticosteroids

Corticosteroids are frequently used to reduce cerebral edema and its ICP consequences in CNS tumors. They have important side effects that can cause impaired glucose tolerance, weight gain, gastrointestinal bleeding, immunosuppression, electrolyte disturbance, osteoporosis and mood changes, most of which need relevant management in the perioperative period.

Antiepileptic Drugs

AEDs are generally continued in the perioperative period unless directed otherwise by the medical or surgical teams. Alternative routes of administration for AEDs should be prescribed if patients are not able to take their oral medications postoperatively.

Antiparkinson Drugs

Drugs for Parkinson's disease are usually continued and the timing of administration is important to prevent rigidity postoperatively. Advice should be sought from the surgical team for patients with resistant Parkinson's disease undergoing deep brain stimulation or other destructive thalamic procedures.

Investigations

Preoperative tests are performed to detect and monitor underlying health conditions and are selected depending on the comorbidities of the patient and grade of surgical severity. UK National and international guidelines on preoperative testing can be used to develop local policies and procedures.

Procedure Specific Preoperative Assessment

Neurosurgical procedures can range from relatively minor to majorly invasive with proportionate perioperative risks. As such, the preoperative assessment will vary considerably depending on the nature of the procedure.

Tumor Surgery

The signs and symptoms of brain tumors vary depending on the size, location, mass effect, edema, and presence of hydrocephalus. The neurological history and examination should be considered in association with neuroimaging findings to help predict likely postoperative neurological function. It is particularly important to check preoperative electrolytes and glucose due to the frequency of sodium disorders and corticosteroid-related hyperglycemia. Pituitary tumors are additionally associated with systemic endocrine and metabolic disorders and a full endocrine evaluation is required.

Neurovascular Surgery

Emergency neurovascular surgery carries significant risks and often precludes a comprehensive preoperative assessment. However, core considerations include evaluating the baseline neurological function and managing associated complications such as hydrocephalus, cardiopulmonary dysfunction, and electrolyte disturbance. In elective neurovascular surgery, a full preoperative assessment is performed with particular focus on associated systemic conditions. The current status of a patient's treatment with anticoagulant and antiplatelet drugs should be established and a perioperative management plan formulated. For interventional neuroradiology procedures, the patient and procedure should be evaluated for suitability of a local anesthetic technique which may need to be considered in certain circumstances.

Functional Neurosurgery

Functional neurosurgery procedures are performed to manage Parkinson's disease, epilepsy, Tourette's syndrome, and severe depression. A full medication history is required preoperatively and a plan made, in conjunction with specialists, regarding drug doses and timings in the perioperative period. The systemic effects and potential interactions with anesthetic agents for each of these drugs should also be evaluated.

Surgery for Traumatic Brain Injury

The formal preoperative process is not possible in head trauma patients. It is particularly important to assess for other injuries, including chest trauma and those that could cause major hemorrhage. These types of injury can affect oxygenation and cerebral perfusion pressure intraoperatively. Every effort should be made to stabilize associated injuries and prevent secondary brain injury during the perioperative period.

Spinal Surgery

Spinal disease can be secondary to congenital conditions, trauma, or ageing. Patients presenting for spinal surgery may be relatively fit and well. However, intraoperative positioning, blood loss, and postoperative analgesia are important challenging issues in relation to this surgery. The focus of preoperative assessment is to determine any movement restrictions, assess current analgesic requirements and develop a comprehensive perioperative plan. A full systems review is required to identify associated medical conditions and ensure that these are adequately managed. A complete airway examination is essential and patients should be counseled if awake fiberoptic intubation is planned.

Preoperative Risk Assessment

Preoperative risk scores aim to predict postoperative morbidity and mortality, inform patient consent and facilitate safe postoperative planning. None of the scoring systems is sufficiently validated in neurosurgery to recommend their routine use in individuals. Simple measures of functional status such as the ASA classification can crudely predict population outcomes in elective cranial neurosurgery. In all patients, comorbid medical conditions should be optimally managed without causing unnecessary delays that may adversely affect surgical outcomes.

Consent

Communication with a neurosurgical patient may be difficult due to disorders of consciousness, language and hearing deficits, or vision abnormalities. A mental capacity assessment is indicated if there is doubt about whether a patient can give consent to treatment. All efforts should be made to communicate effectively with the patient, involving relatives or independent mental capacity advocates as appropriate.

The neuroanesthesia preoperative discussion should cover a plan for anesthesia, use of invasive monitoring procedures, postoperative pain relief and significant morbidity and mortality risks relevant to the patient. Specific risks that need to be mentioned include positioning-related complications such as eye and peripheral nerve damage along with tongue injuries and needle marks related to neurophysiological testing. Awake craniotomy procedures require appropriate patient selection and in-depth discussions to sufficiently prepare patients for this demanding intervention.

Postoperative Planning

Safe and effective postoperative care is planned on the basis of information gathered at the preoperative assessment. Effective analgesic regimes, strategies to prevent and treat postoperative nausea and vomiting, and plans for restarting or modifying the patient's normal medications should be made preoperatively. Elective critical care admission may be needed if invasive monitoring, organ support or ventilation is expected. A small subgroup of patients undergoing neurosurgical interventions may be suitable for day-case surgery.

Further Reading

Association of Anaesthetists of Great Britain and Ireland: Preoperative assessment and patient preparation – The role of the anaesthetist 2, 2010. Available online at www.aagbi.org/sites/default/files/preop2010.pdf, accessed date 18 October 2017.

Barnett, S.R., Nozari, A.: The preoperative evaluation of the neurosurgical patient. *Int Anesthesiol Clin* 2015; **53**:1–22.

Jones, K., Swart, M., Key, W.: Guidance on the provision of anaesthesia services for pre-operative assessment and preparation. *Royal College of Anaesthetists* 2014. Available online at www.rcoa.ac.uk/system/files/GPAS-2014-02-PREOP_2.pdf, accessed date 18 October 2017

Kristensen, S.D., Knuuti, J., Saraste A., et al: 2014 ESC/ESA guidelines on noncardiac surgery: Cardiovascular assessment and management. *Eur Heart J* 2014; **35**:2383–2431.

National Institute for Health and Care Excellence.: Preoperative tests for elective surgery, 2003. Available online at www.nice.org.uk/guidance/cg3, accessed date 18 October 2017.

Reponen, E., Tuominen, H., Korja, M.: Evidence for the use of preoperative risk assessment scores in elective cranial neurosurgery: A systematic review of the literature. *Anesth Analg* 2014; **119**:420–432.

Basic Concepts of Neuroimaging

12

Daniel Scoffings

Key Points

- The majority of neuroimaging for patients on neurointensive care is conducted with computed tomography because of its availability, speed, and high sensitivity to hemorrhage.
- CT is the primary imaging modality for traumatic injuries to the brain and cervical spine and is often used to image the thoracolumbar spine.
- CT angiography and CT venography can be used to look for blunt cerebrovascular injury when certain injury patterns are detected in the head and neck.
- Perfusion CT can be useful in cases of suspected vasospasm after aneurysmal subarachnoid hemorrhage.
- MRI is more sensitive to changes of diffuse axonal injury, ischemia, and spinal cord injury.
- MRI is more difficult and time consuming to perform on intubated patients owing to the requirement for MRI compatible pumps and ventilators.

Abbreviations

3D	Three dimensional
CSF	Cerebrospinal fluid
CT	Computed tomography
CTA	Computed tomography angiography
CTP	Computed tomography perfusion
CTV	Computed tomography venography
DSA	Digital subtraction angiography
EDH	Extradural hematoma
FLAIR	Fluid-attenuated inversion recovery
MRI	Magnetic resonance imaging
SAH	Subarachnoid hemorrhage
SDH	Subdural hematoma
SWI	Susceptibility-weighted imaging

Contents

Introduction

Imaging of patients for elective neurosurgery is performed primarily to assess the position and character of a lesion, mass effect, cerebral edema, and postoperative complications. Imaging of patients who have not undergone neurosurgery is usually performed for cases of trauma and subarachnoid hemorrhage. The primary objectives of imaging focus on defining the extent and prognosis of any intracranial injury and ruling out axial spine instability.

Computed Tomography

Although less sensitive than MRI, CT is often the first imaging modality used for assessing the brain in patients who are admitted to neurointensive care. This is largely due to its wide availability, the relative speed of image acquisition compared to MRI and the lack of requirement for special MRI-compatible pumps and ventilators. Bedside imaging can also be performed with mobile CT scanners in some units, obviating the inherent risks of transporting critically ill patients to the radiology department. The image quality of mobile CT scanners is generally not as good as those of static units but is sufficient for the detection of new hemorrhage, hydrocephalus, brain shift, and large areas of parenchymal edema.

Most brain CT is performed without intravenous contrast, but post-contrast imaging is useful in suspected cases of infection and tumor. Rapid acquisition of a 3D CT dataset during arterial or venous phase after bolus injection of intravenous contrast forms the basis of CTA and CTV, respectively. CTP is performed by repeatedly scanning the head before and then during the first passage of injected contrast through the brain. From this data, it is possible to calculate color maps that show cerebral blood flow, cerebral blood volume, and transit time parameters. CTP is useful in the assessment of patients with suspected vasospasm following SAH, when it can assess areas of infarcted tissue and potentially salvageable ischemia.

Magnetic Resonance Imaging

A number of different MRI sequences are in common use for imaging the brain and spine. *T1-weighted* images show white matter with higher signal intensity than gray matter and CSF of low signal. On *T2-weighted* images, white matter is of lower signal than gray matter and CSF, which have high signal intensity. The FLAIR sequence suppresses CSF signal so that it is of low intensity. For this reason, at first glance FLAIR images can be confused with T1-weighted images; however, FLAIR images have T2 weighting, so white matter is of lower signal than gray matter, which is the opposite of a T1-weighted image.

Diffusion-weighted images are sensitized to the movement of water protons. When diffusion is restricted, such as in acute infarcts and within cerebral abscesses, diffusion weighted images show high signal. These images also contain an element of T2 weighting, which means that high signal on a diffusion-weighted image may also be caused by conditions that cause high signal on T2-weighted images ("T2 shine through"). $T2^*$-*weighted* gradient echo sequences and SWI are highly sensitive to local disturbances of the magnetic field caused by the iron in blood degradation products and are useful in the detection of areas of microhemorrhage after traumatic brain injury.

Spinal Trauma

There is a 5%–10% incidence of cervical spine injury associated with blunt poly-trauma. CT is recommended for imaging the cervical spine in patients who are high risk according to the Canadian C-spine rule (Table 12.1) and for low risk patients who cannot actively rotate their head to 45 degrees on each side. Clearance of the cervical spine in obtunded adult blunt trauma patients has been a contentious area but a recent meta-analysis concluded that a normal high-quality CT of the cervical spine should allow collar removal. Flexion and extension radiographs are not recommended for this purpose. Some patterns of cervical spine injury, such as subluxation and fractures at C1-3 are associated with increased risk of blunt injury to the neck arteries and some centers undertake screening CTA in this context.

Table 12.1 The Canadian C-Spine Rule

High Risk Factors At least 1 of the following	Low Risk Factors At least 1 of the following
• Dangerous mechanism of injury (fall from a height greater than 1 meter or 5 steps, axial load to the head – for example, diving, high-speed motor vehicle collision, rollover motor accident, ejection from a motor vehicle, accident involving motorized recreational vehicles, bicycle collision, horse riding accidents) • Paresthesia in upper or lower limbs	• Involved in a simple rear end collision • Is comfortable in a sitting position • Has been ambulatory at any time since the injury • Has no midline cervical spine tenderness

Table 12.2 Indications for Computed Tomography in Acute Head Injury

Within 1 hour*	Within 8 hours*
• GCS < 13 on initial assessment • GCS < 15 at 2 hours after the injury • Suspected open or depressed skull fracture • Any sign of basal skull fracture • Post-traumatic seizure • Focal neurological deficit • More than 1 episode of vomiting	• Age 65 years or older • Any history of bleeding or clotting disorders • Dangerous mechanism of injury (pedestrian or cyclist struck by a motor vehicle, an occupant ejected from a motor vehicle or fall from a height >1 m or 5 stairs) • >30 mins retrograde amnesia of events immediately before the head injury

* Perform CT within 1 or 8 hours of the risk factor *being identified*

Radiographs remain the primary modality for assessing suspected thoracic and lumbar spine injury, except in patients with abnormal neurological symptoms in whom there is a strong suspicion of thoracic or lumbar spine injury, in which case CT is recommended. Multiple injured patients often undergo CT of the chest, abdomen, and pelvis, and in these cases reformatted images of the thoracic and lumbar spine from the same dataset are sufficient. The main indication for MRI in spinal injury is the assessment of patients with neurological abnormality attributable to spinal cord injury. It also has a role in assessing the integrity of spinal ligaments and intervertebral discs.

Intracranial Trauma

The main aims of CT in head injury are to define the type and site of hemorrhage, to recognize complications such as cerebral edema and brain herniation, and to evaluate depressed skull fractures (Table 12.2).

Skull Fractures

Sensitivity for skull fractures is increased with the use of multiplanar reconstruction of thin-section, multi-slice CT data. When fractures cross the paths of venous sinuses or involve the carotid canals, CTV and CTA, respectively should be considered to look for associated venous thrombosis or blunt arterial injury.

Extradural Hematomas

Traumatic intracranial hemorrhage can be parenchymal, such as contusions or extra-axial, including EDHs or SDHs and subarachnoid hemorrhage. EDHs classically have a biconvex shape and are typically limited by the cranial sutures. They are associated with an adjacent skull fracture in up to 90% of cases. Most EDHs arise from an arterial source, while venous bleeding is less common. Areas of low attenuation within an EDH (the 'swirl sign') suggest the presence of active hemorrhage. A lucid interval after injury is a frequent occurrence, possibly as a result of slow blood loss or initial hypotension.

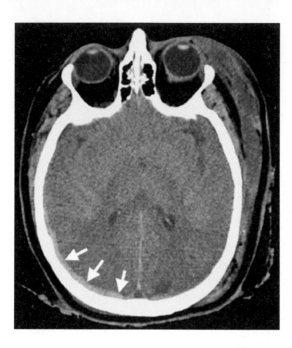

Figure 12.1 Axial computed tomography showing an acute subdural hematoma (arrows) with a typical concave medial margin.

Subdural Hematomas

SDHs are associated with significant head injury and up to 30% of patients with severe head injury will have a subdural collection. They are much more common than EDH and result from shearing of bridging veins. Collections are concave medially and can cross cranial sutures (Figure 12.1). Although in the acute stage blood is hyperattenuating on CT, untreated hematomas become isoattenuating to normal brain before becoming hypoattenuating in the chronic stage. The most common site for SDH is over the cerebral convexities, but they can also occur along the falx cerebri, tentorium, and in the posterior and middle cranial fossae. Bilateral frontal convexity low attenuation subdural hygromas frequently develop in the days after a significant head injury and may be seen on follow-up CT, they typically resolve without needing intervention.

Diffuse Axonal Injury

Diffuse axonal injury is associated with shearing of axons and disruption of white matter tracts. Certain sites are associated with axonal injury, including the subcortical white matter, body and splenium of the corpus callosum, and the brainstem in the region of the superior cerebellar peduncle. Severe hyperextension injuries may result in axonal damage to the cerebral peduncles and at the pontomedullary junction. MRI, in particular SWI, is much more sensitive than CT in identifying the microhemorrhages of diffuse axonal injury.

Subarachnoid Hemorrhage

Spontaneous SAH is most often caused by rupture of an aneurysm or arteriovenous malformation. It is less frequently associated with dural arteriovenous fistulas, hemorrhagic

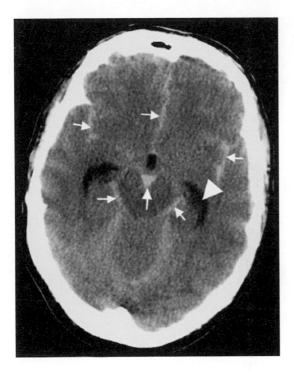

Figure 12.2 Axial computed tomography showing extensive acute subarachnoid hemorrhage in the basal cisterns, anterior interhemispheric fissure and sylvian fissures (arrows). Note dilatation of temporal horn of lateral ventricle, indicating hydrocephalus (arrowhead).

tumor, or bleeding diatheses. SAH is shown by CT as increased attenuation in the subarachnoid spaces (Figure 12.2); however, this is time sensitive. Sensitivity is 99% when CT is done within 6 hours of headache onset but falls to 50% by 7 days. Current practice remains to perform lumbar puncture to look for CSF xanthochromia in cases of CT-negative suspected SAH. The extent and location of blood on the CT scan may indicate the probable source of hemorrhage.

Although DSA remains the reference standard, CTA is now frequently the first-line investigation for detection of aneurysms and has near-equivalent diagnostic accuracy. If CTA is negative, DSA should be performed. DSA is negative in 15%–20% of cases. Repeat angiography approximately 5 to 7 days later may identify an occult aneurysm that may have been tamponaded by local hemorrhage. A negative repeat DSA suggests nonaneurysmal SAH (occurring in up to 15% of cases), which is frequently perimesencephalic. Such hemorrhage is possibly venous in origin and carries a good prognosis. Aneurysms are multiple in up to 20% of patients, and in such cases the presence of an irregular 'teat' on one of them suggests recent rupture.

Raised Intracranial Pressure

Brain imaging can appear normal in cases of raised intracranial pressure so the diagnosis of raised ICP cannot be excluded on the basis of a normal CT or MRI. Conversely, widespread sulcal narrowing, ventricular compression, and narrowing of the basal cisterns indicate diffuse brain swelling and imply the presence of raised ICP (Figure 12.3). Pressure gradients

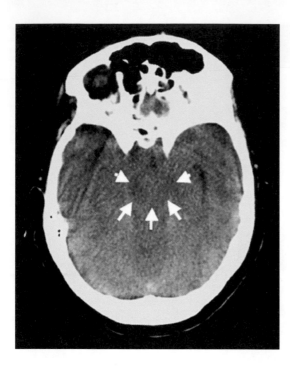

Figure 12.3 Axial computed tomography in a patient with raised intracranial pressure showing complete effacement of the perimesencephalic and quadrigeminal cisterns (arrows).

between different intracranial compartments can result in several patterns of brain herniation such as:

- tonsillar herniation through the foramen magnum
- ascending transtentorial herniation of the cerebellar vermis
- temporal lobe (uncal) herniation
- descending transtentorial herniation
- subfalcine herniation

Mass effect can lead to associated hydrocephalus (e.g., effacement of the fourth ventricle causing dilation of the third and lateral ventricles, as well as subfalcine herniation causing contralateral lateral ventricle dilation).

Intracranial Tumors

A full account of the imaging appearances of intracranial tumors is beyond the scope of this chapter, but some generalizations can be made.

Gliomas

Low-grade infiltrating gliomas typically appear as non-enhancing areas of increased signal intensity in the white matter and cortex on T2-weighted and FLAIR images. Mass effect results in effacement of the sulci and expansion of the gyri. Though sometimes apparently well circumscribed, the tumor extends beyond the abnormality shown by imaging. Glioblastoma multiforme is characterized by an irregular rind of peripheral enhancement around a central region of non-enhancing necrosis that is of low attenuation on CT, low signal on T1-weighted images, and high signal on T2-weighted images. Variable amounts of high T2 signal surround the enhancing part of the lesion and extend into the hemispheric white matter. Though often described as vasogenic edema, this peritumoral signal change represents a combination of edema and tumor cells.

Metastases

Metastases tend to occur at the gray-white matter junction and are solitary in up to 50% of cases. Enhancement, which may be homogeneous or ring shaped, is a characteristic feature, and peritumoral vasogenic edema is often disproportionately extensive for the size of the lesions.

Cerebral Lymphoma

Primary cerebral lymphoma tends to occur in locations that abut the ependyma, leptomeninges, or both. In immunocompetent patients, it appears as well defined masses of relatively low T2 signal that enhance homogeneously after the administration of intravenous gadolinium. In the setting of acquired immunodeficiency syndrome, cerebral lymphoma tends to show more heterogeneous ring enhancement.

Meningioma

The extra-axial location of a meningioma is often shown by a thin rim of CSF signal between the tumor and the brain or by a broad dural base. Homogeneous enhancement is typical, calcification occurs in 20%, and vasogenic edema in the adjacent brain is not unusual. Meningiomas induce hyperostotic change in the adjacent skull in 20% of cases.

Further Reading

National Institute for Health and Care Excellence (2016). *Spinal injury: Assessment and initial management*. NICE Guideline (NG41).

Dreizin, D., Letzing, M., Sliker, C.W., et al: Multidetector CT of blunt spine trauma in adults. *Radiographics* 2014; **32**:1842–1865.

Liang, T., Tso, D.K., Chiu, R.Y., Nicolaou, S.: Imaging of blunt vascular neck injuries: A clinical perspective. *Am J Roentgenol* 2013; **201**:893–901.

Currie, S., Saleem, N., Straiton, J.A, et al: Imaging assessment of traumatic brain injury. *Postgrad Med J* 2016; **92**:41–50.

Mir, D.I., Gupta, A., Dunning, A., et al: CT perfusion for detection of delayed cerebral ischemia in aneurysmal subarachnoid hemorrhage: A systematic review and meta-analysis. *Am J Neuroradiol* 2014; **35**:866–871.

Chapter 13

Neurosurgical Operative Approaches

Michael McDermott

Key Points

- The frontotemporal approach and its modifications is the most common neurosurgical approach for pathology in the anterior and middle cranial fossa.
- The bi-frontal craniotomy can be used for pathologies in the anterior skull base, those that extend into the nasal cavity, and those that extend back to the suprasellar region.
- Transsphenoidal approaches can be sublabial, transnasal, or completely endonasal.
- Posterior fossa approaches can be complicated by transient trigeminal or vagal reflexes that cause profound bradycardia.
- Prior to sitting/semi-sitting procedures, a bubble echocardiogram can help exclude a right to left intracardiac shunt.

Contents

General Principles

The choice of surgical approach largely depends on the location of the lesion, the surrounding anatomy, the characteristics of the tumor, other co-morbidities of the patient, and the experience of the surgeon. We will discuss some of the common neurosurgical approaches used.

The main goal of any approach is to be able to reach the lesion with minimal brain retraction thereby limiting any potential for brain injury. In many instances, this means more bone removal to minimize brain retraction. The amount of exposure that can be gained with each approach is therefore variable and depends upon: (1) the amount of bone removal and (2) arachnoid dissection, which will allow separation of lobes from one another (e.g., frontal from temporal lobe along the Sylvian fissure) along with vessels from the surface of the brain or surrounding nerves. The head should be elevated above the heart to avoid venous congestion. The use of a lumbar subarachnoid or external ventricular drain should also be considered to reduce the volume of the intracranial cavity and thereby the force of retraction necessary for a given exposure.

In craniotomies for lesions involving the venous sinuses, bleeding from inadvertent injury can usually be controlled with direct pressure and the use of hemostatic agents. However, there is potential for considerable blood loss and the possibility of air emboli. In general, the management of intraoperative complications can be facilitated by preoperative discussions between the surgeon and anesthesiologist about position, approach, expected blood loss, and hemodynamic changes (such as bradycardia during coagulation of the tentorium) and by regular intraoperative updates on the course of the surgical intervention.

Unilateral Frontotemporal Approaches

The unilateral frontotemporal approaches are used for unilateral tumors and vascular lesions. Examples of lesions that can be treated via the unilateral frontotemporal approach include small olfactory groove meningiomas, small tuberculum sella meningiomas, anterior circulation aneurysms, and basilar apex aneurysms. Variations of the frontotemporal approach include:

(1) Medial subfrontal approach, where the bone flap is extended to the midline. This approach can be modified to include the orbital rim as a secondary osteotomy bone piece – a cranio-orbital approach.

(2) Lateral frontotemporal approach, the so-called 'pterional' approach (Figure 13.1), where the bone flap extends in a curvilinear manner toward the supra-orbital rim just above the superior temporal line, then parallel to the supra-orbital rim to the frontozygomatic

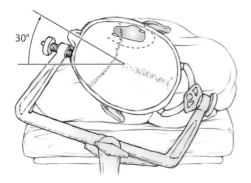

30°

Figure 13.1 Unilateral frontotemporal (pterional) approach showing positioning, skin incision, and bone flap.

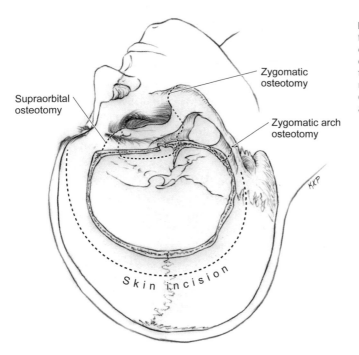

Supraorbital
osteotomy

Zygomatic
osteotomy

Zygomatic arch
osteotomy

Skin incision

Figure 13.2 Right frontotemporal orbitozygomatic craniotomy. In addition to craniotomy for pterional approach there are osteotomies through medial supra-orbital margin, body of zygoma, and zygomatic arch above temporomandibular joint.

process, then below this and posteriorly crossing the sphenoid wing, down into the squamous portion of the sphenoid bone and then back up toward the superior temporal line posteriorly.

(3) The orbitozygomatic approach (commonly referred to as the 'O-Z' approach – Figure 13.2) which includes the pterional approach bone flap followed by removal of the supra-orbital rim, frontozygomatic process, posterior half of the body of zygoma, and the arch of the zygomaen masse in a second osteotomy.

(4) Extended middle fossa approach with removal of the petrous apex between foramen ovale anteriorly, arcuate eminence of the cochlea posteriorly, and the greater superficial petrosal nerve laterally (Kawase approach).

For the medial subfrontal approach, the patient is placed supine the neck flexed on the chest, the head extended on the neck without rotation. For the pterional and 'O-Z' approaches the patient is placed supine on the operating table with ipsilateral shoulder elevation and the head rotated 30 degrees. The frontotemporal craniotomy is usually accompanied by varying degrees of bone removal from the sphenoid ridge, posterior orbital roof, and anterior clinoid and may be extended by removal of the orbital rim with or without the zygoma (cranioorbital and orbitozygomatic approaches). Removal of the orbital rim requires dissection of the periorbita from the orbital roof. During the orbital dissection, the trigemino-ocular reflex may be provoked which consists of bradycardia, hypotension, apnea, and gastric hypermotility. Lesions are often approached by splitting the Sylvian fissure. Structures that are potentially injured include the internal carotid artery, anterior cerebral artery, middle cerebral artery, posterior communicating artery, olfactory nerve, optic nerve, optic chiasm, oculomotor nerve, and pituitary stalk.

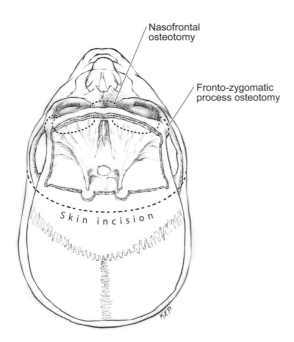

Nasofrontal osteotomy

Fronto-zygomatic process osteotomy

Skin incision

Figure 13.3 Bi-frontal craniotomy using coronal incision from ear to ear. For skull base approaches, bi-lateral supra-orbital osteotomy can be done removing supra-orbital bar in one piece (extended bi-frontal craniotomy).

Bi-Frontal Approach and Extended Bi-Frontal Approach

The bi-frontal approach is used for midline tumors (Figure 13.3). Lesions that are treated via the bi-frontal approach include large olfactory groove meningiomas, large planum sphenoidale meningiomas, tuberculum sellae meningiomas, and some large craniopharyngiomas. A lumbar subarachnoid drain may be placed for large tumors prior to positioning to help with relaxation of the brain. The patient is placed supine on the operating table with the neck flexed on the chest and the head extended at the neck with no rotation. A bi-coronal incision is made from zygomatic arch to zygomatic arch. The scalp is reflected to the point where the supraorbital nerves are seen. Laterally, the temporalis muscle is reflected inferiorly and posteriorly, while preserving the frontal is branch of the facial nerve. A bi-frontal bone flap is elevated taking care to not violate the superior sagittal sinus.

For large tumors that extend superiorly, an extended bi-frontal approach may be necessary. In this approach, dissection is carried out around the orbit so that the orbital bar can be removed. During the orbital dissection, the trigemino-ocular reflex, as previously explained, may be provoked. Other structures that may be injured include the superior sagittal sinus, olfactory nerves, optic nerves/chiasm, and anterior cerebral arteries. Recent experience indicates that despite the extensive bone removal, the incidence of complications is acceptably low and infections are uncommon.

Interhemispheric Approach

The interhemispheric approach is used for lesions at or close to the midline, including distal anterior cerebral artery aneurysms, falcine meningiomas, lesions of the corpus callosum, and lateral and third ventricular lesions (Figure 13.4). A lumbar subarachnoid drain may be placed for large tumors prior to positioning. The patient is placed supine on the operating room table

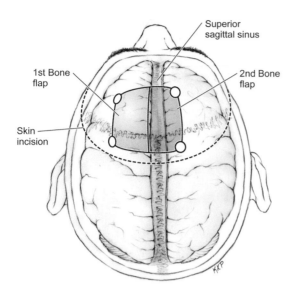

Superior sagittal sinus

1st Bone flap

2nd Bone flap

Skin incision

Figure 13.4 Bi-partite bone flap crossing midline for interhemispheric approach. First portion of bone flap is lateral to midline avoiding risk of injury to venous lakes and superior sagittal sinus. Under direct vision midline dura can then be dissected to the opposite side and second bone piece created.

with the head slightly flexed. In a variation of this approach, the patient is placed semi lateral with the head turned 90 degrees to the table and bent laterally up at a 45-degree angle.

For both positions, the craniotomy involves crossing the superior sagittal sinus. Injury to the sinus may cause an air embolism or large volume blood loss but is usually easily controlled with direct pressure. Other structures that are potentially injured include the distal anterior cerebral artery, sensory, and motor cortex. If a transcallosal transventricular approach is used, there is potential for injury to the thalamus and the deep venous drainage system and the possibility for intraventricular hemorrhage.

Transsphenoidal Approach

The transsphenoidal approach is used for sellar lesions with or without suprasellar extensions or for clival lesions (Figure 13.5). The patient is supine on the operating room table with the body flexed and the head in a sniffing position. A lumbar subarachnoid drain may be placed for lesions with suprasellar extension. Infusion of saline into the lumbar drain is used to help push the tumor inferiorly so that it can be easily reached. Maintaining normal or elevated $PaCO_2$ is also helpful. The drain is sometimes left postoperatively for management or prevention of cerebrospinal fluid leakage. Structures that can be potentially injured during the exposure include the cavernous sinus, internal carotid artery, optic chiasm, and pituitary stalk. Injury to the cavernous sinus can easily be controlled with hemostatic agents. Injury to the internal carotid artery may result in massive blood loss, requiring endovascular intervention.

Currently, sublabial, transnasal, and endonasal transsphenoidal approaches are practiced. For the sublabial approach the labial mucosa just past the gingival crease above the upper central incisors is opened and the nasal cavity accessed via a submucosal dissection. The mucosa is tripped all the way back to the rostrum of the sphenoid and the sphenoid sinus entered with a ronguer. Most experienced surgeons have now moved to the transnasal microsurgical approach where a smaller speculum introduced through a single nostril provides all the visibility and access necessary. The opening can be extended anteriorly up the front wall of the sella to include the tuberculum and planum whereby larger suprasellar

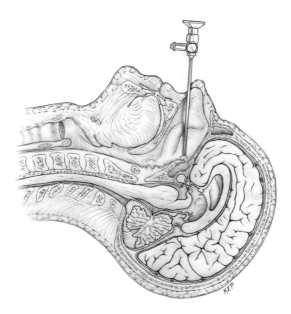

Figure 13.5 Transnasal transsphenoidal approach using endoscope. Same approach can be taken using nasal speculum and microscope (transnasal transsphenoidal microsurgical approach) without need for any sublabial or external incisions.

tumors can be removed, the so-called 'extended transsphenoidal' approach. The endonasal endoscopic approach is the current minimally invasive technique coming to the fore using nothing but the endoscope for visualization and using working instruments up both nostrils.

Petrosal Approach (Retrolabyrinthine-Middle Fossa Approach)

There are a number of approaches in which part of the petrous bone is removed. Here, we describe the retrolabyrinthine-middle fossa approach which is used for lesions that arise on the upper two-thirds of the clivus such as petroclival meningiomas and chordomas (Figure 13.6). Neurophysiologic monitoring of the trigeminal, abducens, facial, and vestibulocochlear nerves is typical. A lumbar subarachnoid drain is often placed. The patient is supine on the operating table with a bolster underneath one shoulder and the head turned 60 degrees. A small temporoparietal craniotomy is done followed by a mastoidectomy/posterior fossa craniectomy, exposure of the sigmoid sinus, and retro-labyrinthine exposure of the presigmoid dura of the posterior fossa and toward the petrous apex below the superior petrosal sinus. The temporal dura and presigmoid dura are opened and the cuts connected with sectioning of the superior petrosal sinus and tentorium. Structures that can be potentially injured include the sigmoid sinus/jugular bulb; the hearing apparatus; cranial nerves IV, V, VI, VII, VIII; brainstem; and vein of Labbé. For larger tumors in this region such as meningiomas, the incidence of new neurological deficits is reported as higher than 50% in some published reports.

Midline Suboccipital Approach

The midline suboccipital approach is used for lesions in the cerebellar hemispheres as well as near the midline in the dorsal medulla and pons (Figure 13.7). For tumors in the pineal region this opening provides access to the superior cerebellar surface for the infratentorial supracerebellar approach. A lumbar drain is not needed here since the cisterna magna is easily accessible for release of cerebrospinal fluid. The patient is prone on the operating

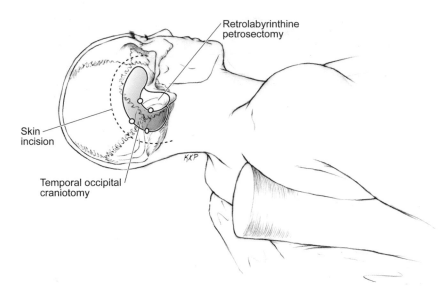

Figure 13.6 Petrosal approach for tumors involving posterior and middle cranial fossa. Temporal craniotomy combined with presigmoid, retrolabyrinthine bone removal. Dura is opened anterior to sigmoid sinus, along floor of middle fossa and tentorium incised.

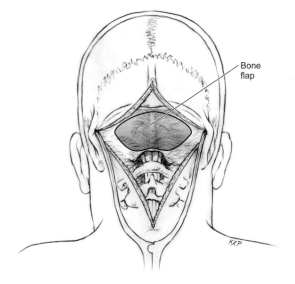

Figure 13.7 Midline suboccipital approach. Craniotomy below transverse sinuses and down to or including lip of foramen magnum.

room table with the head flexed and chin tucked. Patients who are obese, large breasted, or of large size present problems with elevated venous and airway pressures in the prone position that may compromise conditions such that a sitting position may be required. In such a case where the risk of air embolism is higher, a bubble echocardiogram is required to rule out a right to left shunt. Whether prone or sitting, a midline incision is made a few centimeters above the inion and extended down to C3–C4. The craniotomy is carried out superiorly to the transverse sinus and inferiorly to or through the foramen magnum. A C1 laminectomy may also be required for tumors that extend from the fourth ventricle into the upper cervical spine (e.g., ependymoma). The potential danger in this approach is injuring the transverse sinus, posterior inferior cerebellar artery, and brainstem. For large tumors around the confluence of the sinuses (Torcula Herophili) a larger craniotomy may be required including bone over both occipital lobes and the cerebellum.

Retrosigmoid Approach

The retrosigmoid suboccipital approach is mainly used for lesions in the middle third of the clivus such as cerebellopontine angle tumors, microvascular decompression, anterolateral pontine lesion, and anterior inferior cerebellar artery aneurysms (Figure 13.8). A lumbar

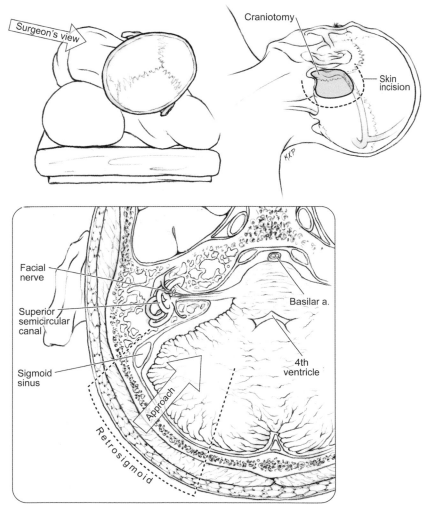

Figure 13.8 Retrosigmoid approach to cerebellopontine angle. Bone over sigmoid sinus drilled off using diamond burr to avoid injury. A common approach for meningiomas, acoustic neuromas, trigeminal neuralgia, and hemifacial spasm.

subarachnoid drain is sometimes placed preoperatively. The patient is semilateral on the operating table with a bolster underneath one shoulder. The head is turned 90 degrees with respect to the floor. The margins of the transverse and sigmoid sinuses are exposed with the craniotomy, often using image guidance. Bleeding from the transverse and sigmoid sinuses can occur during the craniotomy and can usually be controlled with pressure. With opening of the dura, the cerebellum is usually bulging and necessitates release of cerebrospinal fluid from the cisterna magna or the cerebellopontine angle cistern for decompression. Retraction of the cerebellum allows exposure of the brainstem and cranial nerves. Depending on the lesion, neurophysiological monitoring of the cranial nerves may be necessary. Structures that can potentially be injured include the pons and the cranial nerves, mainly the trigeminal, abducens, facial, and vestibulocochlear nerves. For lesions that are lower, the vagus nerve can also be monitored.

Far Lateral Suboccipital Approach

The far lateral approach is used for lesions in the lateral and anterolateral region of the foramen magnum and the lower third of the clivus such as foramen magnum meningiomas, posterior inferior cerebellar artery aneurysms, and medullary cavernous malformations (Figure 13.9). A lumbar subarachnoid drain is not necessary since the cisterna magna is easily accessible for release of cerebrospinal fluid. The patient is in a three-quarters prone park bench position with the head flexed toward the neck, rotated 120 degrees from vertical and laterally flexed 20 degrees. The contralateral arm is secured in a sling over the edge of the top of the table. A suboccipital craniotomy is performed from midline to the sigmoid sinus laterally. The occipital condyle can be drilled down to the hypoglossal canal. A C1

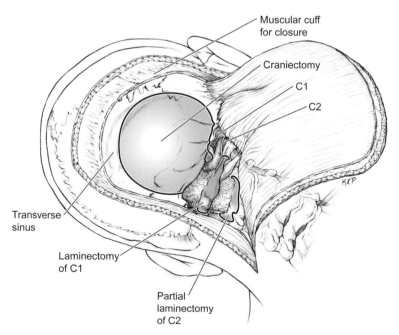

Figure 13.9 Far lateral suboccipital approach. Suboccipital craniotomy extended into posterior one-third of occipital condyle combined with C1 (occasionally C2) hemilaminectomy.

Table 13.1 Neurosurgical Approaches by Intracranial Compartment

Approaches	Compartment	Typical Pathology
Pterional Subfrontal Bi-frontal Extended frontal Orbito zygomatic Extended middle fossa	ACF, MCF ACF ACF ACF ACF, MCF MCF, PCF	Tumors: gliomas, meningiomas, schwannomas, craniopharyngioma, giant pituitary adenomas Vascular: aneurysm, AVM, AV fistula
Interhemispheric	Supratentorial, lateral and third ventricle	Tumors: gliomas, meningiomas, intraventricular tumors Vascular: AVM, ACA aneurysms
Transnasal transsphenoidal	Sphenoid, ethmoid sinuses, sella, clivus, ACF	Tumors: Pituitary adenoma, craniopharyngioma, chordomas, neuroblastoma, meningioma
Petrosal approach	MCF, PCF, CPA, clivus	Tumors: Meningiomas, schwannomas, chordomas Vascular: AVM, basilar trunk aneurysm
Midline suboccipital	PCF, pineal region, fourth ventricle, FM	Gliomas, choroid plexus papilloma, ependymoma, medulloblastoma, pineal tumors Vascular: AVM, rare distal PICA aneurysms
Retrosigmoid	PCF, CPA, FM	Tumor: schwannomas, meningiomas, gliomas, epidermoid cysts
Far lateral suboccipital	PCF, CPA, FM Cervicomedullary junction	Tumors: meningiomas Vascular: PICA aneurysms, medullary CVM

ACF, anterior cranial fossa; CPA, cerebellopontine angle; FM, foramen magnum; MCF, middle cranial fossa; PCF, posterior cranial fossa.

cervical laminectomy is also performed. Structures that can potentially be injured include the vertebral artery, posterior inferior cerebellar artery, the jugular bulb, the lower brainstem, and lower cranial nerves.

Further Reading

Chi, J.H., McDermott, M.W.: Tuberculum sellaemeningiomas. *Neurosurg Focus* 2003; 14(6):Article 6, June.

Chi, J.H., Parsa, A.T., Berger, M.S., Kunwar, S., McDermott, M.W.: Extended bifrontal craniotomy for midline anterior fossa meningiomas: Minimization of retraction-related edema and surgical outcomes. *Neurosurgery* 2006 October; 59(4)(Suppl 2):ONS426–34.

McDermott, M.W., Durity, F.A., Rootman, J., Woodhurst, W.B.: Combined frontotemporal-orbitozygomatic approach for tumors of the sphenoid wing and orbit. *Neurosurg* 1990; 26:107–116.

McDermott, M.W., Parsa, A.T.: Surgical management of olfactory groove meningiomas. Neurosurgical operative atlas. In: B. Behnam, (Ed.) *Neuro-oncology*, 2nd ed. 2007, New York, NY: Thieme, pp. 161–170.

Quinones-Hinojosa, A., Chang, E.F., McDermott, M.W.: Falcotentorialmeningiomas: Clinical, neuroimaging, and surgical features in six patients. *Neurosurg Focus* 2003; **14**(6): Article 11, June.

Quinones-Hinojosa, A., Chang, E.F., Khan, S.A, Lawton, M.T., McDermott, M.W.: Renal cell carcinoma metastatic to the choroid plexus mimicking intraventricular meningioma. *Can J Neurol Sci* 2004; **31**:115–120.

Surgical Positioning

Chanhung Z. Lee and Michael McDermott

Key Points

- Increased intracranial pressure can result from increased abdominal pressure, from venous congestion, and from having the head below the level of the heart.
- Venous congestion can result from venous outflow obstruction caused by hyperrotation or hyperflexion of the neck.
- Increased PEEP and airway compromise can result from kinking of the endotracheal tube caused by neck flexion during long operative procedures.
- Given the high risk of air embolism, all patients undergoing a craniotomy in the sitting position should be considered for a preoperative echocardiogram to rule out a patent foramen ovale.
- In the prone position, bolsters should be adequately placed to minimize the pressure on the abdomen and the thorax.

Abbreviations

PEEP   Positive end-expiratory pressure
PFO   Patent foramen ovale

Contents

- Parkbench or Three-Quarters Prone Positions
  - (Far Lateral Approach)
- Prone Position
  - (Suboccipital Approach)

Introduction

The positioning of patients is critical in neurosurgical procedures. Proper positioning should allow for the most optimal exposure of the lesion with minimal retraction of the brain while ensuring that the position is physiologically and physically safe for the anesthetized patient. In addition, one must also be aware of positions that can result in adverse effects on cerebral blood flow and volume which may lead to increased intracranial pressure. Inappropriate positioning leading to prolonged tissue compression can cause organ damage, airway compromise or skin breakdown while stretching of neural structures can result in neurological deficits.

General Principles

Intraoperative problems can occur from increased intracranial pressure, venous congestion, and airway compromise due to positioning effects alone. Raised intracranial pressure can result from increased extra-abdominal pressure, venous congestion from kinking of the internal jugular vein, and positioning the head below the level of the heart. Venous congestion itself can exacerbate brain swelling and lead to excessive venous bleeding that can hinder the operation. The development of macroglossia, although rare, has also been attributed to venous flow congestion from surgical positioning in the prone or far lateral positions. This can result from insufficient abdominal bolstering, increased PEEP from kinking of the endotracheal tube or venous obstruction from hyper-rotation or hyperflexion of the neck. As a general rule, a distance of one or two fingerbreadths should be maintained between the chin and chest during neck flexion and the use of an armored endotracheal tube can help avoid kinking.

Inadequate protection of pressure points can result in skin breakdown or compression of peripheral nerves. Common pressure points include elbows, heels, iliac crests, breasts, and male genitalia. Peripheral nerve injuries can also occur from stretching of the nerves, particularly the brachial plexus. In general, the patient should be positioned in a way that would be comfortable for a patient who is awake over a prolonged period of time. The American Society of Anesthesiologists has published a practice advisory for the prevention of perioperative peripheral neuropathies. Corneal abrasions should be avoided in all cases usually by maintaining closure of the eyelids by hypoallergenic adhesive tape augmented with ophthalmic ointment or gel. In cases when transcranial stimulation is applied for evoked-potential monitoring, damage to oral tissues especially the tongue and lips may occur even with bite-block placement. In the following sections, we will discuss the specific positioning considerations for common neurosurgical approaches.

Supine Position

(Frontotemporal, Bifrontal, Subfrontal, and Interhemispheric Approaches – Figure 14.1)

The bifrontal, subfrontal, interhemispheric, and other frontotemporal approaches are performed by positioning the patient supine on the operating room table using

Semi-Lateral or Supine Position (petrosal, retrosigmoid, and unilateral frontotemporal approaches)

① Bolster
② Padded arm board
③ Padding between knees and ankles
④ Padding under heals
⑤ Adequate distance between chin and clavicle

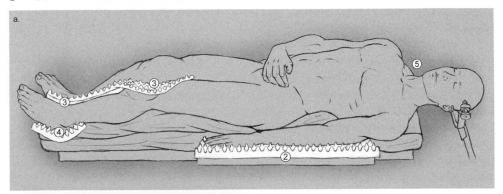

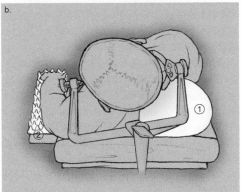

Figure 14.1 Semilateral position (**a**) or supine position with a bolster (**b**). There should not be any excessive traction on the brachial plexus or obstruction of venous drainage in the neck.

occasionally only minimal rotation of the neck. The influence of gravity on the circulation is minimal in this position. The head may be flexed slightly for interhemispheric approaches to the lateral or third ventricles or extended slightly in the subfrontal approaches. Neck flexion or extension in these approaches is generally minimal. The patient may be at an increased risk of air embolism in the reverse trendelenberg position particularly during bifrontal craniotomies when the superior sagittal sinus is traversed and at risk of injury.

In this position, attention must also be paid to the extremities. The upper extremities are usually positioned at the patient's sides. When the arm is tucked or flexed across the body, foam padding should be applied to the elbow and wrist to avoid injury to the ulnar and median nerves. The knees should be elevated to decrease tension on the lower back and the heels should be padded to avoid skin breakdown.

Semilateral or Supine Position with a Bolster

(Petrosal, Retrosigmoid, and Unilateral Frontotemporal Approaches – Figure 14.1)

Petrosal and retrosigmoid approaches, as well as others that requires moderate rotation of the neck, are performed by placing the patient in a supine position with the ipsilateral shoulder elevated. The use of a shoulder bolster is particularly important in elderly patients with less flexible necks and it helps to avoid kinking of the internal jugular vein with neck rotation. In petrosal and retrosigmoid approaches, the elevated shoulder is often pulled down inferiorly with tape to minimize the obstruction to the surgical view. Excessive traction on the shoulder can result in stretch injury to the brachial plexus. Other considerations for this position are similar to that of the supine position.

Sitting Position

(Supracerebellar Infratentorial Approach)

The sitting position is sometimes used for surgery to the posterior fossa using the supracerebellar infratentorial approach. It has the advantage of facilitating surgical exposure, draining blood, and cerebrospinal fluid away from the surgical site, less venous bleeding and lower intracranial pressure. Major complications with this position include the risk of air embolism (occurring in 9%–43% of patients), hypotension, inadequate cerebral perfusion, and postoperative tension pneumocephalus (resulting from air entry into the subdural space). Given the high risk of air embolism, some centers advocate preoperative echocardiogram in all patients undergoing a craniotomy in the sitting position to rule out a PFO. Although case series have revealed that this investigation may be of limited benefit, preoperative identification of a PFO has significant implications for perioperative management. Percutaneous PFO closure can be considered prior to surgery in the sitting position. Monitors such as precordial Doppler, capnography, and right heart transvenous catheters are useful for detecting an air embolism and should be placed preoperatively. Nitrous oxide should be avoided if the likelihood of venous air embolism is a serious concern.

When the sitting position is used for the supracerebellar infratentorial approach, extreme neck flexion may lead to kinking of the endotracheal tube. An armored tube should be utilized and hyperflexion should still be avoided to reduce other risks, including potential cervical spine ischemia. Extreme neck flexion for prolonged periods can also be associated with macroglossia and swelling of the soft palate due to obstruction of venous and lymphatic drainage. Although uncommon, this has the potential to produce postoperative airway obstruction, hypoxia, and hypercapnia.

Lateral Position

(Posterior Parietal or Occipital Craniotomies – Figure 14.2)

The lateral position is often used for posterior parietal or occipital craniotomies. An axillary roll is often used during this position to prevent brachial plexus compression or pressure on the dependent shoulder. It is important to prevent a brachial plexus injury by proper placement of the axillary roll under the upper chest rather than the axilla. To maintain the lateral position, blankets or other forms of padded support should be placed along the patient's back and abdomen. The knees should be flexed with padding placed between them to avoid pressure over the fibular head and peroneal nerve.

Lateral Position (posterior parietal or occipital craniotomies)

① Axillary roll
② Back and abdomen support
③ Bottom knee bent
④ Padding between legs
⑤ Padding under knee and ankle
⑥ Ipsilateral shoulder pulled inferiorly
⑦ Head in neurtral position

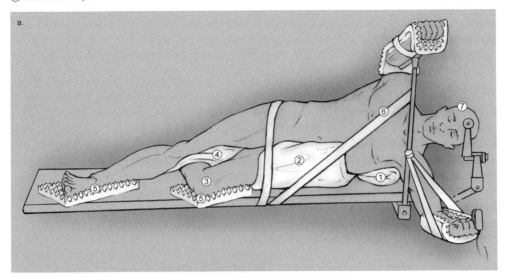

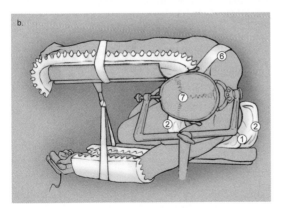

Figure 14.2 (**a**), (**b**) Lateral position. A variation is to place and tape the upper part of the arm along the length of the torso. The lower part of the arm can be folded across the chest with the hand in proximity to the upper part of the shoulder. Note that the axillary roll is placed under the chest to prevent pressure on and injury to the axillary structures.

Parkbench or Three-Quarters Prone Positions

(Far Lateral Approach – Figure 14.3)

The parkbench or three-quarters prone position is used in surgery using a far lateral approach. It involves placing the patient in a lateral position on the operating table, such that the dependent arm is hanging over the top edge of the table and secured with a sling to provide adequate support and protection. Care must be taken to pad all the pressure points. An axillary roll should be placed under the dependent chest for the same reasoning as for the lateral position. The trunk is rotated 15 degrees from the lateral position into a semiprone position and supported with pillows and/or blankets. The ipsilateral shoulder is pulled inferiorly but once again too much tension on the shoulder can result in stretching of the brachial plexus.

The head is flexed at the neck, then rotated 120 degrees from the vertical, and laterally flexed 20 degrees. This results in considerable rotation and flexion of the neck and can result in kinking of the endotracheal tube, as well as the internal jugular vein. The use of a reinforced endotracheal tube should be considered but whichever type is used, it should be meticulously secured and supported to avoid dislodgement as the patient's head may be turned looking toward the floor. The head also needs to be properly positioned to prevent obstruction to cerebral venous outflow.

Prone Position

(Suboccipital Approach – Figure 14.4)

The prone position is used for the suboccipital approach and posterior spinal surgeries. The potential for complications is significant. Turning the patient to a prone position can cause hemodynamic changes and ventilation impairment. Hypotension may result from a decrease in preload and cardiac output, dictated by the patient's volume status and cardiac reserve.

In this position, the patient can be placed on purpose made frames or firm mattresses or by using two bolsters to support the chest wall and pelvis whilst the arms are positioned to the side of the body. To ensure that the abdominal and femoral venous returns are not unduly compromised, as well as to allow for adequate diaphragmatic excursion, the bolsters should be sufficiently far apart and large enough not to cause pressure on the abdomen. Breasts and male genitalia should be checked to minimize any pressure on them, arms and knees should be padded, and the ankles should be elevated so that the toes will hang freely. Because the neck is flexed in the suboccipital approach, there is risk of kinking of the endotracheal tube which can be avoided if a reinforced one is used. Although a rare occurrence, blindness has been reported after surgery in the prone position, particularly in cases with prolonged duration, significant blood loss, hypotension, and in patients with glaucoma. Direct pressure on the eyes must always be avoided.

Parkbench or Three-Quarter Prone Position (far lateral approach)

1. Dependent arm hangs off table
2. Axillary roll
3. Back and abdomen support
4. Bottom knee bent
5. Padding between and under legs
6. Ipsilateral shoulder pulled inferiorly

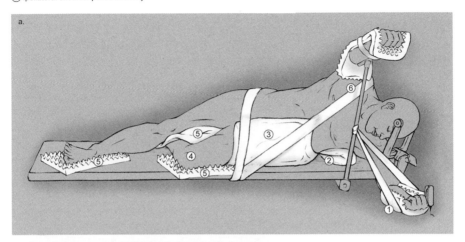

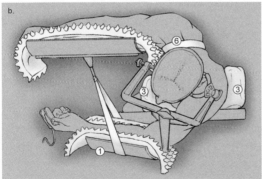

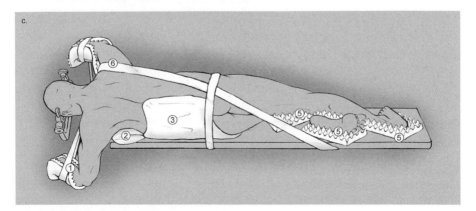

Figure 14.3 (a)–(c) Park bench or three-quarter prone position. A variation is to place and tape the upper part of the arm along the length of the torso. The lower part of the arm can be folded across the chest with hand in proximity to the upper part of the shoulder. Inappropriate flexion and rotation can obstruct venous drainage and ventilation.

Prone Position-A (suboccipital approach)
Head in Mayfield clamp

① Bolster
② Arms down side
③ Avoid pressure on abdomen
④ Avoid pressure on male genital and breasts
⑤ Arm and knee padding
⑥ Chin tucked
⑦ Mayfield head clamp

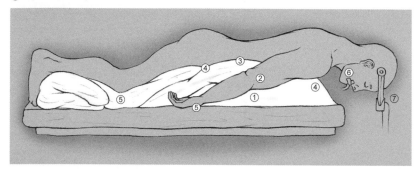

Prone Position-B (suboccipital approach)
Head on face pillow

① Bolsters
② Arms alongside the head
③ Avoid pressure on abdomen
④ Avoid pressure on male genital and breasts
⑤ Arm and knee padding
⑥ Face pillow with eyes and nose free of compression

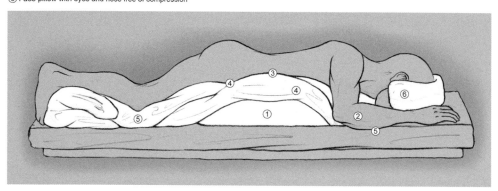

Figure 14.4 Prone position. (**a**) Fixation of the head and cervical spine is needed for suboccipital and upper spine procedures. (**b**) For lower spinal procedures the head is supported in a foam or other device. Care should be taken to ensure that no pressure is placed on the eyes and nose.

Further Reading

American Society of Anesthesiologists Task Force on Prevention of Perioperative Peripheral Neuropathies: Practice advisory for the prevention of perioperative peripheral neuropathies: An updated report by the American Society of Anesthesiologists Task Force on prevention of perioperative peripheral neuropathies. *Anesthesiology* 2011; **114**:741–754.

American Society of Anesthesiologists Task Force on Perioperative Visual Loss: Practice advisory for perioperative visual loss associated with spine surgery: An updated report by the American Society of

Anesthesiologists Task Force on Perioperative Visual Loss. *Anesthesiology* 2012; **116**:274–285.

Casorla, L., Lee, J.W.: Patient positioning and associated risks. In: Miller, R.D., Eriksson, L.I., Fleisher, L.A., Wiener-Kronish, J.P., Young, W.L. (Eds.). *Miller's Anesthesia*, 8th ed. Philadelphia: Elsevier Churchill Livingstone; 2015: 1240–1265.

Ganslandt, O., Merkel, A., Schmitt, H., et al: The sitting position in neurosurgery: Indications, complications and results. A single institution experience of 600 cases. *Acta Neurochi (Wien)* 2013; **155**:1887–1893.

Laban, J.T., Rasul, F.T., Brecker, S.J., Marsh, H.T., Martin, A.J.: Patent foramen ovale closure prior to surgery in the sitting position. *Br J Neurosurg* 2014; **28**:421–422.

Tamkus, A., Rice, K.: The incidence of bite injuries associated with transcranial motor-evoked potential monitoring. *Anesth Analg* 2012; **115**:663–667.

Warner, M.E.: Patient positioning and potential injuries. In: Barash, P.G., Cullen, B.F., Stoelting, R.K., Cahalan, M.K., Stock, M.C., Ortega, R. (Eds.). *Clinical Anesthesia*, 7th ed. Philadelphia: Lippincott Williams & Wilkins; 2013: 803–823.

Anesthesia for Elective Supratentorial Surgery

Anne Booth and Rowan Burnstein

Key Points

- Preoperative assessment aims to assess neurological status, determine the presence of raised intracranial pressure, optimize the underlying disease, and formulate a management plan for the postoperative period.
- Induction of anesthesia should aim for minimal disturbance of physiological parameters.
- Emergence from anesthesia should be smooth and allow for a rapid return of cognitive function and early neurological assessment.
- Total intravenous anesthesia or inhalational agents with muscle relaxation are suitable anesthetic techniques to use.
- Intraoperatively, the aim for anesthesia is to achieve normotension, normothermia, controlled ventilation with normocapnia, and a relaxed brain.
- Pain control after a craniotomy procedure often requires analgesia with opioid agents in addition to blocking scalp nerves with local anesthetic.

Abbreviations

5-ALA	5-amino levulinic acid
CPP	Cerebral perfusion pressure
CSF	Cerebrospinal fluid
CT	Computed tomography
GCS	Glasgow Coma Scale
ICP	Intracranial pressure
MRI	Magnetic resonance imaging
PEEP	Positive end-expiratory pressure

Contents

- The Lesions
- Clinical Presentation
- Surgical Approaches
- Preoperative Management
- Intraoperative Management
  - Induction

- – Positioning
- – Maintenance of Anesthesia
- – Fluid Management
- – Intraoperative Complications
- • Postoperative Management

The Lesions

The area of the brain above the tentorium cerebelli is known as the supratentorial region. Indications for surgery in this area are multiple but generally comprise of space occupying lesions, vascular abnormalities (see Chapter 16), and functional neurosurgery (see Chapter 21). Space occupying lesions can be neoplastic or non-neoplastic. Approximately 60% of supratentorial neoplasms are primary brain tumors, of which gliomas are the most common. Gliomas range from relatively benign pilocytic and well-differentiated astrocytomas to aggressive anaplastic astrocytomas and glioblastoma multiforme. Other common benign tumors include meningiomas and pituitary adenomas.

Glial tumors often disrupt the blood-brain barrier and typically show a significant amount of contrast enhancement on CT and MRI. These lesions are frequently surrounded by large areas of edema, particularly prominent around fast growing tumors, which usually respond to corticosteroids. This edema can persist or even rebound after surgical excision of the tumor. Although tumor blood flow varies, autoregulation is usually impaired within the tumor. Induced hypertension can lead to an increase in tumor blood flow, which can worsen edema and cause bleeding. The surrounding brain tissue may be relatively ischemic, perhaps because of compression.

Meningiomas, which account for 15% of primary brain tumors, are slow growing, and can be very vascular. Vascularity can sometimes be reduced by preoperative embolization. Because of size or location, they may require multiple attempts at resection.

Pituitary adenomas are benign tumors arising from the sella turcica and present with either symptoms relating to disturbed endocrine functions, and/or pressure effects on local structures.

Approximately 35% of supratentorial tumors are secondary neoplasms arising predominantly from the lung (50%) and breast (10%). The incidence of secondary tumors rises with increasing age. Excision of solitary lesions is justified in patients in whom the underlying disease is well controlled.

Other supratentorial lesions include hematomas, cystic lesions, CSF collections, and brain abscesses. The latter may arise because of local spread from sinuses or ear infections and are especially common in immunocompromised or diabetic patients, those with right-to-left cardiac shunts and intravenous drug abusers.

Clinical Presentation

Most brain neoplasms tend to grow slowly and allow adaptive mechanisms to be established such that tumors may become very large before becoming symptomatic. Supratentorial neoplasms may generate generalized or focal symptoms. Symptoms of raised ICP (headaches, nausea, vomiting, ataxia, visual disturbances, and cognitive disturbances) are often insidious in onset, particularly in slowly expanding lesions. Focal symptoms may develop because of the effects of the tumors on adjacent functional areas. New onset of seizures in adults is often the first indication of a supratentorial tumor. Focal neurological deficits and symptoms of raised ICP may respond initially to steroids. Patients may present for surgical diagnosis (biopsy), for debulking or for curative resection.

Surgical Approaches

Biopsy of supratentorial lesions is usually undertaken via a stereotactic approach or a mini craniotomy. Debulking procedures generally favor either a pterional or a frontal craniotomy (see Chapter 13). The former accesses the temporal and parietal lobes and necessitates that the patient's head be turned away from the site of the lesion in the supine position, whereas the latter approach includes bi-frontal craniotomy for bilateral or midline lesions. When intraoperative brain swelling is significant, the bone flap may not be replaced during surgical wound closure. Some months later a cranioplasty using a plate can be used to close the bony defect.

Preoperative Management

Specific preoperative assessment should include an accurate evaluation of the lesion, including its site and size, ease of surgical access, required positioning of the patient, expected blood loss, and changes in ICP, even if it is not evident clinically or radiologically. Accurate clinical assessment of the patient's neurological state should be undertaken, including specific focal neurological signs, level of consciousness using the GCS, as well as a comprehensive review of concurrent disease.

Premedication for anesthesia is not generally necessary but may be prescribed if the patient is particularly anxious and there is no evidence of significant intracranial hypertension. A short-acting benzodiazepine is usually adequate. Medications such as anticonvulsants and steroids should be taken up to the time of operation and continued into the postoperative period.

Intraoperative identification and resection of gliomas can be enhanced by the preoperative administration of 5-ALA which can increase the likelihood of complete resection. This is administered 2–4 hours prior to induction of anesthesia. 5-ALA causes light sensitization and patients should be protected from direct exposure to sunlight and strong ambient light for 24 hours. Up to 25% of patients experience significant intraoperative hypotension that can be difficult to manage and may require norepinephrine or some other vasoconstrictor.

Based on the preoperative assessment, a plan should be made regarding postoperative management including whether the patient is likely to require management in a high-dependency or critical care setting.

Intraoperative Management

The aims of general anesthesia are:
- Smooth induction
- Hemodynamic stability (hypotension can lead to ischemia in areas of impaired autoregulation, and hypertension may increase the risk of hemorrhage and vasogenic edema)
- Brain relaxation (for optimal surgical access and to reduce the risks of retractor damage)
- Timely and smooth emergence from anesthesia to allow early neurological assessment

Induction

Induction of anesthesia should be achieved with an intravenous anesthetic agent of choice, usually propofol or thiopental, combined with an opiate and a non-depolarizing muscle relaxant. Normotension should be maintained by anticipating hemodynamic responses. The hypertensive response to laryngoscopy can be obtunded by an additional bolus of induction agent, a short-acting opioid or intravenous lidocaine.

Standard routine monitoring is suitable for most patients during induction of anesthesia. Continuous intra-arterial blood pressure monitoring is used for major craniotomies and should be sited prior to induction in patients with co-morbidities, especially hypertension and ischemic heart disease. Advanced hemodynamic monitoring or central venous access may be indicated for cardiopulmonary disease or when large blood loss or fluid shifts are anticipated. Core temperature should be monitored and a urinary catheter should be inserted especially if hyperosmolar agents are to be administered intraoperatively. Other neuromonitoring, such as electroencephalography (see Chapter 50), somatosensory and motor-evoked potentials (see Chapter 49), trans-cranial doppler ultrasound (see Chapter 51), and jugular bulb catheterization (see Chapter 46) can be used in specific circumstances.

Once all monitoring is established, skull pins are generally applied. This is a potent stimulus and the hypertensive response can be obtunded in a fashion similar to the response to laryngoscopy. Scalp infiltration with local anesthetic prior to pin insertion is also effective.

Positioning

A neutral head position, elevated up to 30 degrees, is recommended to decrease ICP by improving venous drainage. Flexing or turning of the head may obstruct cerebral venous outflow and lead to dramatic elevation of ICP, which resolves on resumption of a neutral head position. However, a skilled surgeon should be able to position and turn the head for surgical access without obstructing venous return. Lowering of the head impairs cerebral venous drainage and results in an increase in ICP. Application of PEEP, especially >10 cmH$_2$O, especially can potentially increase ICP or venous oozing.

Maintenance of Anesthesia

The choice of anesthetic agents in largely at the discretion of the anesthetist, and either a total intravenous technique with propofol or an inhalational agent (sevoflurane, desflurane, and isoflurane) in combination with a short-acting opioid and muscle relaxant may be used. The technique used should not increase ICP or decrease CPP and should allow rapid emergency at the end of surgery. Unless there is a need to monitor cranial nerve function or motor responses, continuous muscle relaxation should be used and monitored with a nerve stimulator. The patient's ventilation should be controlled to maintain normocapnia, and body temperature should be maintained at normothermia.

Fluid Management

Maintenance and resuscitation fluids in routine neurosurgical patients are provided with glucose-free iso-osmolar crystalloid solutions to prevent increases in brain water content from hypo-osmolality. Glucose-containing solutions are avoided in all neurosurgical patients with normal glucose metabolism. These solutions can potentially exacerbate ischemic damage and cerebral edema. Both hypoglycemia and hyperglycemia must be

---

BOX 15.1 Management of Intraoperative Cerebral Edema

Optimize oxygenation

Maximize venous drainage: ensure an adequate head-up position (15- to 30-degree tilt)

Reduce oxygen metabolism: deepen anesthesia, bolus intravenous anesthetic agents, or lidocaine

Reduction in brain extracellular fluid volume with mannitol or hypertonic saline; furosemide may be used as an adjunct

Cerebrospinal fluid drainage

Consider hypocapnia

Consider hypothermia (not proven)

Consider anticonvulsants

---

avoided because both have been demonstrated to potentiate cellular damage. "Tight glycaemic control", however, has been associated with reduced brain glucose availability and increased cerebral metabolic distress. Blood glucose should be monitored and maintained between 5.0 and 10 mmol/L (90 and 180 mg/dl).

Intraoperative Complications

Severe complications include hemorrhage, intraoperative cerebral edema, and air embolism. Management of air embolism is covered in Chapter 17. Blood products should be readily available in the event of major bleeding with a goal of resuscitation to a hematocrit of 30%. Thromboplastin release causing disseminated intravascular coagulopathy may occur, and clotting factors should be given early. Acute cerebral edema requires aggressive management, as presented in Box 15.1.

Postoperative Management

Patients whose preoperative level of consciousness was depressed should be managed in a critical care setting. These patients may be electively ventilated postoperatively, but the decision to do so will be based on preoperative and intraoperative factors along with discussions with neurosurgeons and intensivists.

Patients with a high preoperative GCS are usually extubated once they open their eyes to command and have a gag reflex. The overall aim is to achieve smooth emergence with minimal coughing or straining to avoid an increase in ICP as a result of a rise in cerebral venous pressure. Hypertension in the postoperative period is most often due to inadequate analgesia. Other possible causes include hypothermia, hypercarbia, hypoxia, hypo-osmolality, anemia, brain manipulation, emergence phenomena, sympathetic stimulation or the effects of adrenaline-containing local anesthesia. If possible, the likely cause of the hypertension needs to be identified then treated. Hypertension can be managed with a short-acting beta blocker such as metoprolol, labetalol, or esmolol. Direct acting vasodilators can raise ICP and should be avoided. Blood pressures of >160 mmHg systolic or 110 mmHg mean are associated with a higher incidence of post-craniotomy hematomas.

Careful attention to adequate postoperative analgesia is important. The analgesic effects of strong opiates need to be balanced against their sedative effects. Good analgesia can be effected with the use of multimodal agents. A combination of local anesthesia, paracetamol or acetaminophen, intraoperative magnesium, and judicious use of medium- to long-acting opiates can be used in combination to achieve this.

Further Reading

Au, K., Bharadwaj, S., Venkatraghavan, L., Bernstein, M. (2016). Outpatient brain tumor craniotomy under general anesthesia. *Journal of Neurosurgery*, **125**(5), 1130–1135. https://doi.org/10.3171/2015.11 .JNS152151.

Batra, A., Verma, R., Bhatia, V. K., Chandra, G., Bhushan, S. (2017). Dexmedetomidine as an Anesthetic Adjuvant in Intracranial Surgery. *Anesthesia, Essays and Researches*, **11**(2), 309–313. https://doi.org/10.4103/0259-1162.194555.

Gruenbaum, S. E., Meng, L., Bilotta, F. (2016). Recent trends in the anesthetic management of craniotomy for supratentorial tumor resection. *Current Opinion in Anaesthesiology*, **29**(5), 552–557. https://doi.org/10.1097/ ACO.0000000000000365.

Gupta, A., Sattur, M. G., Aoun, R. J. N., et al (2017). Hemicraniectomy for Ischemic and Hemorrhagic Stroke: Facts and Controversies. *Neurosurgery Clinics of North America*, **28**(3), 349–360. https://doi.org/10.1016/j .nec.2017.02.010.

Ruggieri, F., Beretta, L., Corno, L., et al (2017). Feasibility of Protective Ventilation During Elective Supratentorial Neurosurgery: A Randomized, Crossover, Clinical Trial. *Journal of Neurosurgical Anesthesiology*. https://doi.org/ 10.1097/ANA.0000000000000442.

Chapter 16

Anesthesia for Intracranial Vascular Lesions

Manuel Aliaño Hermoso, Ram Adapa, and Derek Duane

Key Points

- Aneurysmal SAH usually occurs after 40-years of age with a female bias of 3:2.
- The 30-day mortality is approximately 50% while morbidity in survivors can reach 30%.
- Most aneurysms arise from the anterior circulatory cerebral vasculature.
- SAH may cause significant cardiovascular, pulmonary, and metabolic complications that need to be optimized before surgical or endovascular treatment.
- Perioperative blood pressure management is crucial to prevent rebleeding or cerebral ischemia secondary to vasospasm.
- Inhalational or total intravenous techniques are suitable for anesthesia during cerebral aneurysm surgery.
- High-dependency care for hemodynamic and neurological monitoring is preferred for most neurovascular patients.
- An AVM is an abnormal collection of dysplastic vessels. Up to 10% of patients have an associated aneurysm.
- During arterio-venous malformation surgery, uncontrollable venous hemorrhage is a significant risk.
- Hyperemic complications of cerebral edema or hemorrhage are responsible for most of the postoperative morbidity and mortality in patients with an AVM.

Abbreviations

AVM   Arteriovenous malformation
CBF   Cerebral blood flow
CPP   Cerebral perfusion pressure
CSF   Cerebrospinal fluid
CSW   Cerebral-induced salt wasting
CT   Computerized tomography
CTA   Computerized tomographic angiography
DSA   Digital subtraction angiography
EEG   Electroencephalography
GCS   Glasgow Coma Scale
ICP   Intracranial pressure

MAP   Mean arterial pressure
SAH   Subarachnoid hemorrhage
SIADH   Syndrome of inappropriate antidiuretic hormone secretion
TIVA   Total intravenous anesthesia
TPG   Transmural pressure gradient

Contents

- Aneurysmal Subarachnoid Hemorrhage
  - Epidemiology
  - Pathophysiology of Cerebral Aneurysms
  - Diagnosis and Investigations
  - Treatment of Cerebral Aneurysms
- Anesthetic Management
  - Preoperative Assessment
  - Monitoring
  - Induction of Anesthesia
  - Maintenance and Emergence
  - Postoperative Anesthetic Care
  - Management of Intraoperative Aneurysm Rupture
- Arteriovenous Malformations
  - Pathogenesis and Epidemiology
  - Diagnosis and Treatment
  - Anesthetic Management and Complications
- Further Reading

Aneurysmal Subarachnoid Hemorrhage

Epidemiology

The incidence of SAH secondary to rupture of a cerebral aneurysm is 8–10 cases per 100,000 per year which represents about 10% of all cerebrovascular accidents. It is more common between the ages of 40 and 60 years and it presents in females more than males with a ratio of 3:2. Up to 80% of spontaneous SAHs are due to a rupture of a cerebral aneurysm while the remaining causes are non-aneurysmal (Box 16.1).

The prehospital mortality rate is almost 10% and approximately 25% of inpatients die within the first 2 weeks despite treatment. The 30-day mortality rate is close to 45%, whereas the incidence of moderate to severe neurological morbidity can reach 30%. A good outcome after management is seen only in about 30% of cases while without treatment, re-rupture is close to 50% within 6 months.

Mortality and morbidity is related to (1) the overwhelming neuronal damage after the initial bleed; (2) rebleeding, (2–4% of untreated patients in the first 24 hours and 20% within 2 weeks); (3) ischemic brain damage from cerebral vasospasm (radiological signs can be found in up to 40%–60% of cases); (4) seizures; and (5) myocardial ventricular dysfunction.

BOX 16.1 Causes of Non-Aneurysmal Subarachnoid Hemorrhage:

Trauma
Arteriovenous malformations (AVMs)
Arterial dissection
Dural venous sinus thrombosis
Coagulation disorders
Pituitary apoplexy
Cocaine Abuse

BOX 16.2 Predisposing Factors Related to Aneurysm Formation

Family history of the disease
Atherosclerosis
Hypertension
Excess alcohol consumption
Smoking
Obesity
Coarctation of the aorta
Polycystic kidney disease
Fibromuscular dysplasia
Estrogen deficiency
Ehlers-Danlos syndrome
Marfan's syndrome.

Outcome is adversely affected by older age, low coma score on admission, intracerebral or intraventricular hemorrhage, and rebleeding.

Pathophysiology of Cerebral Aneurysms

Degenerative changes in the cerebral arterial wall induced by turbulent blood flow at a vessel's branching point contribute to the formation of aneurysms. This susceptibility to hemodynamic stress may be related to structural abnormalities in these arteries produced by several predisposing factors (Box 16.2).

The commonest type of aneurysm is described as saccular (berry-like) while other types such as fusiform, dissecting, traumatic, and mycotic types are less common. Most saccular aneurysms are less than 12 mm in diameter and classified as "small" while giant aneurysms (>24 mm in diameter) are found in less than 5% of all cases. Multiple aneurysms can occur in about 15%–20% of patients.

Aneurysms arise on the anterior cerebral artery (40%), posterior communicating artery (25%), and the bifurcation of the middle cerebral artery (25%). Only 10% of aneurysms develop in the vertebrobasilar system, mostly on the basilar artery.

The pathophysiologic changes that occur when an aneurysm ruptures include:

- A sudden large increase in ICP
- A decrease in CBF, which may help stop further bleeding
- Cerebral vasoconstriction
- Loss of cerebrovascular autoregulation
- A decrease in CPP
- Spread of blood through the subarachnoid space causing inflammation

Direct neural destruction by the force of extravasated blood, cerebral ischemia, and sympathetically mediated cardiac dysfunction are primarily responsible for the morbidity and mortality. The likelihood of aneurysm rupture depends on its size (more likely if >6 mm), morphology, location, and any previous history of SAH. During the initial bleeding, blood can spread through the subarachnoid space, but with rebleeding, intracranial hemorrhage is more common and can be intraparenchymal (20%–40%), intraventricular (10%–20%), or subdural (5%).

Diagnosis and Investigations

The clinical manifestations of SAH include: sudden severe headache with vomiting, neck pain (meningismus), photophobia, seizures, cranial nerve signs, focal neurologic deficits, transient loss of consciousness, or prolonged coma. An urgent, non-contrast-enhanced, high-resolution CT head scan will diagnose SAH in more than 95% of patients.

To define the exact size, location, and configuration of cerebral aneurysms, the invasive procedure of DSA is the "gold standard" investigation. Contrast-enhanced CTA, which involves three-dimensional reconstruction of cerebrovascular images after intravenous injection of dye, is now commonly used prior to surgery. This investigation has a sensitivity and specificity of over 80% both of which increase with larger aneurysms.

If the initial CT scan is negative for SAH a lumbar puncture can be performed to examine the CSF for xanthochromia, which is caused by the released haem moiety of red blood cells degrading to bilirubin.

Treatment of Cerebral Aneurysms

Grading systems help stratify the degree of clinical impairment, assess the likelihood of complications, and guide prognosis. The Hunt and Hess scale (Box 16.3) grades the clinical presentation of the aneurysm patient from zero (unruptured aneurysm) to 5 (deep coma). The World Federation of Neurological Surgeons Grading Scale ranks presentation according to GCS score and motor deficit; (I-15/Absent; II-14–13/Absent; III-14–13/Present; IV-12–7/ Present or Absent; V-6–3/Present or Absent). The Fisher grading system groups patients in relation to the radiological appearance of the amount of blood on the CT head scan: (1-no subarachnoid blood; 2-diffuse; 3-localized clot; 4-Intracerebral or intraventricular clot with diffuse or no SAH). In general, patients with a good neurological status prior to intervention and minimal intracranial blood on imaging have a better outcome.

Surgical or endovascular treatment within 1 to 3 days of rupture minimizes the risk of rebleeding and vasospasm. Patients who are Hunt and Hess grade I or II may undergo prompt treatment, whereas patients whose GCS score is less than 8 often have their intervention delayed until neurologic improvement occurs. Some centers provide early treatment for patients graded III to IV to allow aggressive management of vasospasm with induced hypertension.

> **BOX 16.3** Hunt and Hess Grading Scale (Journal of Neurosurgery 1968; 28 (1):14–20)
>
> Grade 0   Grade 0 Unruptured aneurysm
> Grade 1   Asymptomatic or minimal headache and slight nuchal rigidity
> Grade 2   Moderate to severe headache, nuchal rigidity no neurological deficit other than the cranial nerve palsy
> Grade 3   Drowsiness, confusion, or mild focal deficit
> Grade 4   Stupor, moderate to severe hemiparesis, possible early decerebrate rigidity, vegetative disturbances
> Grade 5   Deep coma, decerebrate rigidity, moribund appearance

Surgical treatment of aneurysms involves the application of a vascular clip across the aneurysm's neck. Other surgical techniques can involve complex flow diversion procedures or simply wrapping the aneurysm sac in muslin gauze. Morbidity and mortality for operative intervention is determined by the experience of the surgeon, size and location of the aneurysm, and the presence of cerebral edema and intracerebral hemorrhage.

Nowadays, most cerebral aneurysms can be treated by endovascular platinum coil occlusion with or without balloon remodeling or by using stent-like flow diverters. The benefits of these techniques include a less invasive procedure, greater suitability for patients with significant comorbidity, and a better outcome for posterior circulation aneurysms. Results from the International Subarachnoid Aneurysm Trial indicated that despite a greater incidence of rebleeding, there was a significant reduction in poor outcome at early and late follow-up of patients undergoing coil embolization versus surgical clipping. Repeat angiography is undertaken for these patients to identify if further embolization procedures are required to treat aneurysm recurrence.

Anesthetic Management

The goals of anesthetic management, whether for a surgical or endovascular embolization procedure, involve: (1) avoiding aneurysm rupture from increases in the TPG (MAP minus local ICP); (2) maintaining adequate CPP and cerebral oxygenation; and (3) limiting brain swelling from cerebral edema or vascular engorgement. In general, the same basic principles govern the conduct of anesthesia whether operative or radiological interventions are used to secure the aneurysm (see Chapter 28).

Preoperative Assessment

Patients need to be assessed for the presence and extent of all intracranial and extracranial complications of a SAH (Boxes 16.4–16.5). These complications are discussed in more detail in Chapter 35. Patients who are Hunt and Hess grade I or II often show minimal disturbance in cerebral hemodynamics, whereas those graded III and IV can show loss of cerebrovascular autoregulation and responsiveness to carbon dioxide.

The preoperative assessment should include a complete history, physical examination with special focus on the neurological evaluation, and a review of important imaging studies. It is essential to optimize cardiac, pulmonary, and metabolic function before induction of anesthesia. This may involve treatment of: (1) dysrhythmias, (2) hypovolemia

---

BOX 16.4 Intracranial Complications of Subarachnoid Hemorrhage

Rebleeding
Vasospasm leading to cerebral ischemia/infarction
Hydrocephalus
Expanding intracerebral hematoma
Seizures

BOX 16.5 Extracranial Complications of Subarachnoid Hemorrhage

Myocardial dysfunction
Arrhythmias
Hypoxemia secondary to neurogenic pulmonary edema
Dysnatraemias secondary to SIADH or CSWS
Gastric hemorrhage

---

to minimize vasospasm, (3) hypotension secondary to ventricular dysfunction, (4) hypoxia resulting from neurogenic pulmonary edema, and (5) dysnatremias caused by SIADH or CSW.

Medical therapy for coexisting conditions should be continued, and patients should be maintained on nimodipine and anticonvulsant medications throughout the perioperative period or according to local practice.

Baseline investigations should include a complete blood count, electrolyte studies, cardiac troponin levels, coagulation profile, blood group determination, 12-lead electrocardiograph, echocardiography when indicated, and a chest radiograph. Premedication may be appropriate in good-grade patients but should be avoided in general.

Monitoring

In addition to routine cardiac, respiratory, urine output, and nasopharyngeal temperature monitoring, direct measurement of intra-arterial blood pressure is essential and for some patients is appropriate before induction. Invasive and non-invasive hemodynamic monitoring may be necessary to guide vascular filling, especially if myocardial dysfunction is suspected. More specialized intraoperative cerebral monitoring can be performed including; jugular bulb or cerebral oximetry, transcranial doppler measurement of CBF velocities, EEG, and evoked potentials. Blood analysis for levels of oxygen, carbon dioxide, acidemia electrolytes, lactate, glucose, and hemoglobin should be performed intermittently throughout the case.

Induction of Anesthesia

Intravenous induction of anesthesia via a large-bore cannula is the most common technique used. Wide swings in either MAP or ICP will alter the TPG (TPG = MAP – ICP) across the aneurysm and may cause it to rupture. Unfortunately, this event is associated with a high mortality. Laryngoscopy, intubation, and the application of skull pins are potent hypertensive stimuli which should be anticipated and prevented. Intravenous or topical lidocaine, β-blockers, short-acting opiates or intravenous induction agents can be used to facilitate this. MAP should then be maintained within 20% of the patient's normal preoperative level to achieve an adequate CPP. Poorer-grade patients with intracranial hypertension will tolerate only minimal changes to their cerebral hemodynamics and require particular attention to ICP and MAP control at induction.

Maintenance and Emergence

Cerebral aneurysm surgery can be performed using inhalational agents or TIVA. Short-acting drugs such as propofol, fentanyl, remifentanil or sufentanil are commonly used. When using inhalational agents, mild hypocapnia will avoid their dose-related effect on cerebral vasodilation. Methods to reduce the volume of intracranial contents by using hyperosmolar agents (mannitol or hypertonic saline), moderate hyperventilation, and drainage of CSF may adversely alter the TPG and should be initiated slowly or ideally, delayed until the dura is open.

During surgery, temporary proximal occlusion of the parent (feeding) vessel is often performed to facilitate dissection and clipping of the aneurysm. Beyond 15–20 minutes of temporary occlusion, the risk of ischemia increases so the MAP is usually augmented to improve collateral circulation. Good evidence is lacking for the use of hypothermia, barbiturates, propofol, and extra doses of mannitol to extend the duration of occlusion. Once the aneurysm has been clipped, mild to moderate hypertension is permitted to improve cerebral perfusion. To assess aneurysm occlusion and adequacy of blood flow in the surrounding cerebral vessels, intraoperative fluorescent angiography using indocyanine green may be performed.

At the end of uneventful aneurysm surgery, patients should be extubated with minimal coughing and hemodynamic fluctuations. Uncontrolled hypertension or persistent hypotension requires treatment to prevent adverse cerebral or cardiac sequelae.

Postoperative Anesthetic Care

Neurovascular patients should be managed in a neurosurgical high-dependency or intensive care unit to ensure continued hemodynamic monitoring, adequate oxygenation, optimum fluid and electrolyte management, and early detection of complications. Analgesics, including small doses of opiates, are used to treat postoperative pain. Patients who fail to return to their preoperative GCS or who develop a focal neurological deficit require urgent clinical assessment by the neurosurgeon to decide if further imaging, surgical intervention or hypertensive management is appropriate. In patients at increased risk of cerebral vasospasm, a 10%–20% increase in MAP above preoperative baseline values may be of benefit.

Management of Intraoperative Aneurysm Rupture

The Incidence of intraoperative aneurysm rupture for non-elective cases is between 5 and 10%. It can occur during dissection or when the clip is applied and is related to surgical experience, state of the cerebral vessels as well as the size and location of the aneurysm. The patient's survival depends on rapidly controlling the bleeding while maintaining adequate cerebral perfusion. Effective communication with the neurosurgical team is essential (Box 16.6).

BOX 16.6 The Anesthetic Management of Intraoperative Rupture

- Ventilation with 100% oxygen
- Transient induction of hypotension (MAP to 50 mmHg as tolerated)
- Hemodynamic interventions to maintain adequate CPP
- Restoration of intravascular volume with blood, clotting products, and crystalloid solutions
- Propofol, thiopental, or etomidate can be considered to achieve electroencephalographic burst suppression thus reducing cerebral metabolic rate and blood flow requirements
- Hyperosmolar therapy with either Mannitol (0.5–1 g/kg) or hypertonic saline (2 ml/kg of 5% NaCl) to help reduce cerebral edema
- Mild hypothermia (34–35 $^\circ$C)
- Once the aneurysm is secured, restore CPP to normal levels

Arteriovenous Malformations

Pathogenesis and Epidemiology

An AVM is an abnormal collection of dysplastic vessels, the majority of which present as supratentorial lesions. This vascular mass normally has a center (nidus) surrounded by dilated draining veins. In the nidus, blood flows directly from dilated arteries to veins with no intervening capillary bed or neural parenchyma and there may be associated flow aneurysms in up to 10% of cases. Most AVMs are high-flow low-resistance shunts whose mean transmural pressure is much less than MAP. Hence, rupture is not related to acute rises in MAP unless the AVM is small and there is higher pressure within the feeding artery. AVMs are congenital lesions occurring with an incidence of <1% in the general population and associated with Osler-Weber-Rendu disease and Sturge-Weber syndrome. They usually manifest before the age of 40 as cerebral hemorrhage (risk of 2%–4% per year), seizures, symptoms of a mass effect, raised ICP, or neurologic signs secondary to cerebral ischemia (steal effect).

Diagnosis and Treatment

Diagnosis of this condition is by investigation with cerebral angiography, CTA and/or magnetic resonance imaging. Treatment options include: (1) surgical excision, (2) endovascular embolization, and (3) staged stereotactic radiosurgery. These interventions can be useful alone or in combination. Surgical outcome is related to the AVM grade (Spetzler-Martin AVM Grading System), which takes into account size, eloquence of adjacent brain, and pattern of venous drainage.

Anesthetic Management and Complications

For surgical resection of an AVM, the anesthetic management follows the same general principles as outlined for SAH. In the preoperative assessment, the presence of an associated aneurysm should be noted, as well as symptoms suggestive of cerebral ischemia or a mass effect. Because large shunts can produce ischemia in non-autoregulating surrounding brain tissue, blood pressure management during induction is essential to avoid rupturing an associated aneurysm or producing ischemic changes in hypoperfused areas. Intraoperative MAP is usually maintained at 20% below what is normal for the patient.

During AVM surgery, severe bleeding can occur and may be associated with malignant cerebral edema. Care should be taken to avoid any rise in venous pressure. The use of deliberate hypotension to decrease blood loss may risk cerebral ischemia and venous outflow thrombosis.

Hyperemic complications of cerebral edema and hemorrhage are responsible for most of the postoperative morbidity and mortality. Hyperemia and its consequences can be caused by:

1. Normal perfusion pressure breakthrough – believed to be due to loss of autoregulation in previously hypoperfused brain tissue unable to deal with restored normal perfusion.
2. "Occlusive hyperemia" – venous outflow obstruction produced by surgical ligation of veins in adjacent normal brain or in the AVM with incomplete occlusion of arterial feeders.

Intracerebral hemorrhage may also occur from an inaccessible or unidentified residual AVM. Therefore, during emergence from anesthesia and in the postoperative period, hypertension should be treated with β-blockers or some other suitable agent to avoid this complications. Because the risk of seizures after this surgery is 40% to 50%, patients may need prophylactic anticonvulsants. All patients after AVM surgery should have hemodynamic and neurological monitoring in a high-dependency area to allow for early identification of complications.

Further Reading

Connolly, E.S.J., Rabinstein, A.A., Carhuapoma, J.R., et al: Guidelines for the management of aneurysmal subarachnoid hemorrhage: A guideline for healthcare professionals from the American Heart Association/American Stroke Association. *Stroke* 2012; **43**(6):1711–1737, https://doi.org/10.1161/STR.0b013e3182587839.

Fisher, C.M., Kistler, J.P., Davis, J.M.: Relation of cerebral vasospasm to subarachnoid hemorrhage visualized by computerized tomographic scanning. *Neurosurg* 1980; **6**(1):1–9.

Gross, B.A., Du, R.: Natural history of cerebral arteriovenous malformations: A meta-analysis. *J Neurosurg* 2013; **118**(2):437–443, https://doi.org/10.3171/2012.10.JNS121280.

Hunt, W.E., Hess, R.M.: Surgical risk as related to time of intervention in the repair of intracranial aneurysms. *J Neurosurg* 1968; **28**(1):14–20, https://doi.org/10.3171/jns.1968.28.1.0014.

Larsen, C.C., Astrup, J.: Rebleeding after aneurysmal subarachnoid hemorrhage: A literature review. *World Neurosurg* 2013; **79**(2):307–312, https://doi.org/10.1016/j.wneu.2012.06.023.

Li, H., Pan, R., Wang, H., et al: Clipping versus coiling for ruptured intracranial aneurysms: A systematic review and meta-analysis. *Stroke* 2013; **44**(1):29–37, https://doi.org/10.1161/STROKEAHA.112.663559.

Mohr, J.P., Kejda-Scharler, J., Pile-Spellman, J.: Diagnosis and treatment of arteriovenous malformations. *Curr Neurolog Neurosci Rep* 2013; **13**(2):324, https://doi.org/10.1007/s11910-012-0324-1.

Report of World Federation of Neurological Surgeons Committee on a Universal Subarachnoid Hemorrhage Grading Scale. *J Neurosurg* 1988; **68**(6):985–986.

Spetzler, R.F., Martin, N.A.: A proposed grading system for arteriovenous malformations. *J Neurosurg* 1988; **65**(4):476–483, https://doi.org/10.3171/jns.1986.65.4.0476.

Spetzler, R.F., McDougall, C.G., Zabramski, J. M., et al: The barrow ruptured aneurysm trial: 6-year results. *J Neurosurg* 2015; **123**(3):609–617, https://doi.org/10.3171/2014.9.JNS141749.

Steiner, T., Juvela, S., Unterberg, A., et al: European Stroke Organization guidelines for the management of intracranial aneurysms and subarachnoid haemorrhage. *Cerebrovasc Dis* 2013; **35**(2):93–112, https://doi.org/10.1159/000346087.

Vlak, M.H.M., et al: Lifetime risks for aneurysmal subarachnoid haemorrhage: Multivariable risk stratification. *J Neurol Neurosurg Psychiatry* 2013; **84**(6):619–623.

Anesthesia for Posterior Fossa Lesions

Rosemary Ann Craen and Hélèe Pellerin

Key Points

- Preoperative neurologic evaluation is crucial to guide perioperative management.
- Be prepared to treat raised intracranial pressure and cardiac arrhythmias.
- Prevention is the cornerstone in the management of venous air embolism.
- Delayed extubation should be considered if brainstem/cranial nerve injuries are anticipated.
- Postoperatively, close monitoring is necessary for early detection of airway compromise and for neurologic deterioration.
- Good blood pressure control in the postoperative period is important.

Abbreviations

BAER	Brainstem auditory evoked response
CSF	Cerebrospinal fluid
ICP	Intracranial pressure
MEP	Motor evoked potentials
PETN$_2$	End-tidal nitrogen tension
PETCO$_2$	End-tidal CO_2 tension
PFO	Patent foramen ovale
SSEP	Somatosensory evoked potentials
TCD	Transcranial doppler
TEE	Transesophageal echocardiography
VAE	Venous air embolism

Contents

- Introduction
- Pathology
- Preoperative Evaluation
- Positioning
- Intraoperative Management

    - Monitoring
    - Induction and Maintenance

- Dysrhythmias
- Emergence
- Venous Air Embolism
  - Monitoring
  - Preoperative Considerations
  - Treatment
- Conclusion
- Further Reading

Introduction

The posterior cranial fossa is part of the intracranial cavity, located between the tentorium cerebelli and the foramen magnum. It contains structures responsible for the vital control of respiratory and cardiovascular systems and therefore presents unique challenges to the anesthesiologist.

Pathology

Pathologies can be classified by tissue of origin (Box 17.1). Tumors are the most common posterior fossa lesions requiring surgical intervention. In children, posterior fossa tumors represent approximately 60% of all brain tumors. In adults, tumors are less frequent and include acoustic neuromas, metastases (mainly from lung and breast cancers), meningiomas, and hemangioblastomas.

An acoustic neuroma is a benign lesion arising from the vestibular portion of cranial nerve VIII in the cerebellopontine angle and can cause hearing loss, tinnitus, vertigo, and hemifacial spasm. Small acoustic neuromas can be removed via a retromastoid approach. Large ones involve a suboccipital approach which can be a long procedure but is intended to preserve facial and cochlear nerve function.

There are two types of Chiari malformations. Chiari I is characterized by descent of the cerebellar tonsils into the cervical spinal canal and causes cough-induced headache, nuchal pain, and lower cranial nerve dysfunction in young adulthood. Chiari II malformation is more complex in which the inferior vermis herniates through the

---

BOX 17.1 Classification of Pathologies in the Posterior Fossa

Meninges	• Tumor meningioma
Brain	• Tumor
	• Chiari malformation
Vascular	• Arteriovenous malformation
	• Cavernoma
	• Venous infarct
	• Cerebral aneurysm
Cerebrospinal fluid	• Cystic lesion
Cranial nerves	• Schwannoma
	• Vascular compression of nerves

foramen magnum, and may be associated with spina bifida, hydrocephalus, and syringomyelia. Lower cranial nerve dysfunction can cause stridor, respiratory distress, dysphagia, and aspiration. Spasticity and quadriparesis are progressive if untreated. Even with aggressive treatment, the condition is fatal in 30% of symptomatic infants. Both Chiari malformations are treated with suboccipital craniectomy and upper cervical laminectomy. Treatment of the associated hydrocephalus may require a shunt procedure for cerebrospinal diversion.

Trigeminal neuralgia, or tic douloureux, is a pain syndrome where small vessels, most commonly arteries, compress the roots of the cranial nerve causing neuralgia. Patients have paroxysmal episodes of excruciating and lancinating pain over the ipsilateral trigeminal distribution. Surgical decompression of the cranial nerves is performed by removing the offending lesion or placing a muscle pad or Teflon sponge between the artery and root entry zone often producing pain relief. Patients with these conditions should have their chronic pain syndrome evaluated to guide pain management postoperatively.

Preoperative Evaluation

In addition to the usual preoperative assessment, a detailed neurologic examination is crucial to plan perioperative management (Box 17.2). Preoperative evaluation may guide the type of intraoperative neuromonitoring required. Imaging should be reviewed and discussed with the neurosurgeon to understand size of the lesion, amount of edema, vascularity of the lesion, presence of hydrocephalus, presence of uncal herniation or foramen magnum compression, and if the transverse sinus is patent or invaded by tumor. Additional information includes success of preoperative embolization and the need for intraoperative CSF lumbar drainage. Meticulous preoperative evaluation and planning will help anticipate and prepare for major intraoperative complications such as raised ICP, significant blood loss and VAE, and for postoperative complications such as neurologic injury and airway compromise.

Patients with posterior fossa lesions, especially in the presence of raised ICP, are more sensitive to sedatives and analgesics, and these agents should be used with caution preoperatively.

BOX 17.2 Characteristics to Look for during the Preoperative Evaluation	
Signs of raised intracranial pressure	• Altered state of consciousness • Nausea and vomiting • Papilloedema
Signs of brainstem dysfunction	• Altered respiratory pattern • Sleep apnea
Signs of cranial nerve dysfunction	• Dysphagia • Absent gag reflex • Changes in phonation
Signs of cerebellar dysfunction	• Ataxia • Dysmetria

Positioning

Posterior fossa surgery can be performed in the prone, semi-prone (park bench, far lateral) position and, less commonly, in the sitting position (see Chapter 14). Use of the sitting position has dramatically declined in recent years due to the increased risks associated with this position, including significant hemodynamic instability, VAE, and spinal cord compression with severe neck flexion. A modified semi-sitting position has been adopted however, as it allows a bloodless surgical field by improving venous and CSF drainage. The incidence of postoperative pneumocephalus is more frequent in this position, but its clinical impact is debatable.

Intraoperative Management

Monitoring

Routine monitoring includes electrocardiography, pulse oximetry, capnography, temperature, urine output, and neuromuscular blockade. An intra-arterial catheter allows invasive monitoring of systemic blood pressure, cerebral perfusion pressure and assessment of arterial tension of carbon dioxide ($PaCO_2$). The decision to insert a central venous line should be dictated by the patient's medical status, the size and the nature of the pathology, the expected degree of blood loss, and the risk for VAE. Electrophysiological monitoring (MEP, SSEP, BAER, cranial nerve monitoring) should be tailored to the site of surgery and the location of the lesion (see Chapter 49).

Induction and Maintenance

No specific anesthetic technique has been identified as the most effective. Goals of anesthesia include maintenance of cerebral perfusion pressure and avoidance of coughing, straining, and hemodynamic instability. Techniques that decrease ICP and facilitate brain relaxation should be used to ensure the best surgical conditions (Box 17.3).

There is some question about whether osmotic diuretics are as effective in decreasing raised ICP in the infra-tentorial compartment as compared to the supratentorial compartment. However, it is still commonly used. Drainage of CSF may be necessary and can be achieved by use of a lumbar drain or a ventriculostomy procedure.

Dysrhythmias

Cardiac dysrhythmias are common during manipulation of the brainstem. Bradycardia is the most frequent and is due to the stimulation of the trigemino-cardiac reflex. Bradycardia

---

BOX 17.3 Treatment of Intracranial Hypertension

- Head-up position
- Free venous drainage
- Hyperventilation
- Drainage of cerebrospinal fluid
- Reduce volatile anesthetic
- Change to intravenous anesthetic
- Give mannitol or hypertonic saline

> **BOX 17.4 Features to Evaluate before Extubation**
>
> - Level of consciousness
> - Airway and gag reflex
> - Face and tongue edema
> - Airway edema
> - Respiratory pattern (respiratory rate, tidal volume)
> - Stable vital parameters (blood pressure, pulse oximetry, core temperature)
> - Absence of residual neuromuscular blockade

usually subsides with cessation of stimulus. Treatment with glycopyrrolate, atropine, or ephedrine may be indicated. Severe hypertension and associated bradycardia reflecting pain is often associated with manipulation of the cranial nerve entry zone during a microvascular decompression procedure.

Emergence

The aim should be early awakening to allow evaluation of neurological function. Patient factors (baseline neurologic dysfunction, airway/tongue edema) and surgical factors (nature, extent, and duration of the surgery) should be carefully evaluated to prevent failed extubation (Box 17.4). A "leak test" around the endotracheal tube with the cuff deflated is used by some, especially after prolonged prone positioning. Delaying extubation may be required to allow the edema to resolve and airway reflexes to return. and afterwards, close monitoring is necessary for early detection of airway compromise and/or neurologic deterioration.

Hypertension should be avoided in the early postoperative phase because it contributes to postoperative brain edema and increases the risk for postoperative intracranial hemorrhage. Scalp blocks or infiltration of the incision with local anesthetics at the end of surgery, or both, will reduce the need for postoperative opiates.

Venous Air Embolism

Factors that increase the risk for VAE include operative site above the level of the heart and the presence of non-collapsible veins. Both are usually present during posterior fossa surgery, especially in the sitting position. The incidence of VAE in posterior fossa surgery varies widely in the literature depending on the monitoring used. If air entrainment is stopped immediately after detection, the effects can be short-lived and insignificant with low morbidity.

The pathophysiology of VAE can be evidenced by an elevation in pulmonary vascular pressure leading to impaired gas exchange, hypoxemia, and CO_2 retention. Mechanical obstruction of pulmonary capillaries and increased intrapulmonary shunting result in a decrease in $ETCO_2$. Bronchoconstriction may occur, and further air entrainment will lead to progressive decreases in cardiac output, hypotension, arrhythmias, and myocardial ischemia or failure. The sudden entry of a large bolus of air into the right heart can have a dramatic effect by causing an airlock that blocks the right ventricular outflow tract and leads to a sudden cardiovascular collapse or cardiac arrest.

PFO is present in 25% of the adult population and increases the risk of paradoxical air embolism when air travels to the systemic circulation through an intracardiac shunt and results in myocardial and cerebral ischemia. It is recommended that any patient scheduled for surgery in the sitting position undergo echocardiography to rule out PFO. However, the sensitivity of echocardiography is low for the detection of PFO (<50%). Therefore, the risk for intraoperative paradoxical air embolism must always be considered, although the clinically observed incidence is low (<2%).

A less invasive test to preoperatively detect PFO is the use of TCD ultrasound. However, the sensitivity and specificity of TCD in detecting PFO are comparable to that of echocardiography. PFO is therefore considered a contraindication to the sitting position. However, recent reports of modified semi-sitting neurosurgical procedures in this population showed no increase in morbidity when a strict protocol was followed (modifying the position to elevate the legs, vigilant monitoring with TEE, manual intermittent jugular compression to detect bleeding, and the use of evoked potential monitoring). There is also an argument for closure of PFO prior to surgery.

Monitoring

Precordial Doppler ultrasonography is the standard monitor, and the probe is placed along the right parasternal border at the fourth intercostal space. It can detect as little as 0.25 ml of air. TEE is the most sensitive of all monitors and can detect paradoxical embolism. However, it is less readily available, is more invasive, and requires special expertise, and its safety with prolonged use in the presence of neck flexion is not well established. In addition, it is still uncertain whether the use of intraoperative TEE for detection of VAE decreases morbidity. Capnography will show an abrupt decrease in $PETCO_2$, whereas an increase in $PETN_2$ is more specific for VAE but can be difficult to monitor. Pulmonary artery pressure monitoring is as sensitive as capnography but seldom used. Monitors that measure the decrease in blood pressure and cardiac output are least sensitive. In summary, precordial doppler ultrasound and capnography remain the recommended monitors for VAE during posterior fossa surgery and should allow detection before clinical signs occur.

Preoperative Considerations

Box 17.5 outlines simple preventive steps to avoid VAE. To allow potential aspiration of air, a right heart multilumen central venous catheter should be positioned 2 cm below the junction of the superior vena cava and the atrium and a single-lumen catheter positioned 3 cm above this junction. Good placement can be confirmed by radiography, monitoring of intravascular pressure, portable ultrasound, or intravascular electrocardiography, in which the presence of a biphasic P-wave in lead two will confirm mid-atrial placement of the tip of

---

BOX 17.5 Prevention of Venous Air Embolism

- Decrease the gradient between the heart and the site of surgery
- Maintain normovolemia to hypervolemia
- Apply bone wax during surgery

BOX 17.6 Treatment of Venous Air Embolism

- Notify the surgeon to flood the surgical site and stop entrainment of air
- Stop N_2O administration if used
- Give 100% O_2
- Lower the operative site
- Perform aspiration through a central venous line
- Consider compression of the jugular veins
- Provide cardio-pulmonary support (fluids, pressors, inotropes)

---

the catheter or the proximal orifice if a multilumen catheter is used. The key is to have a well-established plan for monitoring and treatment of VAE, as well as good communication between the surgeon and anesthesiologist.

Treatment

Notifying the surgeon to prevent further air entrainment is the first step in treatment (Box 17.6). The jugular vein can be compressed temporarily to increase venous pressure and may facilitate localization of site of air entrainment. Flooding the surgical area with saline may help reduce further air entrainment. The addition of positive end-expiratory pressure to the ventilator settings should be avoided because it can increase right atrial pressure and potentiate the risk for paradoxical embolism by reversing the gradient between the atria.

Conclusion

Anesthesia for posterior fossa surgery requires an understanding of the anatomy and pathophysiology involved. Perioperative management includes preoperative evaluation, especially for brainstem and cranial nerve dysfunction, meticulous attention to positioning, and adequate monitoring for the prevention of VAE. Careful assessment of the patient before extubation and good control of blood pressure are of paramount importance.

Further Reading

Cata, J.P., Saager, L., Kurz A., Avitsian, R.: Successful extubation in the operating room after infratentorial craniotomy: The Cleveland clinic experience. *J Neurosurg Anesthesiol* 2011; **23**:25–29, https://doi.org/10.1097/ANA.0b013e3181eee548.

Cavallone, L.F., Vannucci, A.: Extubation of the difficult airway and extubation failure. *Anesth Analg* 2013; **116**:368–383, https://doi.org/10.1213/ANE.0b013e31827ab572.

Chowdhury, T., Mendelowith, D., Golanov, E., et al: Trigeminocardiac reflex: The current clinical and physiological knowledge.

J Neurosurg Anesthesiol 2015; **27**:136–147, https://doi.org/10.1097/ANA.0000000000000065.

Engelhardt, M., Folkers, W., Brenke, C., et al: Neurosurgical operations with the patient in sitting position: Analysis of risk factors using transcranial Doppler sonography. *Br J Anaesth* 2006; **96**:467–472, https://doi.org/10.1093/bja/ael015.

Gracia, I., Fabregas, N.: Craniotomy in sitting position: Anesthesiology management. *Curr Opin Anesthesiol* 2014; **27**:474–483, https://doi.org/10.1097/ACO.0000000000000104.

Hindman, B.J., Palecek, J.P., Posner, K.L., et al: Cervical spinal cord, root, and bony spine injuries: A closed claims analysis. *Anesthesiology* 2011; **114**:782–795, https://doi.org/10.1097/ALN.0b013e3182104859.

Jian, M., Li, X., Wang, A., et al: Flurbiprofen and hypertension but not hydroxyethyl starch are associated with post-craniotomy intracranial haematoma requiring surgery. *Br J Anaesth* 2014; **113**:832–839, https://doi.org/10.1093/bja/aeu185.

Manninen, P.H., Cuillerier, D.J., Nantau, W.E, Gelb, A.W.: Monitoring of brainstem function during vertebral basilar aneurysm surgery. The use of spontaneous ventilation. *Anesthesiology* 1992; 77:681–685.

Chapter 18

Anesthesia for Cerebrospinal Fluid Diversion and Endoscopic Neurosurgical Procedures

Dean Frear

Key Points

- CSF diversion procedures are performed in a wide variety of patients often with complex co-morbidities.
- Most procedures redirect the CSF for absorption in alternate body cavities.
- Endoscopic techniques are increasingly used in the management of ventricular and periventricular pathology.

Abbreviations

CSF	Cerebrospinal fluid
ETV	Endoscopic third ventriculostomy
ICP	Intracranial pressure
IIH	Idiopathic intracranial hypertension
NICU	Neonatal intensive care unit
NPH	Normal pressure hydrocephalus
NSAIDS	Non-steroidal anti-inflammatory drugs
PEEP	Positive end expiratory pressure
TIVA	Total intravenous anesthesia
VP	Ventriculo-peritoneal

Contents

- Introduction
- Cerebrospinal Fluid Dynamics
    - Congenital
    - Acquired
    - Other
- Surgical Procedures
    - Cerebrospinal Fluid Diversion
    - Shunt Assessment
    - Endoscopy

- Anesthetic Considerations
  - Preoperative Evaluation
  - Intraoperative Management
  - Positioning
  - Maintenance
  - Postoperative Analgesia
- Further Reading

Introduction

Procedures to divert CSF are frequently used for the treatment of hydrocephalus and IIH. A diverse range of patients are treated by such procedures, from neonates to the elderly, either with or without multiple co-morbidities. Symptoms of raised ICP such as headache, visual disturbance, and drowsiness are usual for those patients presenting with an obstructed ventricular system. However, some patients can have an insidious onset of gait disturbance, mental decline, and urinary incontinence which are features of NPH. In this syndrome, the ventricles are dilated (ventriculomegaly) but CSF pressure is normal.

While an open diversion procedure is mostly used for the management of pathology resulting in CSF obstruction, more recently, ventricular endoscopic techniques, have seen their scope extended to manage many other conditions. The perceived advantages include reduced tissue trauma from dissection and retraction while improved access to specific areas of the brain can lead to shorter procedures and reduced length of hospital stay.

Cerebrospinal Fluid Dynamics

CSF is continually produced by the choroid plexus (60%–70% of volume) as well as being exuded from vessels within the pia mater. It then circulates within the ventricles and subarachnoid space and is primarily reabsorbed from arachnoid villi which protrude into the cranial venous sinuses (Figure 18.1). In adults, the volume of the ventricular system is 100–150 ml and about 500 ml of CSF is produced per day. Interference with the free flow of CSF or its reabsorption results in hydrocephalus and the development of raised ICP.

Hydrocephalus is commonly classified into communicating and non-communicating types. Non-communicating hydrocephalus can be considered "obstructive" when an internal (e.g., congenital malformation) or external (e.g., tumor) mechanism obstructs the ventricular system preventing the flow of CSF (Box 18.1). Since production continues unabated, CSF accumulates producing a dilated ventricular system. In communicating hydrocephalus, no fixed obstruction exists, but rather flow dynamics and reabsorption are disrupted for a variety of reasons. The two theories relating to the development of hydrocephalus include (1) the CSF bulk flow theory which suggests there is an imbalance between CSF formation and absorption and (2) the hydrodynamic theory where reduced cerebral compliance is implicated. Newer theories, however, have been proposed in which minor CSF pathways may play a significant role in the development of congenital hydrocephalus.

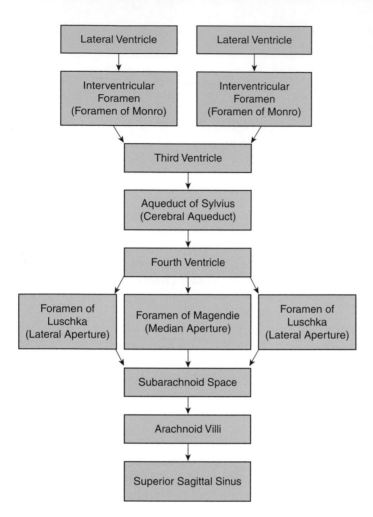

Figure 18.1 Circulation of cerebrospinal fluid.

Surgical Procedures

Cerebrospinal Fluid Diversion

CSF diversion by shunting is the main surgical technique for the management of hydro-cephalus. The aim is to divert the CSF into a high-capacity body cavity from which it can be reabsorbed. In general, the proximal end of a catheter is introduced into the ventricular system via a burr hole and connected to a valve placed beneath the galea. Access to the peritoneal cavity, the pleural space or the right atrium (via the external jugular vein in the neck) is then achieved and the distal end of the catheter is tunneled to this point. Although contraindicated in cases of obstructive hydrocephalus, an alternative is a lumbar-peritoneal shunt, where access to the subarachnoid space is achieved in the lumbar region and a catheter tunneled around to the abdominal incision where it is placed in the peritoneal cavity.

BOX 18.1 Causes of Hydrocephalus

Congenital

Chiari malformations
Aqueductal stenosis
Neural tube defect
Arachnoid cysts
Dandy-Walker syndrome

Acquired

Infections (causes communicating hydrocephalus)
Meningitis
Cysticercosis

Post-hemorrhagic (causes communicating hydrocephalus)
Subarachnoid hemorrhage
Intraventricular hemorrhage
Traumatic brain injury

Secondary to space-occupying lesions (causes obstructive hydrocephalus)
Vascular malformations
Tumors and cysts

Other

NPH
Hydrocephalus ex vacuo (due to brain atrophy)

Shunt Assessment

Whilst shunt procedures are successful in many cases, there remains a high complication rate. The need for a shunt revision varies but can be as high as half of all shunts by two years. Identification of a malfunctioning shunt is not always easy. Intermittent malfunction, over-drainage, or under-drainage may give vague clinical signs and symptoms. Diagnosis can be improved using CSF infusion studies which measure pressures and system compliance to assess shunt and valve performance. Cannulation of either the ventricular system or the shunt via its integral reservoir enables in vivo pressure measurements to be taken. In adults, this may be possible under local anesthesia but for pediatric patients a general anesthetic is often required.

Endoscopy

Preformed spaces such as the ventricular system, the subarachnoid space, or cystic lesions provide ideal conditions for the use of endoscopes. ETV was used initially in cases of obstructive hydrocephalus to avoid some of the complications of long term shunt insertion. The procedure involves creating a hole in the floor of the third ventricle using an endoscope inserted into the ventricular system via a burr hole. By creating a communication between the ventricular system and the subarachnoid cisterns, CSF can bypass the Aqueduct of Sylvius and the IVth ventricle. ETV has also been used with varying success in the treatment of NPH and communicating hydrocephalus.

An endoscopic approach may also be used to fenestrate intraventricular septations in cases of loculated hydrocephalus, guide shunt revision by allowing release of adhesions around the choroid plexus or obstructed catheters, and aid the optimal placement of a ventricular catheter.

Intraventricular tumors may be accurately and safely biopsied using endoscopy, and where they are causing obstruction, an ETV can be performed at the same time. Complete endoscopic resection of such tumors is possible but dependent on their size relative to that of the endoscope. Endoscopic resection of colloid cysts is also possible along with the management of arachnoid cysts by fenestration of the cyst wall into the ventricular system or subarachnoid cisterns.

Anesthetic Considerations

Preoperative Evaluation

Neonatal patients often have multiple co-morbidities including poor lung compliance, immature hepatic and renal function, and the risk of postoperative apnea. Issues associated with the transfer of these patients between theatre and the NICU need to be considered along with the requirement for post-operative ventilation in pre-term infants and those with significant lung pathology.

Older children who often have had multiple shunt revisions, need to be assessed for co-existing chronic childhood diseases such as epilepsy, recurrent chest infections related to cerebral palsy, and gastric reflux. Hydrocephalus may be a feature of specific pediatric syndromes and their associated organ anomalies.

A preoperative assessment in older patients should focus on their underlying disease and co-morbidities. Specific neurosurgical issues to consider would include the presence of raised ICP, altered level of consciousness, and the risk of aspiration. Sedative pre-medication is generally best avoided.

Intraoperative Management

General anesthesia is used for CSF diversion procedures and induction may be undertaken using either intravenous or inhalational agents. For patients with impaired consciousness or at risk of aspiration, rapid sequence induction should be considered. Intubation with reinforced endotracheal tubes is one safe technique for these cases. Neck extension and rotation to facilitate tunneling during shunt insertion can dislodge supra-glottic airways and may cause standard endotracheal tubes to kink. Supra-glottic airways may be used when shunt infusion studies are performed as a stand-alone procedure.

Routine monitoring with electrocardiography, pulse oximetry, capnography, and non-invasive blood pressure measurement is required. Invasive arterial pressure monitoring is not routinely used unless indicated by associated co-morbidities. Temperature control can be particularly challenging in children with the greatest heat loss occurring during positioning and preparation as a significant surface area is exposed and cleaned with cold surgical antiseptic solution. Use of a forced air warmer and temperature monitoring is therefore essential.

Positioning

Ventriculo-peritoneal, ventriculo-pleural, and ventriculo-atrial shunts require supine positioning, with some degree of neck extension and rotation (greatest for VP shunts) to facilitate insertion of the tunneling device. Lumbar-pleural shunts are performed in a lateral position and a wide area of the back and abdomen is surgically prepared and draped. Endoscopic procedures are typically performed supine, slightly head-up with the neck flexed.

Maintenance

TIVA or an inhalational agent can be used for maintenance in the normal manner. Ventilation to normocarbia is especially relevant for shunt infusion studies where a stable end-tidal carbon dioxide level is required for interpretation of the results. Systemic antibiotics as per local guidelines should be administered at induction to reduce the risks of shunt infection.

The most stimulating event during a shunt insertion procedure is typically advancement of the tunneling device and attention should be paid to analgesia and depth of anesthesia during this period. Trauma to surrounding structures is uncommon but remains a potential risk. During ventriculo-pleural shunts ventilation may be halted for a short period to facilitate the distal catheter insertion. Ventilatory recruitment maneuvers and PEEP may assist in minimizing the resulting pneumothorax.

During endoscopic procedures, a continuous flow of irrigation fluid is used to optimize the field of view but this may introduce complications including acute increases in ICP and dysrhythmias including bradycardia and even cardiac arrest. These normally respond to repositioning or removal of the endoscope, but may require pharmacological therapy. Intra-arterial blood pressure monitoring is essential during these cases. Hypothermia has also been reported in small children which is often related to the large volumes of cold irrigation fluid.

Postoperative Analgesia

Intraoperative analgesia with paracetamol and NSAIDS supplemented with a short acting opiate such as fentanyl is typically sufficient. Patients quickly return to eating and drinking enabling oral analgesia to be used in the postoperative period. Chest pain following a pleural shunt may be more significant and require management with moderate to strong opiates.

Further Reading

Garton, H.: Cerebrospinal fluid diversion procedures. *J Neuroophthalmol* 2004; 24(2):146–155.

Kestle, J.R.W., Drake, J.M., Cochrane, D.D., et al: Lack of Benefit of endoscopic ventriculoperitoneal shunt insertion: A multicenter randomized trial. *J Neurosurg* 2003; 98:284–290, https://doi.org/10.3171/jns.2003.98.2.0284

Rigamonti, D. (Ed.) 2014. *Adult Hydrocephalus.* Cambridge: Cambridge University Press, ISBN 978-1-107-03177-7.

Schroeder, H., Gabb, M.: Intracranial endoscopy. *Neurosurg Focus* 1999; 6(4):Article 1.

Symss, N.P., Oi, S.: Theories of cerebrospinal fluid dynamics and hydrocephalus: Historical trend. *J Neurosurg Pediatr* 2013; 11(2):170–177, https://doi.org/10.3171/2012.3.PEDS0934.

Chapter 19

Anesthesia for Epilepsy Surgery

Claas Siegmueller

Key Points

- The mainstay of epilepsy treatment involves AED therapy with the goal of controlling seizures without affecting normal brain activity while minimizing side effects.
- Approximately 70% of epilepsy patients achieve remission with AEDs and many do so with single-agent therapy.
- The side effects and interactions of anti-epileptic medications must be taken into account in the perioperative period.
- The general principles of epilepsy surgery are either resection of the epileptogenic focus or interruption of pathways along which seizure propagation occurs.
- Different anesthetic techniques are used depending on whether the patient requires electrocorticography and/or functional mapping during surgery.
- Anesthetic agents should be chosen carefully to allow intraoperative recording of epileptiform activity.
- Surgical treatment is associated with a risk for intraoperative and postoperative seizures.

Abbreviations

AED	Anti-epileptic drug
CT	Computed tomography
DCS	Direct cortical stimulation
DRE	Drug-resistant epilepsy
ECoG	Electrocorticography
EEG	Electroencephalography
fMRI	Functional magnetic resonance imaging
GABA	Gamma-aminobutyric acid
MAC	Minimal alveolar concentration
MEP	Motor-evoked potentials
MRI	Magnetic resonance imaging
MRS	Magnetic resonance spectroscopy
PET	Positron emission tomography
SPECT	Single-photon emission computed tomography

Contents

Epidemiology, Classification, and Etiology of Epilepsy

Epilepsy is one of the most common neurological diseases, second only to stroke, and affects about 1% of the world's population. Around 1 in 25 people will develop epilepsy with a higher incidence in young children and older adults. Epilepsy is a group of related disorders characterized by a transient occurrence of the signs and symptoms of seizures which are due to abnormal, excessive, or synchronous neuronal activity in the brain.

The latest classification distinguishes between "generalized" and "focal" (formerly called "partial") seizures and a third "unknown" category (Box 19.1). Other previously used terms such as "simple partial", "complex partial", or "secondarily generalized" have been abandoned for lack of precision.

Generalized seizures originate within bilaterally distributed cortical and subcortical networks across which they rapidly spread. Focal seizures start in networks limited to one hemisphere, but can spread contra-laterally.

In over 60% no underlying cause can be identified. The remainder are due to hypoxic or traumatic brain injury, stroke, tumor, inflammation (meningitis, encephalitis) as well as

BOX 19.1 Epilepsy Classification (from ILAE Commission on Classification and Terminology, 2011–2013)	
Generalized seizures	Tonic-clonic (in any combination)
	Typical, atypical
	Absence, absence with special features
	Myoclonic absence
	Eyelid myoclonia
	Myoclonic, myoclonic atonic, myoclonic tonic
	Clonic, atonic, tonic
Focal seizures	
Unknown	Epileptic spasms

certain genetic diseases and metabolic derangements. While epilepsy during childhood and adolescence is predominantly associated with genetic and congenital abnormalities, tumors are a common cause in older adults, and cerebrovascular disease is the predominant trigger for epilepsy developing in the elderly. Trauma and infection as causes occur in any age group.

Treatment of Epilepsy

Medical Treatment

The mainstay of epilepsy treatment continues to be AED therapy with the goal of controlling seizures without affecting normal brain activity while minimizing side effects. Traditional AEDs generally work via the following three mechanisms:

- Increase of (inhibitory) GABA neurotransmitter activity
- Reduction of cation flux (Na^+, Ca_2^+) through voltage-gated channels
- Decrease of excitatory neurotransmitters (glutamate, aspartate)

Potentially serious side effects and interactions are characteristic for AEDs as a drug class, especially older drugs, commonly requiring close patient monitoring and dose adjustments. A number of second-generation AEDs such as vigabatrin, gabapentin, lamotrigine, topiramate, or levetiracetam have been introduced, targeting novel drug action sites like synaptic vesicle proteins or voltage-gated potassium channels. While generally superior to older AEDs with regard to pharmacokinetics, side effect profiles and drug interactions, they do not offer great advantages regarding effectiveness. Approximately 70% of epilepsy patients achieve remission with AEDs, meaning freedom from seizures for ≥5 years, and 40% do so with single-agent therapy.

Approximately 30% of patients who do not achieve remission despite optimal medical therapy have DRE, also called refractory or intractable epilepsy. Drug resistance may develop years after the onset of epilepsy and can have a marked psychological and social impact. In addition, the mortality rate of patients with DRE is around five times that of the general population.

Surgical Treatment

About half the patients with DRE are suitable for surgery. Surgery is also appropriate for a smaller group in which epilepsy may be relatively well controlled, but where features suggest it might be curative. Although the spectrum of patients being considered for surgery has expanded the surgical option is still under-utilized for treating epilepsy.

The general principles of epilepsy surgery are either resection of the epileptogenic focus or interruption of pathways along which seizure propagation occurs. A third group of interventions comprises neurostimulation techniques such as vagus nerve and deep brain stimulation (Box 19.2).

Over 40% of patients achieve complete long-term seizure freedom with surgery. Temporal lobectomy for an epileptic focus with an anatomical correlate such as mesial temporal sclerosis has the highest success rate and is the most common operation. Successful surgery is also likely to improve psychosocial function and halt the cognitive decline associated with long-term DRE.

BOX 19.2	Types of Epilepsy Surgery	
Resective surgery	Anterior temporal lobectomy Extratemporal (parietal, occipital, frontal) cortical excision Selective laser amygdalohippocampectomy	(Potentially) curative
Interruptive surgery	Corpus callosotomy Multiple subpial resections Hemispherectomy	Palliative
Neurostimulation techniques	Vagus nerve stimulation Deep brain stimulation (centromedian thalamic nucleus, cerebellar)	

Diagnostic Workup for Seizure Surgery

The presurgical assessment aims to answer whether the patient suffers from generalized or focal seizures, whether these originate in the temporal lobe or are extratemporal, and whether a structural lesion can be imaged. In addition, it is important to determine the "eloquence" of cortical areas considered for resection, i.e., to establish to what degree they contribute to language, motor, or sensory function (functional mapping).

Electroencephalography

EEG, in combination with video-recording, is still the most important diagnostic tool for patient evaluation before surgery. Continuous video-EEG monitoring, often over several days, allows EEG interpretation focused on seizure events. EEG recordings particularly at the beginning of a seizure yield the most valuable data with regard to localizing an epileptic focus.

Neuroimaging

MRI, due to its superior spatial resolution, is the most accurate anatomical imaging tool for the presurgical evaluation. PET and SPECT allow functional imaging revealing epilepsy foci as hypermetabolic during and hypometabolic in between seizures. MRS can visualize altered concentrations of specific metabolites such as excitatory neurotransmitters in an epileptogenic brain area. Functional MRI is used to for mapping "eloquent" cortex. The patient performs specific tasks during the scan and the fMRI shows changes in regional blood flow and oxygenation.

Neuropsychological Assessment

Neuropsychological testing aims to detect cognitive deficits related to the planned epileptic focus resection area. The goal is to predict possible deficits after surgery and establish a baseline for comparison. To test whether the hemisphere contralateral to the lesion can support language and memory function after resection, a Wada test is performed. This involves injection of amylobarbitone (or propofol) into the internal carotid artery on the side of the lesion, usually via femoral catheterization. During isolated hemispherical anesthesia a number of speech and memory tests are then performed.

BOX 19.3 Types of Electrodes Used for Electrocorticography

Epidural electrodes		Rarely used
		Less precise than subdural electrodes
		Placement through burr holes
		Lower infection risk
Subdural electrodes	Strip electrodes (placed through burr holes)	Covers relatively wide surface area
	Rectangular grid electrodes (requiring craniotomy; unilateral placement only)	Higher infection and hemorrhage risk
		Also used for extraoperative functional cortical mapping if awake surgery not tolerated
Intracerebral depth electrodes		Stereotactic placement with CT, MRI, and angiography guidance
		Targets seizure foci in hippocampus, amygdala, cingulate gyrus, frontal-temporal regions

Extraoperative Electrocorticography

Several types of intracranial electrodes can be placed as part of the surgical workup before resection (Box 19.3). These devices can monitor areas of the brain that are not easy to assess with the standard surface EEG and do so with a higher spatial resolution and lower signal-to-noise ratio. After electrode implantation, ECoG data is analyzed postoperatively (extraoperative ECoG) for several days for spike activity during seizures and interictal epileptiform activity in between, precisely locating the epileptic focus and surrounding irritative area. The patient then returns to the operating room for electrode removal and definitive resection of the epileptogenic tissue. This approach is indicated in about 20% of patients where other investigations have failed to precisely locate the epileptic focus or have yielded conflicting data.

Subdural grid electrodes (Figure 19.1) can be used extraoperatively not just for seizure focus localization but also functional mapping by applying currents between the implanted electrodes. This is valuable in patients who are unable to tolerate an awake craniotomy for functional mapping, for example, children.

Anesthesia Techniques for Epilepsy Surgery

Without Electrophysiological Monitoring

Different anesthetic techniques are used depending on whether the patient requires ECoG and/or functional mapping during surgery. When these techniques are not required, patients will have had the epileptic focus clearly localized and exclusion of involvement of eloquent areas during the presurgical assessment. Under these circumstances, a general anesthetic applying basic neuroanesthesia principles is suitable. General anesthesia is also appropriate for diagnostic surgery, i.e., electrode implantation for extraoperative ECoG.

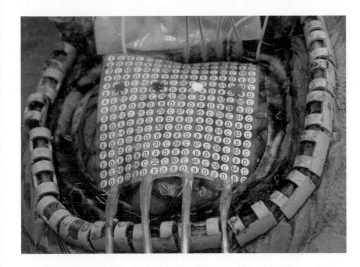

Figure 19.1 Subdural grid electrodes in-situ

It is important to avoid seizures around the time of surgery. Factors to consider include: the need to withhold AEDs during preoperative starvation, sleep deprivation, pro-convulsant anesthesia-related medications, and the pharmacokinetic and pharmacody-namic interactions between AEDs and anesthetic drugs. Volatile anesthetics have the potential to induce epileptiform activity during fluctuating concentrations which is why the risk for inducing seizures is highest during induction or emergence. This is particularly true for enflurane and sevoflurane which should therefore be avoided. Etomidate also causes epileptic EEG patterns and is equally unsuitable. To reduce the perioperative seizure risk, prophylactic administration of a benzodiazepine is advisable.

Intraoperative Electrocorticography

Intraoperative ECoG is used to identify the epileptic focus during surgery and delineate resection margins. A focus in close proximity to eloquent cortical regions such as the bilateral temporal motor and parietal sensory cortices, bilateral occipital visual areas, mesial-temporal areas for memory, or the left frontal-temporal lobes for speech and language capacity will require functional mapping.

To localize an epileptogenic focus demands that drugs influencing EEG activity are avoided when possible. Therefore, perioperative AEDs and benzodiazepine premedication are commonly omitted, even if, this increases the risk of perioperative seizures. These patients can either undergo awake surgery or have a general anesthetic which minimizes adverse effects on ECoG. Most anesthetic drugs have been shown to have pro- as well as anti-convulsant effects at different doses ranges although no clear dose-response relation-ship exists. Low concentrations of enflurane and sevoflurane have been used to facilitate cortical EEG recording as have intraoperative boluses of etomidate and methohexital. Volatile agents, in a concentration normally used to provide general anesthesia, suppress EEG activity significantly. Dexmedetomidine, which does not alter spike rate in most patients, can be used as part of a balanced anesthetic in combination with nitrous oxide and a potent opioid such as alfentanil or remifentanil. The latter do not affect ECoG adversely and indeed can induce epileptiform activity through an unclear mechanism.

Lower doses of propofol also have no significant suppressive effect on focus activity but increase background EEG activity.

Intraoperative Functional Mapping

This is usually carried out by DCS with a hand-held stimulator delivering a current to a small area of the brain surface. The anesthesia technique required depends on which cortical function is being assessed. Mapping of speech and language clearly requires an awake craniotomy with local anesthesia. These cortical areas are identified if DCS causes, for example, dysarthria or expressive aphasia. Localizing eloquent areas for motor function can be done either awake or under general anesthesia. With a general anesthetic DCS is used to trigger MEPs. Since MEPs are easily suppressed by volatile anesthetics, their administration needs to be limited, usually to ≤0.3 MAC. Muscle relaxants obviously have to be avoided.

Because there is a lack of published evidence as to which method of general anesthesia is superior with regard to facilitating ECoG and functional mapping while ensuring patient comfort, techniques are often empiric and institution-specific. Our hospital uses a nitrous oxide/low-dose vapor inhalational anesthesia with a remifentanil infusion for motor mapping under general anesthesia and substitutes the vapor with a dexmedetomidine infusion if ECoG is required.

Further Reading

Berg, A.T., Berkovic, S.F., Brodie, M.J., et al: Revised terminology and concepts for organization of seizures and epilepsies: Report of the ILAE Commission on classification and terminology, 2005–2009. *Epilepsia* 2010; **51** (4):676–685, https://doi.org/10.1111/j.1528-1167.2010.02522.x.

Perks, A., Cheema, S., Mohanraj, R.: Anaesthesia and epilepsy. *Br J Anaesth* 2012; **108**(4):562–571, https://doi.org/10.1093/bja/aes027.

Téllez-Zenteno, J.F., Dhar, R., Wiebe, S.: Long-term seizure outcomes following epilepsy surgery: A systematic review and meta-analysis.

Brain 2005; **128**(Pt 5):1188–1198, https://doi.org/10.1093/brain/awh449.

Tisi, J.de, Bell, G.S., Peacock, J.L., et al: The long-term outcome of adult epilepsy surgery, patterns of seizure remission, and relapse: A cohort study. *The Lancet* 2011; **378**(9800):1388–1395, https://doi.org/10.1016/S0140-6736(11)60890-8.

Voss, L.J., Sleigh, J.W., Barnard, J.P.M., Kirsch, H.E. The howling cortex: Seizures and general anesthetic drugs. *Anesth Analg* 2008; **107** (5):1689–1703, https://doi.org/10.1213/ane.0b013e3181852595.

Wiebe, S., Jetté, N. Epilepsy surgery utilization: Who, when, where, and why? *Curr Opin Neurol* 2012; **25**(2):187–193, https://doi.org/10.1097/WCO.0b013e328350baa6.

Chapter 20

Perioperative Management of Awake Craniotomy

Lingzhong Meng

Key Points

- Awake cranial surgery is associated with beneficial outcomes.
- The goal of anesthetic care is patient safety and comfort, facilitation of surgery, and awake testing.
- Monitored anesthesia care without airway instrumentation and general anesthesia with a laryngeal mask airway are two popular anesthetic techniques used during the pre-awake phase.
- Anesthetic agents with a rapid onset/offset and minimal neuropsychological effects are typically used to facilitate the transition from pre-awake to awake phase.

Abbreviations

ECoG	Electrocorticography
EtCO$_2$	End-tidal carbon dioxide
GA	General anesthesia
LMA	Laryngeal mask airway
MAC	Monitored anesthesia care
TCI	Target controlled infusion

Contents

- – Airway Management
- – Pre-awake Phase
- – Analgesia
- – Intravenous Anesthetic Agents
- – Awake Phase
- – Managing Intraoperative Complications
- – Post-awake Phase
- • Postoperative Care
- • Further Reading

Introduction

Awake craniotomy is the conduct of at least part of an open intracranial procedure in a patient who is awake. The intraoperative care can be divided into three sequential phases based on how the anesthetic is managed, i.e., (1) the pre-awake phase, (2) the awake phase, and (3) the post-awake phase. Awake craniotomy is primarily used to resect brain tumors or epileptic foci that are in close proximity to or reside within the eloquent brain (i.e., language or motor areas) for the purpose of achieving a greater resection while avoiding functional impairment. Accumulating evidence shows some beneficial effects associated with awake brain tumor resection, such as greater extent of resection, fewer late neurological deficits, shorter hospital stay, and longer survival. The goal of anesthetic care is to ensure patient safety and comfort, facilitate awake testing, maintain appropriate brain operating conditions, and improve the outcomes that matter to patients.

Preoperative Care

Patient Selection

At present, there is no consensus on medical conditions that would contraindicate an awake procedure. There are reports of awake craniotomy procedures in patients who have had chronic heart failure with a poor ejection fraction and those in the latter stages of twin pregnancy. The age of patients who have had an awake craniotomy also varies widely from teenagers to octogenarians. Overall, a patient's refusal is arguably the only non-surgical contraindication to an awake craniotomy. However, relative contraindications include conditions that could lead to excessive intraoperative coughing, inability to remain still, obesity, and mood instability.

Establishing Patient Rapport

Compared to surgery under GA, the preoperative interview is an even more important step because of the constant face-to-face interactions between the patient and anesthetist during the awake phase. Gaining the patient's trust is a key requirement for the success of the procedure. Visiting the patient prior to surgery is mandatory. Details including positioning, urinary catheter placement, noise related to craniectomy, and various mapping-related tasks should be carefully explained. Reassurance and empathy are anxiolytic and should not be ignored.

Pre-medication

The only pre-medications that are routinely given are anticonvulsants and corticosteroids. The medications that have the potential to impair neurocognitive function or contribute to emergence delirium during the intraoperative wake up phase are normally avoided.

Intraoperative Care

Monitoring

Routine monitoring should be applied and an intra-arterial catheter and pulse oximetry are preferably placed on the arm that will not be used for motor mapping, i.e., ipsilateral. Respiratory rate and $EtCO_2$ can be monitored via a sampling line integrated into the nasal cannula or connected to the breathing circuit depending on the method of airway management. A urinary catheter is normally placed following intravenous sedation and sterile intra-urethral viscous lidocaine gel application.

An experienced neurophysiologist is normally present for the intraoperative stimulation mapping of language and/or sensorimotor localization. Electrical stimulation of the cortex allows recognition of motor, sensory, and speech areas and when combined with neuropsychological assessment, determination of language areas. Cortical mapping assists the neurosurgeon in determining resection margins and is particularly important for dominant-hemisphere mass lesions where optimal tumor resection can be performed with minimal risk of postoperative neurological deficits. Despite the use of cortical mapping, the majority of neurosurgeons prefer to complete the entire resection with the patient awake so that any infringement on eloquent areas can be recognized immediately. During epilepsy surgery, intraoperative ECoG may be used to identify the extent of the epileptogenic focus and when used in combination with sensorimotor mapping, allows safe resection of epileptic foci whose margins impinge on eloquent areas. Although awake techniques minimize the effects of anesthetic agents on ECoG, specific general anesthetic techniques can also permit minimal interference with this monitoring modality.

Positioning

The operating table is typically turned so that the patient faces the anesthesia workstation allowing ease of airway management if needed and face-to-face interaction during the awake phase. The patient can be positioned supine, laterally on an axillary roll, or semi-laterally with the back of the patient resting on a round longitudinal pillow. The semilateral position is normally preferred because it enhances the patient's positional endurance while facilitating the surgeon's access to the side of the brain and makes direct face-to-face interaction possible (Figure 20.1). It also facilitates ventilation by improving respiratory effort compared to the supine position. The patient's head is secured in a Mayfield frame with the three pin sites infiltrated with local anesthetic.

Semilateral A

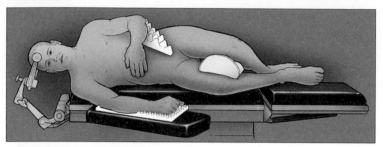

Semilateral B

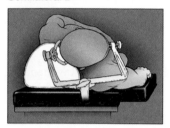

Semilateral C

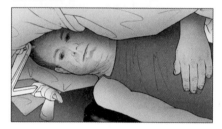

Figure 20.1 (a) Semilateral position for awake craniotomy; (**b**) the surgeon's view; and (**c**) the Anesthesiologist's view.

Airway Management

Under MAC, oxygen administration via nasal cannulae (2–4 L/min) is used along with EtCO$_2$ sampling. A nasopharyngeal airway is normally not needed but can be placed when necessary under propofol sedation. Using MAC, the patient breathes throughout the procedure but there is the risk of hypercapnia due to hypoventilation especially when propofol and remifentanil are used.

Another technique (asleep-awake) is to use an LMA placed during the pre-awake mapping phase then removed during the awake phase and normally not reinserted for the post-awake phase. Even though an LMA offers better airway control, it does not always guarantee satisfactory mechanical ventilation.

Pre-awake Phase

The anesthetic procedure during the pre-awake phase can be either a GA or MAC. The transition from asleep to awake can be lengthy and unpredictable if choosing GA. Patients may wake up drowsy or confused with the potential for causing self-injury or jeopardizing meaningful awake testing. On the contrary, the patient under light sedation may move, talk, and distract the surgeon thus making the procedure more difficult. At present, there is no consensus on the superiority between these two techniques due to the lack of comparative studies.

Analgesia

The provision of adequate local anesthesia using regional, field, and dural blocks is essential. Because the skin, scalp, pericranium, and periosteum of the outer table of the skull all have extensive sensory innervation, subcutaneous infiltration with local anesthetic in the manner of a field block or over specific sensory nerve branches effectively blocks afferent input from all layers of the scalp. The skull can be drilled and opened without discomfort to the patient because it has no sensation itself. However, the dura has extensive innervation and must be anesthetized by a local anesthetic nerve block around the nerve trunk running with the middle meningeal artery, as well as by a field block around the edges of the craniotomy. Relatively large doses of local anesthetic may be required, and therefore caution must be exercised to avoid toxicity. Intravenous opioid boluses are rarely required but a low rate remifentanil infusion (0.05 mcg/kg/min) can be used for its rapidly titratable analgesic and sedative effects.

Intravenous Anesthetic Agents

The ideal drug for an awake craniotomy should have a fast onset/offset of action, no neurological effect after termination and minimal cardiovascular or respiratory depressant effects. Unfortunately, there is currently no such agent and every anesthetic drug used for an awake craniotomy has its own drawbacks. As different patients have different sensitivities to the same drug, invariable sedation protocols have limited use, and a flexible approach based on the response of each individual patient is advocated.

A frequently used sedative regimen is low dose propofol (20–50 mcg/kg/min – or an equivalent TCI) and remifentanil (0.02–0.06 mcg/kg/min) infusions titrated to make the patient drowsy yet arousable without causing airway obstruction. Dexmedetomidine (0.2–0.5 mcg/kg/h) can be added to augment sedation or used as a sole agent to limit the risk of airway obstruction and hypoventilation-related hypercapnia. If an LMA is used, either intravenous (propofol 50–80 mcg/kg/min and remifentanil 0.1–0.2 mcg/kg/min) or inhalational (sevoflurane or desflurane < 0.5 minimum alveolar concentration) agents can be used to affect a rapid transition from asleep to awake states.

Awake Phase

The surgeon normally gives a time estimate to wake up the patient. All sedative or hypnotic agents are typically discontinued at the moment when the bone flap is removed. The goal is to wake up the patient smoothly and rapidly without agitation and confusion. An alternative approach, is to continue with a very low-dose remifentanil infusion to facilitate a smooth transition. The goal is to have the patient engaged, cooperative, pain-free, and comfortable. A swab soaked with ice-cold water can be used to wet the patient's lips and mouth for comfort. Patients frequently need help with opioid-related itching of the nostrils. Most patients will need to move their hips/legs/arms due to positional discomfort. It is important to instruct the patient not to move the head and shoulders when making positional adjustments. The room temperature should be adjusted for patient's comfort and an air blanket can be used as needed to provide either warm or cool air. Empathy, handholding, and reassurance offer great support to patients and should always be used during the awake phase. Ongoing encouragement, coaching, and conversation are very useful.

Managing Intraoperative Complications

Awake procedures have very low complication rates (Box 20.1) and are generally well tolerated by patients. However, the depth of sedation required can be associated with respiratory depression, airway obstruction, apnea, and brain swelling. Facilities for emergency airway control should always be available. To manage an airway problem, one should alert the surgeon, call for help, stop all infusions, mask ventilate the patient with 100% oxygen using a jaw thrust supplemented if necessary by an oral or nasal airway. In anticipation of such a life-threatening event, there should always be an LMA to hand while some anesthesiologists also like to have an endotracheal tube and video laryngoscope ready. Placement of an LMA should be attempted if mask ventilation fails. These can be difficult to position in a patient who is semilateral with their head slightly turned and secured in a Mayfield frame. The maneuver of pulling the tongue out using a gauze swab or Magill forceps may facilitate the LMA placement. If insertion fails, intubation using a flexible fiberoptic instrument or a video laryngoscope can be attempted.

The reported incidence of intraoperative seizures ranges from 3% to 16%. It frequently occurs during mapping-related stimulation. The first line treatment is ice-cold crystalloid irrigation onto the cortex by the neurosurgeon (repeated if necessary). Most seizures can be stopped by iced cortical spray. However, if ineffective, intravenous propofol (30–50 mg) should be administered and repeated as necessary. The patient needs to be closely observed for seizure recurrence or airway compromise. Most intraoperative seizures are resolved without adverse consequences although apnea and cardiac arrest can occur. Airway instrumentation is normally not needed, unless excessive amounts of propofol are administered.

Hypertension, hypotension, and tachycardia are more common during awake techniques than during general anesthesia. These hemodynamic changes can be appropriately treated when recognized early and rarely result in adverse outcomes.

BOX 20.1 Complications of Awake Craniotomy

Uncooperative patient
Cardiovascular (hypertension, hypotension, tachycardia)
Excessive sedation
Respiratory depression
Loss of control of the airway
Brain swelling
Seizures
Pain
Local anesthetic toxicity

Post-awake Phase

Once the awake stimulation mapping and surgical resection is complete, sedation can be restarted and the case can usually be finished without an LMA even if it was used during the pre-awake phase. Patients frequently require lower infusion rates of sedatives in this phase than the pre-awake phase for comparable levels of sedation. This may be due to the fatigue from the awake phase or the lower level of painful stimuli during skull closure compared to opening. The goal of sedation is to keep the patient drowsy without causing airway obstruction.

Postoperative Care

Some institutions admit the patient to a neurointensive care area for overnight monitoring after an awake craniotomy. On average, patients are discharged home within 1 to 5 days after awake brain tumor resection while some discharge patients home on the same day of surgery.

Further Reading

Hervey-Jumper, S.L., Li, J., Lau, D., et al: Awake craniotomy to maximize glioma resection: Methods and technical nuances over a 27-year period. *J Neurosurg* 2015; **123**:325–339, https://doi.org/10.3171/2014.10.JNS141520.

Meng, L., Berger, M.S., Gelb, A.W.: The potential benefits of awake craniotomy for brain tumor resection: An anesthesiologist's perspective. *J Neurosurg Anesthesiol* 2015; **27**:310–317, https://doi.org/10.1097/ANA.0000000000000179.

Meng, L., Weston, S.D., Chang, E.F., Gelb, A.W.: Awake craniotomy in a patient with ejection fraction of 10%: Considerations of cerebrovascular and cardiovascular physiology. *J Clin Anesth* 2015; **27**:256–261, https://doi.org/10.1016/j.jclinane.2015.01.004.

Meng, L., Han, S.J., Rollins, M.D., Gelb, A.W., Chang, E.F.: Awake brain tumor resection during pregnancy: Decision making and technical nuances. *J Clin Neurosci* 2016; **24**:160–162, https://doi.org/10.1016/j.jocn.2015.08.021.

Serletis, D., Bernstein, M.: Prospective study of awake craniotomy used routinely and nonselectively for supratentorial tumors. *J Neurosurg* 2007; **107**:1–6, https://doi.org/10.3171/JNS-07/07/0001.

Chapter 21

Anesthesia for Stereotactic and Other Functional Neurosurgery

Darreul P. Sewell and Alana M. Flexman

Key Points

- Stereotactic neurosurgery is used to treat and diagnose a wide variety of diseases of the nervous system.
- Stereotactic neurosurgery is based on the use of three-dimensional localization of specific areas of the human nervous system acquired by neuroradiologic imaging techniques.
- Most commonly, stereotactic neurosurgery is performed with a stereotactic system that includes a head frame fixed to the patient's skull.
- Bilateral stimulation of the subthalamic nucleus with a deep brain stimulator is one of the most effective treatments of advanced Parkinson's disease.
- Many stereotactic neurosurgery procedures are performed under low-dose sedation, without general anesthesia.

Abbreviations

CT   Computed tomography
MRI   Magnetic resonance imaging
DBS   Deep brain stimulation
IPG   Impulse generator
PD   Parkinson's disease
LMA   Laryngeal mask airway
MER   Microelectrode recording
VAE   Venous air embolism

Contents

Introduction

Stereotactic neurosurgery involves locating surgical targets relative to an external frame of reference which is applied to the patient's cranium. Stereotactic neurosurgery is accomplished in one of two ways:

Frame-Based
A rigid stereotactic frame is applied to the patient's head followed by either CT or MRI. Based on further analysis of this data, the surgical target is located and the trajectory planned.

Frameless
Special markers (fiducials) are pasted onto the patient's scalp before imaging. The fiducials are incorporated into the MRI imaging. In the operating room, the patient's head is secured to the operating table with a three-point pin fixation clamp that includes a neuronavigation reference attachment. Using a special pointer, the fiducials on the patient's head will be cross-referenced with the MR images, which will be used to direct the image-guided procedure.

Functional neurosurgery refers to the surgical management of disorders with no gross anatomical or surgical target in the brain. It is used to treat movement disorders related to PD essential tremors and dystonias while it is also used in the management of chronic pain and depression. The overall goal of this type of surgery is to provide symptomatic relief and improve a patient's quality of life. Functional neurosurgery may involve making permanent lesions in specific areas of the brain or placing electrodes for reversible stimulation of targeted areas. It is essential for the anesthesiologist to have a thorough understanding of the patient's disease process, the surgical procedure involved and the unique anesthetic demands that these interventions require.

Closed Brain Biopsy

Closed brain biopsy can be either frame-based (CT guided with stereotactic frame) or frameless (stealth-guided). A small burr hole is created in the skull followed by insertion of a biopsy needle. Stealth-guided brain biopsy requires a high degree of accuracy and a motionless patient.

These procedures can be performed under general anesthesia or local anesthesia depending on the comorbidities and the anticipated cooperation of the patient. If local anesthesia is used, over-sedation should be avoided given the risks of airway compromise and movement. Hyperventilation and osmotic diuretics are not typically required and the patient's blood pressure should be managed to avoid unexpected hypertensive peaks that could precipitate intracranial bleeding. If a patient fails to wake up, further imaging is warranted to investigate for hemorrhage, cerebral edema, or pneumocephalus.

Deep Brain Stimulation

DBS involves the disruption and modulation of dysfunctional neuronal pathways to remove or improve brain function without destroying critical structures. Deep brain stimulators are implantable devices consisting of electrodes placed in discrete areas of the brain attached to an IPG located in a remote part of the body (analogous to a cardiac

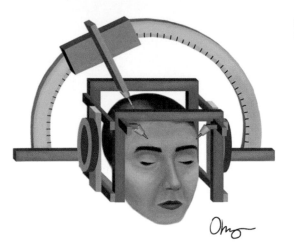

Figure 21.1 Patient in a typical frame used for deep brain stimulation.

pacemaker). Stimulation of brain centers can be adjusted to achieve the greatest benefit while minimizing side effects.

The treatment of PD that is refractory to medical therapy with DBS is now more common. The anatomical targets include the subthalamic nucleus (most common), globus pallidus and ventralis intermedius nucleus. The procedure is effective in relieving the motor symptoms although the disease remains chronic and progressive. DBS has several benefits compared to direct lesioning of targeted brain structures including reversibility, titration of stimulation, and a better safety profile.

Surgery for DBS involves the insertion of electrodes into the brain followed by the implantation of the IPG at a remote site. Both phases are usually completed in a single procedure. Once the stereotactic frame is applied to the patient's head (Figure 21.1), an MRI is performed to identify the relevant target brain structures and to allow intraoperative planning for accurate placement of the electrodes. The patient is then transferred from the radiology suite to the operating room and positioned in a semi-recumbent position with their head frame fixed to the operating table. Electrodes are inserted through a burr hole into the brain under stereotactic guidance, supplemented by imaging and MERs. After successful electrode placement, the leads are internalized, tunneled, and connected to the IPG implanted in the upper chest. The IPG is typically not activated for several days or weeks after the procedure to allow resolution of edema.

Anesthetic Management

Preoperative Evaluation

The insertion of the DBS electrodes is often done with the patient awake. As such, adequate preparation and management of expectations is important. A thorough airway assessment is essential to ensure an appropriate management plan is available while the patient is in the frame.

Patients that present for DBS surgery will often have longstanding PD that is resistant to medical therapy. On the day of surgery, patients may have been asked to reduce or stop their anti-Parkinson medications. These patients can present with severe motor symptoms including akinesia, tremor, and rigidity. The muscle rigidity can increase the risk of airway complications due to pulmonary aspiration and laryngospasm. In addition to other co-morbidities, patients with PD may have sleep apnea, impaired respiratory reserve, impaired airway reflexes, and autonomic dysfunction, leading to orthostatic hypotension and delayed gastric emptying.

Intraoperative Management

The patient will commonly need to be awake and cooperative during prolonged phases of the surgery in order to participate in neurological testing. The aim during this time is to help the patient remain comfortable, calm and cooperative.

Initially, a compatible head frame is applied to the patient using either local or regional anesthesia (scalp block) with a small amount of anxiolytic medication (e.g., midazolam 1–2 mg intravenously) prior to imaging. Occasionally, general anesthesia is required prior to application of the head frame for patients with dystonia, severe anxiety, or other psychiatric concerns. The airway can be managed with either an endotracheal tube or an LMA if appropriate. The anesthesiologist should ensure the necessary MRI-compatible monitors are used and emergency equipment is available in the radiology suite.

Once the imaging is complete, the patient is transported to the operating room, carefully positioned on the table to which the head frame is also attached. Allowing a small degree of flexion at the lower cervical spine and extension at the atlanto-occipital junction may facilitate emergent airway management if required. Routine monitoring, including electro-cardiography, non-invasive blood pressure, pulse oximeter, and capnography, is used throughout the procedure. Invasive arterial blood pressure may be indicated depending on patient co-morbidities and supplemental oxygen is always provided.

After infiltration of local anesthetic, burr holes are drilled into the skull to allow placement of the stimulating electrodes. Varying degrees of sedation may be used for this portion of the procedure depending on institutional practice. During electrode placement, the patient ideally should be fully awake to allow testing for symptomatic improvement and the detection of any neurological side effects. As the electrode is advanced into the thalamus and subthalamic regions of the brain, the electrical activity of individual neurons is monitored, producing MERs. Specific nuclei are identified from characteristic MERs and once positioned at the desired site, the clinical effects of electrode stimulation are confirmed. Electrode placement may also be facilitated and confirmed using intraoperative fluoroscopy or stereotactic navigation.

In the final stage of the procedure, the leads must be tunneled and connected to the IPG implanted in the upper chest. There is no requirement for the patient to be awake for this part of the surgery. General anesthesia is typically induced once the head frame has been removed and the airway can be safely manipulated. Once the procedure is complete, the patient is woken up and transferred to the post-anesthesia care unit.

Several sedation strategies are employed for DBS procedures. Regardless of the technique used, over-sedation leading to respiratory depression and airway compromise must be avoided given the limited access to the airway. In addition, the use of sedation carries a risk of disinhibition and loss of patient cooperation. Benzodiazepines and beta-blockers (e.g., labetalol) can reduce tremor and their use should be minimized as appropriate. All anesthetic agents have the potential to interfere with neurologic testing and MERs and a fully awake patient is preferred for the testing portion of the procedure. During other phases, a combination of sedatives with a short half-life (e.g., propofol, remifentanil) may be used for comfort. Dexmedetomidine may also be used as it allows the patients to be easily roused and cooperative. In low doses, dexmedetomidine does not appear to interfere with MERs. General anesthesia may be necessary for a small minority of patients who cannot tolerate the procedure or who have severe uncontrolled movements. The use of general anesthesia does not allow accurate interpretation of MERs and the surgeon is unable to assess the clinical response to stimulation of the electrodes during placement. In these cases, lead placement may be facilitated using MRI guidance.

Complications

Up to 16% of patients experience intraoperative complications. Of major concern to the anesthesiologist is the potential for airway and respiratory complications. These may occur due to over-sedation or intracranial events such as seizure or hemorrhage and are hazardous as the head frame restricts access to the airway. In emergency situations, an LMA may be useful to help manage the airway and avoid hypoxia. In addition, patients with advanced PD may suffer aspiration from bulbar dysfunction, and hypotension from autonomic dysfunction.

Surgical complications include intracranial hemorrhage, neurological changes, seizures, and (VAE). Intracranial hypertension occurs in approximately 2%–4% of patients and those with intraoperative hypertension are at higher risk. Consideration should be given to keeping the systolic blood pressure less than 140 mmHg, either with antihypertensive medication or appropriate analgesia, anxiolytics, or sedation, if required.

Neurological complications can include either focal weakness or speech deficits and these usually occur during electrical stimulation of the leads. Seizures are commonly partial in nature and usually do not require treatment but occasionally small doses of propofol or midazolam are required. Due to the head-up position, VAE is a rare but potentially life-threatening complication. Coughing during opening of the skull is often the first sign of VAE and late signs include hypotension and hypoxemia.

Long-term complications are generally related to the implanted hardware. These include infection, lead migration, lead fracture, generator malfunction, and skin erosion over the IPG.

Further Reading

Bekker, A., Eloy, J.: Anesthesia for functional neurosurgery. *Austin J Anesthe Analg* 2014; 2(3):1016.

Braun, M., Winkler, D., Wehner, M., Busch, T., Schwarz, J. Deep brain stimulation and general anesthesia. *Basal Ganglia* 2011; 1(2):79–82.

Fabregas, N., Craen, R.A.: Anaesthesia for minimally invasive neurosurgery. Best Practice & Research. *Clinical Anaesthesiology* 2002; 16(1), 81–93.

Fabregas, N., Hurtado, P., Garcia, I., et al: Anesthesia for minimally invasive neurosurgery. *Colomb J Anesthesiol* 2015; 43:15–21.

Matta, B., Menon, D., Smith, M. (2011) Core Topics in *Neuroanaesthesia and Neurointensive Care*. Cambridge: Cambridge University Press.

Miocinovic, S., Somayajula, S., Chitnis, S., Vitek, J.L.: History, applications and mechanisms of deep brain stimulation. *JAMA Neurol* 2013;

70(2):163–171, https://doi.org/10.1001/2013
.jamaneurol.45.

Osborn, I.P., Kurtis, S.D., Alterman, R.L.:
Functional neurosurgery: Anesthetic
considerations. *Int Anesthesiol Clin* 2015;
53(1):39–52, https://doi.org/10.1097/
AIA.0000000000000040.

Ostrem, L., Ziman, N., Galifianakis, N.B.,
et al: Clinical outcomes using clear point
interventional MRI for deep brain
stimulation lead placement in Parkinson's
disease. *J Neurosurg* 2016; 23 (4):
908–916. https://doi.org/10.3171/2015.4
.JNS15173.

Chapter 22

Anesthesia for Pituitary Surgery

Xinying Chen and Arun Gupta

Key Points

- Patients undergoing pituitary surgery should be evaluated for possible mass effect and/or syndromes of hormonal hypersecretion. These have significant anesthetic implications and require careful preoperative evaluation and perioperative management.
- Preoperative examination should include a careful examination to identify a potentially difficult airway. Airway adjuncts should be prepared and awake fiberoptic intubation should be considered. Obstructive sleep apnea is common and the patient may benefit from a short period of postoperative non-invasive ventilation.
- Perioperative steroid supplementation is routinely administered for surgical stress because most patients have maximal baseline steroid secretion. Liaison with an endocrinologist will be ideal for perioperative management and postoperative follow-up.
- Transsphenoidal or endonasal approaches to pituitary tumors have superseded intracranial approaches as they are safer but they can be associated with significant complications.
- Inhalational or total intravenous anesthetic techniques are appropriate.
- Postoperative complications include disorders of water and salt balance such as diabetes insipidus, syndrome of inappropriate antidiuretic hormone secretion, or cerebral salt-wasting syndrome. Careful monitoring of fluid balance and electrolytes is required.

Abbreviations

ACTH   Adrenocorticotrophic hormone
CSF   Cerebrospinal fluid
CSW   Cerebral salt wasting
CT   Computed tomography
DI   Diabetes insipidus
ETT   Endotracheal tube
GH   Growth hormone
ICP   Intracranial pressure
MRI   Magnetic resonance imaging

NIV	Non-invasive ventilation
OSA	Obstructive sleep apnea
SIADH	Syndrome of inappropriate antidiuretic hormone
TSH	Thyroid stimulating hormone

Contents

Anatomy

The pituitary gland is located in the sella turcica of the sphenoid bone at the base of the skull. Of importance, the optic chiasm, hypothalamus, and 3rd ventricle lie above the sella and the cavernous sinus, internal carotid arteries, 3rd, 4th, and 6th cranial nerves lie on the lateral wall.

Physiology

The pituitary gland consists of an anterior and posterior lobe both of which are of different embryological origins. The anterior pituitary (adenohypophysis) comprises two thirds of the gland and synthesizes six hormones. The secretion of hormones by the anterior pituitary is under feedback control of the hypothalamus via the hypophyseal portal system, which runs in the hypophyseal stalk.

The posterior pituitary (neurohypophysis) is anatomically continuous with the hypothalamus via the hypothalamo-hypophyseal nerve tract and it stores and releases hormones secreted from the hypothalamus (vasopressin and oxytocin). The hormones secreted by the pituitary gland are summarized in Tables 22.1 and 22.2.

Table 22.1 Anterior Pituitary Hormones

Hormone	Hypothalamic Feedback	Target Organ and Function	Clinical Disease
Growth hormone	GHRH, somatostatin (inhibitory)	Musculoskeletal system: anabolic effects on bone and muscle. Increase protein synthesis and lipolysis, decrease insulin sensitivity	Acromegaly
ACTH	CRH	Adrenal glands: stimulates the glands to produce glucocorticoids and aldosterone	Cushing's disease
Prolactin	PRH, dopamine (inhibitory)	Mammary glands: stimulates the glands to produce milk Ovary: inhibits the actions of gonadotropins on the ovary	Prolactinoma
TSH	TRH	Thyroid gland: increased blood flow and production of thyroid hormones	Hyperthyroidism
FSH, LH	LHRH	Gonads: stimulate the testes to produce sperm and testosterone, and the ovaries to produce eggs and estrogen	

Table 22.2 Posterior Pituitary Hormones

Hormone	Clinical Effects
Antidiuretic hormone	Kidneys: regulates the amount of water excreted by the kidneys and maintains water balance in the body
Oxytocin	Uterus: contracts the uterus during childbirth and immediately after delivery Mammary glands: stimulates contractions of the milk ducts in the breast

Pituitary Pathology and Clinical Features

Pituitary tumors represent 10% of all intracranial neoplasms. The majority are pituitary adenomas which can be locally invasive but do not metastasize.

Pituitary adenomas are broadly classified according to size and functional status. Microadenomas are less than 1 cm in size while macroadenomas exceed this. Tumors of the anterior pituitary can be "functioning" (hormone-secreting) or "non-functioning" (non-secreting).

Common manifestations include:

1. **Mass effect:** This is more common with macroadenomas. They commonly present with headache and subtle visual field defects. Larger tumors can cause hypopituitarism, cranial nerve palsies, hydrocephalus, and raised ICP due to blockage of third ventricle outflow.
2. **Hormonal excess from functioning adenomas:** The most common type is a prolactinoma (usually macroadenomas) and GH secreting adenomas causing acromegaly. Cushing's disease and thyrotoxicosis are rare but clinically significant.
3. **Pituitary hypofunction:** Intrasellar growth can result in compression of adjacent normal pituitary tissue causing pituitary hypofunction. It can also be caused by previous radiotherapy, surgery, or hemorrhage in the area.
4. **Nonspecific symptoms:** Includes infertility and epilepsy.

Preoperative Diagnosis and Management

Diagnosis of pituitary disease requires a combination of clinical suspicion, elevated hormone levels, and imaging. MRI is superior in identifying microadenomas whereas CT is better at detecting bony invasion.

Preoperative Assessment

Preoperative assessment of patients scheduled for pituitary surgery should focus on identification and management of raised ICP and the effects of hormonal hypersecretion and/or hyposecretion.

Syndromes of Hormonal Hypersecretion

Acromegaly

Acromegaly is a chronic, progressive, multisystem disease caused by hypersecretion of GH from a functioning pituitary macroadenoma; therefore, patients present with local mass effect and excess of GH. The insidious progression leads to a late diagnosis and the disease is usually advanced at presentation.

The clinical features that are of anesthetic concern are those that involve the upper airway along with the cardiac and respiratory systems. Upper airway changes include prognathism, macroglossia, hypertrophy of the uvula, and epiglottis and aryepiglottic folds leading to a reduction in size of the glottic opening. Hoarseness of voice should prompt investigation for laryngeal stenosis or recurrent laryngeal nerve injury. Awake fiberoptic intubation or videolaryngoscopy should be considered for a potentially difficult airway.

Up to 70% of patients have significant OSA because of soft tissue enlargement of the upper airway. This is associated with airway difficulties, cardiac instability, and postoperative cardiorespiratory failure. Respiratory function may be additionally compromised by kyphoscoliosis and proximal myopathy.

Cardiac issues include refractory hypertension with eccentric left ventricular hypertrophy, ischemic heart disease, arrhythmias, heart block, cardiomyopathy, and bi-ventricular dysfunction. Preoperative transthoracic echocardiography is useful to assess left ventricular size and performance. Diabetes mellitus and other endocrine pathologies may also be present.

Cushing's Disease

The term Cushing's disease is reserved for an excess of glucocorticoid due to hypersecretion of ACTH from a pituitary corticotrophic adenoma. Surgical excision is the definitive management, but medical treatment may reverse much of the effects of excess glucocorticoid and considerably reduces perioperative risk. The typical habitus is one of truncal obesity, moon facies, and thin extremities.

Patients may have a difficult airway due to obesity and an increased incidence of OSA. Cardiac issues include hypertension, left ventricular hypertrophy, diastolic dysfunction, and congestive cardiac failure. A Transthoracic Echocardiogram may be considered to assess cardiac function. Other anesthetic issues include coagulation abnormalities, osteoporosis, thin skin, glucose intolerance, or diabetes mellitus.

Preoperative Hormonal Optimization

Perioperative Steroid Supplementation

Most patients will require hydrocortisone at induction of anesthesia and two additional divided doses over 24 hours followed by a tapering regimen. Patients with hypopituitarism will also need regular hormonal supplementation continued on the day of surgery. This may differ from center to center and should be advised by an endocrine specialist.

Preoperative Control of Thyroid Function

Hyperthyroidism caused by TSH producing adenomas should be aggressively treated with somatostatin analogues, antithyroid medications, and beta-blockade as indicated before surgery.

Surgical Approach and Intraoperative Considerations

Most surgical resections of pituitary adenomas are now performed extracranially via an endonasal transsphenoidal approach. The advantages of this approach are minimal surgical trauma and blood loss, direct access to the gland, minimal patient discomfort, and decreased incidence of hypopituitarism and DI. In some patients, fat is harvested from the abdomen and used to seal the intranasal opening to prevent CSF leak.

A lumbar intrathecal catheter is occasionally used to aid visualization of pituitary tumors in selected cases with suprasellar extension. Injection of normal saline increases CSF pressure, which pushes the tumor towards the surgical field facilitating surgery. The patient is positioned supine with head up tilt. Local anesthetic with vasoconstrictor is instilled into the nostrils to improve surgical conditions. A very small minority of patients require excision of pituitary tumors via craniotomy.

Anesthetic Management

The general aims of anesthesia for transsphenoidal pituitary surgery are: (1) optimization of cerebral oxygenation, (2) maintaining hemodynamic stability, (3) providing conditions that facilitate surgical exposure, and (4) rapid smooth emergence. For this surgery, patients are usually positioned supine with a 30-degree head up tilt.

Airway Management

A potential difficult airway should be anticipated and carefully evaluated in patients with acromegaly and Cushing's disease. Airway adjuncts, long blades, and video laryngoscopies could all be useful in these cases. Awake fiberoptic intubation may be a prudent option.

An armored or south-facing oral ETT is frequently used for endonasal pituitary surgery. A throat pack is often required to minimize aspiration of blood and must be removed prior to extubation. An alternative to a throat pack is an oro-gastric tube to suction out blood from the stomach. Intranasal mucosal application of a vasoconstrictor (such as epinephrine) or cocaine paste is often employed by the surgeon to reduce blood loss.

Anesthetic Technique

Intravenous or inhalational techniques are both appropriate. Either technique must be responsive to the high levels of stimulation during the transsphenoidal dissection, and much lower levels of stimulation whilst operating on the sellar tumor. The use of remifentanil is useful during periods of intense stimulation and allows the flexibility of rapid adjustment of analgesic requirements.

Routine monitoring including temperature is required. Invasive arterial monitoring may be justified depending on co-morbidities and/or if hormonal abnormalities exist but is not routinely needed.

Postoperative Care and Complications

Smooth emergence is ideal to prevent dislodgement of nasal packs. Airway obstruction is not uncommon and is usually due to blood in the nasopharynx or the abnormal airway morphology associated with acromegaly. Postoperative nausea and vomiting is common hence routine pharmacological prophylaxis should be administered. Postoperative pain is moderate and requires adequate multimodal analgesia.

Hormonal replacement therapy will be required in all patients after surgery. Steroid replacement therapy is administered in a standardized reducing regime, and additional replacement therapy is defined by patients' postoperative hormonal function. Close liaison with endocrinologists should be sought for all replacement therapy.

Surgery is usually associated with minimal blood loss. However, injury of the cavernous sinus and carotid artery can cause massive blood loss. Cavernous sinus injury is more common and can cause persistent venous oozing. Persistent CSF leak is also a potential complication and a Valsalva maneuver may be used at the end of surgery to identify such leakage. In the case of a significant leak, the surgeon will seal the sella with autologous fat and fascia, usually harvested from the patient's thigh or abdomen.

Postoperative neuroendocrine abnormalities can occur after pituitary surgery. DI causing polyuria and hypernatremia usually develops within the first 24 hours and resolves spontaneously in about a week. If persistent, DI is treated with parenteral or intranasal desmopressin. Hyponatremia can be caused by excess desmopressin administration or rarely, due to SIADH) or CSW. Management of these syndromes includes fluid restriction or steroids such as fludrocortisone.

Further Reading

Aziz, M.: Airway management in neuroanesthesiology. *Anesthesiol Clin* 2012; **30**(2):229–240.

Bharadwaj, S., Venkatraghavan, L.: Dexamethasone and hypothalamic-pituitary-adrenal axis suppression after transsphenoidal pituitary surgery. *J Neurosurg Anesthesiol* 2015 April; **27**(2):181.

Bhatia, N., Ghai, B., Mangal, K., Wig, J., Mukherjee, K.K.: Effect of intramucosal infiltration of different concentrations of adrenaline on hemodynamics during transsphenoidal surgery. Journal of anaesthesiology, *Clin Pharmacol* 2014; **30**(4):520–525.

Dunn, L.K., Nemergut, E.C.: Anesthesia for transsphenoidal pituitary surgery. *Curr Opin Anaesthesiol* 2013; **26**(5):549–554.

Dyer, M.W., Gnagey, A., Jones, B.T., et al: Perianesthetic Management of Patients with Thyroid-Stimulating Hormone-Secreting Pituitary Adenomas. *J Neurosurg Anesthesiol* 2016; **29**(3): 341–346.

Gopalakrishna, K.N., Dash, P.K., Chatterjee, N., Easwer, H.V., Ganesamoorthi, A.: Dexmedetomidine as an anesthetic adjuvant in patients undergoing transsphenoidal resection of pituitary tumor. *J Neurosurg Anesthesiol* 2015; **27**(3):209–215.

Laws, E.R., Wong, J.M., Smith, T.R., et al: A checklist for endonasal transsphenoidal anterior skull base surgery. *J Neurosurg* 2016; **124**(6):1634–1639.

Salimi, A., Sharifi, G., Bahrani, H., et al: Dexmedetomidine could enhance surgical satisfaction in Trans-sphenoidal resection of pituitary adenoma. *J Neurosurg Sci* 2017; **61**(1):46–52.

Chapter

23

Anesthesia for Patients with Head Injury

Poppy Aldam and Vaithy Mani

Key Points

- Secondary injury must be avoided. The anesthetic technique must allow early detection and prompt treatment of factors that may exacerbate such injury.
- Cerebral perfusion pressure must be maintained at greater than 60 mm Hg.
- The principles of anesthesia for patients with head injury apply from the time of the injury, including transfer from the scene to a neurosurgical center and the perioperative period.
- Associated injuries in polytrauma patients can cause significant physiologic derangements. In particular, chest injuries may cause hypoxia, as well as hypotension (secondary to blood loss, myocardial contusion, or acute valvular lesions).
- Post-operative high-dependency or intensive care with intracranial pressure monitoring and assessment of neurologic status is essential.

Abbreviations

ATLS	Advanced trauma life support
$CMRO_2$	Cerebral metabolic rate of oxygen
CPP	Cerebral perfusion pressure
GCS	Glasgow Coma Scale
ICP	Intracranial pressure
MAC	Minimum alveolar concentration
TBI	Traumatic brain injury
TIVA	Total intravenous anesthesia

Contents

- Pre-operative Assessment
  - History and Examination
  - Investigations
- Intraoperative Management
  - Induction
  - Airway management
  - Vascular Access and Catheters
  - Monitoring
  - Maintenance of Anesthesia
  - Ventilation
  - Blood Pressure Management
  - Hyperosmolar Therapy
  - Hyperglycemia
  - Hypothermia
  - Thromboprophylaxis
  - Intraoperative Treatment of Raised Intracranial Pressure
- Post-operative Management
- Further Reading

Introduction

Head injury is amongst the commonest causes of death and disability in people aged 5 to 40 years worldwide. Falls, assaults, and road traffic accidents make up the majority of etiologies of head injury, with road traffic accidents accounting for a greater proportion of severe head injuries.

Classification

Severity of head injury is classified using the GCS:

- Mild head injury: GCS score of 13 to 15
- Moderate head injury: GCS score of 9 to 12
- Severe head injury: GCS score 8 or less

Modification of the above classification is needed in the presence of drug or alcohol intoxication. Reversible causes contributing to a reduction in GCS such as hypoxia, hypovolemia, drugs, and alcohol should be considered and corrected. In head injured patients, up to 5% are categorized as severe with an associated mortality of nearly 20%.

Pathophysiology

Primary injury occurs at the time of the initial physical insult and is irreversible. Little can be done to limit primary injury except for public health interventions and safety messages.

Secondary injury results from further physiological processes triggered by the primary injury. It occurs in the hours to days following the primary injury and involves damage to neurons unaffected by the primary injury. Secondary brain injury is a cause of major morbidity and mortality in head injured patients. The perioperative management of these patients should focus on minimizing development of a secondary brain injury.

Table 23.1 Factors Causing Secondary Brain Injury

Intracranial	Systemic
Hematoma	Hypotension
Hydrocephalus	Hypoxia
Cerebral edema	Hypercapnia
Seizures	Hyperglycemia
Vasospasm	Hyperthermia

Morphology of Injury

Intracranial hematomas can be classified by their location. These include:

(1) Extradural Hematoma

Injury to the middle meningeal artery secondary to a skull fracture causes arterial bleeding which collects between the skull and the dura mater, often in the parieto-temporal area. A characteristic lucid interval may occur between injury and onset of neurological symptoms.

(2) Subdural Hematoma

Tearing of cortical bridging veins between the dura and pia mater can cause venous blood to accumulate.

(3) Subarachnoid Hemorrhage

Traumatic subarachnoid hemorrhage is caused by an arterial injury, and associated with the same complications (such as hydrocephalus and secondary vasospasm) as aneurysmal subarachnoid hemorrhage.

(4) Intracerebral Hematoma

This usually affects the white matter or basal ganglia. The prognosis is related to the size of the hematoma and degree of mass effect caused.

(5) Cerebral Contusion

These cause multiple bilateral areas of hemorrhage that usually affect the grey matter of the temporal and frontal lobes. There is often marked associated edema around the lesions. Causes of secondary brain injury are outlined in Table 23.1

Indications for Surgical Management

Only 1–3% of all patients with head injury who are admitted to hospital in the United Kingdom for observation will go on to require neurosurgery. However, this number can increase to almost 30% in patients with severe head injury. Pathologies that require urgent neurosurgical intervention include:

- Depressed skull fracture greater than skull thickness
- Intracranial mass lesions with signs of impending herniation
- Acute extradural or subdural hematomas
- Intracerebral hematomas
- Subarachnoid hemorrhage with hydrocephalus
- Elevated ICP refractory to medical management

Pre-Operative Assessment

History and Examination

Many patients may already be intubated and ventilated when received in the operating room or neurosurgical center. A checklist for a transferred patient should include:

- Mechanism and time of injury
- Initial GCS score at the scene of the incident
- GCS score prior to intubation
- Size and reactivity of pupils
- Induction drugs, maintenance, and drugs given before or during transfer
- Grade of laryngoscopy and equipment used
- Sites of intravenous access and monitoring
- Cardiorespiratory stability during transfer
- Results of any investigations in referring center
- Any known or suspected associated injuries
- Any known allergies, past medical history, or medications

A primary survey encompassing airway, breathing, and circulation should be repeated on receipt of the head injured patient. There should be careful assessment and documentation of GCS score, pupil size, reactivity, and presence of pre-existing neurological deficits.

Head injury often occurs in the context of polytrauma. Life-threatening injuries should be managed as a priority before neurosurgical intervention as this approach can help maintain adequate CPP. If the patient is relatively stable, then priority is given to neurosurgical interventions that are required.

Spinal precautions must be instigated in the head injured patient and should remain in situ until the spine has been formally cleared in accordance with local practice and national guidelines. Cervical spine injury should be considered in patients with severe head injuries as its occurrence is typically around 5%.

There is a strong association between head injury and alcohol consumption or recreational drug use. This may have significant implications for perioperative management and should be enquired from the history.

Investigations

Apart from routine biochemical and hematological tests, analysis of clotting function and the availability of cross-matched blood are particularly important prior to neurosurgery. Further investigations relevant to the trauma patient should have been carried out in accordance with ATLS protocols and the results noted.

Intraoperative Management

Induction

Propofol and thiopentone are the most commonly used induction agents in these patients, because they can significantly reduce ICP by causing cerebral vasoconstriction and as a result of a reduction in $CMRO_2$. In hemodynamically compromised patients, ketamine or etomidate could be used. Suxamethonium is the more frequently used drug to facilitate rapid muscle relaxation for intubation. With the availability of sugammadex, rocuronium is gaining popularity as the muscle relaxant of choice for rapid sequence induction. Neither of them have any clinically significant effect on ICP.

Airway Management

Many patients with head injury are already intubated, but some patients may be conscious, when they present for surgery. Airway management in these patients is complicated by the urgency of surgery and the potential for cervical spine injury. All patients should be considered to have a full stomach and must undergo rapid sequence induction. Manual in-line stabilization as part of the airway management technique should be used in case of cervical spine injury unless this has been explicitly ruled out. If the patient has a cervical collar, the front portion may be opened to facilitate cricoid pressure and mouth opening. It is crucial to have a backup plan in case of difficult intubation, as inadequate ventilation can lead to a severe increase in ICP due to hypoxia and hypercapnia.

Vascular Access and Catheters

Invasive arterial blood pressure monitoring is essential in these cases and it allows for regular blood gas measurements. Central venous access is preferred especially in patients with hemodynamic instability, but this should not unduly delay surgery. If urgently required, vasopressors can be used via large peripheral veins in dilute concentrations until central venous access can be established. It is usual practice to insert a urinary catheter in these patients as they receive hyperosmolar therapy. Body temperature needs to be monitored to avoid extremes of hypo/hyperthermia.

Monitoring

Suggested monitoring for patients with severe TBI in the intraoperative phase includes:
- Electrocardiography
- Invasive blood pressure
- SpO_2
- Temperature
- Urine output
- Neuromuscular monitoring
- ICP

Maintenance of Anesthesia

The major goals of anesthetic management are to:
- Maintain adequate CPP (see Table 23.2). In the head injured patient with no ICP monitoring in situ assume an ICP of 20 mmHg.
- Provide optimal surgical conditions and treat raised ICP by using propofol, hyperosmolar therapy, and short-term hyperventilation if appropriate.
- Provide adequate analgesia.
- Avoid secondary injury by preventing hypoxia, hypercapnia, hyperglycemia, and hyperthermia.

Table 23.2 Cerebral Perfusion Pressure-Targets for Various Age Groups

Age Range	Target CPP (mm Hg)
Under 1 year old	40
1–5 years old	45–50
6–17 years old	50–60
Adults	60

TIVA using infusions of propofol and remifentanil is a widely used technique. If volatile anesthesia is preferred, sevoflurane at a concentration of less than 1 MAC is suggested while nitrous oxide should be avoided. Patients are kept paralyzed with neuromuscular blocking agents to facilitate controlled ventilation to normocapnia, and avoid coughing or straining by the patient, which can cause an increase in ICP. Neuromuscular junction monitoring is recommended in all patients when using these agents.

Ventilation

Ensure adequate oxygenation (PaO_2 of more than 11 kPa) and normocapnia ($PaCO_2$ 4–4.5 kPa). Hyperventilation with hypocapnia can be judiciously used for short-term control of raised ICP but prolonged hypocapnia can cause cerebral ischemia and should be avoided.

Blood Pressure Management

It is important to maintain adequate CPP of at least 60 mmHg in adults. Targets for various age group is summarized in Table 23.2. Non-glucose containing crystalloids are commonly used both for resuscitation and maintenance, and there is no evidence that colloids offer any more benefit. Once fluid resuscitation is adequate and bleeding is excluded as the cause for hypotension, vasopressors (metaraminol, noradrenaline, or phenylephrine) can be used to maintain target CPP of around 60 mmHg. There is little evidence to support the use of one vasopressor over the another to maintain cerebral perfusion.

Hyperosmolar Therapy

Due to osmotic diuresis, which can result in hypovolemia and hypotension, hyperosmolar therapy is recommended only when there are signs of transtentorial herniation or progressive neurological deterioration not attributable to extracranial causes. Mannitol can be used at a dose of 0.25–1 g/kg.

Hypertonic saline is used as an alternative agent or in patients who are refractory to mannitol treatment. It is available in different concentrations, although 5% hypertonic saline is commonly used in the United Kingdom at a dose of 2–3 ml/kg.

Hyperglycemia

Hyperglycemia after TBI is associated with increased morbidity and mortality, by potentiating secondary brain injury. Hence it is important to monitor and maintain normal blood glucose levels.

Hypothermia

There is some evidence to show slightly more favorable Glasgow outcome scores in patients who had hypothermia, even though there is no difference in mortality, as compared to patients who had normothermia.

Thromboprophylaxis

Intraoperative thromboprophylaxis prevention should be instituted which includes graduation compression stockings and intermittent pneumatic calf compression devices.

Intraoperative Treatment of Raised Intracranial Pressure

The following measures may be used to treat an acute intraoperative rise in ICP

- Reverse Trendelenburg position (head up to 30 degrees)
- Treat hypotension, hypercapnia, hypoxia
- Transient hyperventilation to cause hypocapnia (4 kPa)
- Increase anesthetic depth with intravenous agents
- Hyperosmolar therapy

Post-Operative Management

Post-operative management is dependent on the preoperative GCS score and the presence of other injuries. Patients with severe injuries and ongoing depressed level of consciousness will require sedation and ventilation on a specialist neuro-intensive care unit. There may be a need for monitoring of ICP in these patients.

Patients suitable for extubation immediately after surgery should be closely monitored in a high dependency setting by staff familiar with care of the neurosurgical patient in the post-operative period. Adequate analgesia and anti-emetic therapy are vital in the post-operative period.

Post-operative seizures and thromboembolic events are not uncommon after neurosurgical interventions in the polytrauma patient. Prophylactic treatment for seizures in certain circumstances may be appropriate for up to 1 week. Pharmacological thromboprophylaxis should be commenced when considered safe by the neurosurgical team.

Further Reading

Allen, B.B., Chiu, Y.-L., Gerber, L.M., Ghajar, J., Greenfield, J.P.: Age-specific cerebral perfusion pressure thresholds and survival in children and adolescents with severe traumatic brain injury. *Paediatr Crit Care Med: A Journal of the Society of Critical Care Medicine and the World Federation of Pediatric Intensive and Critical Care Societies* 2014; **15**(1):62–70.

Carney, N., Totten, A.M., O'Reilly, C., et al: Guidelines for the management of severe traumatic brain injury, fourth edition. *Neurosurgery* 2017; **80**(1), 6–15.

Cooper, D.J., Ackland, H.M.: Clearing the cervical spine in unconscious head injured patients – the evidence. *Crit Care Resusc: Journal of the Australasian Academy of Critical Care Medicine* 2005; 7(3):181–184.

Coles, J.P., Fryer, T.D., Coleman, M.R., et al: Hyperventilation following head injury: Effect of ischaemic burden and cerebral oxidative metabolism. *Crit Care Med* 2007; 35(2):568–578.

Chapter 24

Anesthesia for Spinal Surgery

Eschtike Schulenburg

Key Points

- Patients undergoing cervical spinal surgery often present with a difficult airway making preoperative assessment of the airway essential.
- To prevent both peripheral nerve and eye injuries, careful prone positioning is essential.
- An intravenous anesthetic technique interferes less with intraoperative neurophysiological monitoring.
- Current guidelines on the management of cardiac arrest in the prone position should be followed.
- Multimodal analgesia regimes facilitate effective postoperative pain control, mobilization, and early discharge.

Abbreviations

CPR	Cardiopulmonary resuscitation
ECG	Electrocardiogram
ETT	Endotracheal tube
FOI	Fiberoptic intubation
FRC	Functional residual capacity
GABA	Gamma-aminobutyric acid
IV	Intravenous
MEP	Motor evoked potential
NMDA	N-methyl-D-aspartate
NSAID	Non-steroidal anti-inflammatory drug
PCA	Patient controlled analgesia
PEA	Pulseless electrical activity
SSEP	Somatosensory evoked potential
TIVA	Total intravenous anesthesia

Contents

- Introduction
- Preoperative Assessment
  - Airway Assessment

Introduction

Patients present for spinal surgery because of trauma, degenerative changes in the spinal column, malignancy, myelopathy, and infections. Spondylosis, a degenerative osteoarthritis of spinal joints, is frequently encountered along with spondylolisthesis (a forward displacement of a vertebra), disc space narrowing and acute disc prolapse. Younger patients with scoliosis and kyphotic conditions require complex and lengthy surgical correction while a growing number of elderly patients with complex medical co-morbidities frequently require major spinal surgery.

Preoperative Assessment

A comprehensive review of a patient's general medical history, medication, and general physical health is required prior to surgery. A systems approach to the preoperative assessment ensures all co-morbidities are thoroughly reviewed.

Airway Assessment

Difficulty in airway management is common in patients presenting for cervical and upper thoracic surgery. When assessing the airway, particular emphasis should be placed on previous difficulty with intubation, cervical spine instability, cord compression, pre-existing arthritis, previous cervical surgery, and restricted neck movement. Awake or asleep FOI or videolaryngoscopy should be considered because it minimizes movement of the cervical spine during airway manipulation.

Respiratory System

Spinal surgery patients can frequently present with altered respiratory function and limited pulmonary reserve. Scoliosis can lead to restrictive lung function, reduced vital, and total lung capacities. Significant thoracic trauma with multiple rib fractures and flail segments often require ventilation. Preoperative lung function tests and arterial blood gas analysis can guide management.

Cardiovascular System

Autonomic dysreflexia with severe hypertension is a common manifestation in patients with chronic spinal cord injury and known triggers should be avoided. Elderly patients with significant cardiac co-morbidity require careful clinical examination, including an ECG and echocardiogram, if appropriate. Exercise testing is often difficult due to existing spinal pathology such that a dobutamine stress echocardiogram may be required.

Neurological System

A neurological assessment should include documentation of any pre-existing focal neurology. Patients with known neuromuscular diseases such as muscular dystrophy, may be at risk for aspiration and postoperative respiratory failure.

Hematological System

Anticoagulation with warfarin, aspirin, and clopidogrel is common in the elderly population. The preoperative administration of these drugs is contraindicated in elective spinal surgery due to the risk of bleeding and hematoma formation with subsequent spinal cord compression. This is particularly relevant in anterior cervical surgery as a neck hematoma may lead to significant and rapid airway compression. Major spinal surgery such as scoliosis correction requires blood to be cross-matched for transfusion.

Intraoperative Management

Maintenance of hemodynamic stability and normotension is essential to ensure adequate spinal cord perfusion. Further neurological deterioration can result from poor patient positioning, hypoxia related to intubation difficulty and intraoperative hypotension. All inhalational anesthetic agents can reduce the amplitude of MEPs in a dose-dependent manner and therefore a TIVA technique is preferable when intraoperative neurophysiological monitoring is used.

The choice of airway management (FOI, video, or direct laryngoscopy) depends on any associated cervical cord concerns but a reinforced, properly secured ETT is the airway of choice in the prone position. Some centers use a non-reinforced ETT which avoids the need to exchange it if the patient is admitted to the intensive care unit after surgery. Large bore IV access should be established and safeguarded to prevent dislodgement when turning prone. Invasive arterial monitoring is often useful in obese patients, those with significant medical co-morbidities and where there is potential for major intraoperative blood loss. Central venous access and cardiac output monitoring is also commonly used in high risk procedures. Urinary catheterization is required in patients with pre-existing spinal cord trauma and when lengthy procedures are anticipated. Eyes are routinely closed with tape to prevent corneal abrasions and additional padding is recommended. Temperature monitoring and the use of a forced air warming device are routine during spinal surgery. Cell salvage should be considered when major hemorrhage is likely. Tranexamic acid reduces transfusion requirements during major spinal surgery and does not seem to be associated with an increase in deep venous thrombosis or myocardial infarctions.

Prone Positioning

Safe prone positioning in spinal surgery requires the selection of the correct equipment and having sufficient members of staff available for moving and handling the patient. A minimum of six people should be routine but when patients are obese or require log-rolling, greater numbers will be required to assist. Patients with unstable cervical spine injuries sometimes require an awake fiberoptic intubation followed by awake prone positioning. Routinely, patients are positioned after general anesthesia has been induced, followed by radiological examination or MEP monitoring to confirm spinal canal alignment.

Various frames (e.g., Wilson, Allen), tables (e.g., Jackson), and mattresses (e.g., Montreal) can be used to position the patient correctly for a given spinal procedure. The arms should be abducted no further than 90-degrees and slightly internally rotated to reduce strain on the brachial plexus. Common peripheral nerve injuries include those to the brachial plexus, ulnar, median, lateral cutaneous, common peroneal, and sciatic nerves. Direct compression in the axilla must be avoided and the elbows should be well padded. Pressure related injuries are of concern during long procedures and careful attention should be paid to adequately padding body pressure points, especially in the obese population. Poor positioning can expose patients to the risk of abdominal organ ischemia, resulting in an unexplained metabolic acidosis.

Prone positioning can lead to significant changes to the cardiovascular and respiratory systems. If the abdomen is free and unimpeded, both arterial partial pressure of oxygen and FRC are slightly increased with minimal changes in lung compliance. However, a poorly positioned patient with a reduced FRC can develop hypoxia. An impeded abdomen will result in a significant increase in intra-abdominal pressure leading to congestion of the venous system, a bloody surgical field and increased blood loss. A decrease in cardiac output on turning prone is the result of a decrease in preload and hence stroke volume. Hypovolemia in the prone position may lead to hypoperfusion and organ ischemia.

Visual Loss

Visual loss after spinal surgery (1:30000) is a devastating complication. Risk factors include reduced ocular perfusion pressure, long duration of surgery (>6 hours), significant intraoperative blood loss, hypotension, non-neutral head positioning, the incorrect use of horseshoe head rests and patient specific factors. Mechanisms include ischemic optic atrophy, cortical ischemia, and central retinal artery occlusion with reduced retinal perfusion.

Spinal Cord Monitoring

Intraoperative neurophysiological monitoring combining MEP and SSEPs can reduce the incidence of intraoperative cord and nerve damage in complex spinal surgery (see Chapter 49).

SSEPs monitor the sensory pathways along a peripheral nerve (e.g., posterior tibial nerve), the dorsal column, and the sensory cortex. A decrease in the signal amplitude of >50% and an increase in latency >10% is significant.

MEPs are achieved by placing electrodes on the scalp over the motor cortex. Needle electrodes are also placed into muscles in all four limbs to elicit compound muscle action potentials. Typically, abductor polices brevis, hypothenar muscles, tibialis anterior, abductor halluces, deltoids, and biceps are used depending on the specific surgical procedure. These monitoring modalities are described in greater detail in Chapter 49.

Volatile anesthetics can significantly affect both somatosensory and evoked potentials. The use of propofol and narcotic infusions with short acting muscle relaxants for intubation are preferable. Continued muscle paralysis may preclude adequate monitoring of MEPs.

Cardiopulmonary Resuscitation

During a cardiac arrest in neurosurgery, it is currently recommended that a smaller initial starting dose of Adrenaline (50–100 mcg) is given and then incremented. Once a total of 1 mg has been given, all subsequent doses of Adrenaline should be 1 mg when managing PEA during a cardiac arrest.

If a patient is undergoing surgery in the prone position, CPR can begin with the patient in this position without immediate need to turn the patient supine. All surgical instruments should immediately be removed and the wound covered with saline soaked swabs and a clear dressing. If chest compressions are ineffective (as guided by end-tidal carbon dioxide and an arterial waveform traces), the patient should be turned to the supine position without delay.

When a patient is fixed in the Mayfield clamp, chest compressions will result in the thorax moving whilst the head is fixed to the operating table. This may result in injury to the cervical spine, skull, and the scalp. The Mayfield clamp should therefore be released from the operating table without removing the head pins prior to commencing either chest compressions or defibrillation. This will enable the surgeon to hold the head and neck in a stable position during CPR. However, during defibrillation, the surgeon should not be in direct contact with the patient. There is a theoretical risk of burns to the scalp at the pin site during defibrillation but this has not yet been reported in the literature. A horse shoe type head rest should be attached to the bed to support the patient's head during defibrillation, or alternatively, the patient may be moved down the bed once released from the Mayfield clamp.

Emergency repositioning of a patient undergoing surgery in the prone position will require excellent team work and clear allocation of roles. Frequent simulated practice is highly recommended.

Postoperative Management

Tracheal extubation should be carefully planned. Airway complications are common following lengthy surgery in the prone position, especially after cervical surgery requiring both an anterior and a posterior approach, and these patients should be considered for overnight ventilation on the intensive care unit. Extubation is appropriate if there is an audible leak upon deflation of the cuff. Anterior cervical surgery may lead to a neck hematoma and rapid compromise of the airway. After spinal surgery, any new motor deficits should prompt immediate neurosurgical review which may lead to urgent imaging or exploratory surgery.

Pain Management

Minimally invasive surgical techniques result in less postoperative pain and an earlier discharge from hospital. Multi-level spinal surgery, as well as scoliosis, are associated with significant postoperative pain and require a multimodal approach to its management.

Opioid analgesia, using morphine or oxycodone, given orally, intravenously or via a PCA device have proven effective but are associated with side effects such as respiratory depression, nausea, constipation, and pruritus.

Regular paracetamol as part of a multimodal analgesia regimen is effective in managing mild postoperative pain, especially where the use of NSAIDs are contraindicated due to bleeding concerns, renal impairment, or asthma.

Epidural analgesia can be delivered via catheters placed by the surgeon intraoperatively which result in superior pain relief. New neurological deficits or a motor block should always prompt rapid surgical review and an immediate cessation of the infusion.

Gabapentin and pregabalin are efficacious in reducing opioid requirements and post-operative pain in lumbar spinal surgery. Gabapentin is an amino acid with a chemical structure similar to the neurotransmitter GABA. Gabapentin reduces central sensitization by lowering posterior horn neuron hyperexcitability. Common side effects include somno-lence, dizziness, weight gain, peripheral edema, and ataxia. Pregabalin has greater bioavailability.

Clonidine and dexmedetomidine are both emerging as new and effective options in the management of pain following spinal surgery. Ketamine as an NMDA receptor antagonist reduces the development of hyperalgesia and opioid tolerance. The widespread use of ketamine postoperatively is, however, limited by its side effect profile but these are less frequent with low-dose infusions.

Further Reading

Bajwa, S. J. S., Haldar, R. (2015). Pain management following spinal surgeries: An appraisal of the available options. *Journal of Craniovertebral Junction & Spine*, **6**(3), 105–110.

Cheriyan, T., Maier, S. P. 2nd, Bianco, K., et al (2015). Efficacy of tranexamic acid on surgical bleeding in spine surgery: a meta-analysis. *The Spine Journal: Official Journal of the North American Spine Society*, **15**(4), 752–761.

Chowdhury, T., Petropolis, A., Cappellani, R. B. (2015). Cardiac emergencies in neurosurgical patients. *BioMed Research International*, **2015**, 751320.

Chui, J., Craen, R. A. (2016). An update on the prone position: Continuing professional development. *Canadian Journal of Anaesthesia = Journal Canadien D'anesthesie*, **63**(6), 737–767.

Kitaba, A., Martin, D. P., Gopalakrishnan, S., Tobias, J. D. (2013). Perioperative visual loss after nonocular surgery. *Journal of Anesthesia*, **27**(6), 919–926.

Moghimi, M. H., Reitman, C. A. (2016). Perioperative complications associated with spine surgery in patients with established spinal cord injury. *The Spine Journal: Official Journal of the North American Spine Society*, **16**(4), 552–557.

Park, J.-H., Hyun, S.-J. (2015). Intraoperative neurophysiological monitoring in spinal surgery. *World Journal of Clinical Cases*, **3**(9), 765–773.

Chapter 25

Airway Management and Cervical Spine Disease

Jane Sturgess

Key Points

- Cervical spine disease can be acute or chronic and both conditions present unique challenges.
- Concerns during airway management in patients with cervical spine disease include confirmation of the degree of instability, planning for the possibility of a failed intubation or ventilation and preventing secondary neurological injury due to airway manipulation.
- Cervical spine immobilization is essential during airway maneuvers and may involve removal of the rigid hard collar with the application of manual in-line stabilization.
- Awake or asleep intubation techniques using a variety of equipment are appropriate for airway management.

Abbreviations

ASA	American Society of Anesthesiologists
BMV	Bag mask ventilation
CT	Computed tomography
DAS	Difficult airway society
LMA	Laryngeal mask airway
MILS	Manual In-line stabilization
MRI	Magnetic resonance imaging
OAA	Occipito-Atlanto-Axial

Contents

- Airway Management Techniques
- Cervical Spine Movement with Bag Mask Ventilation
- Cervical Spine Movement with Cricoid Pressure
- Cervical Spine Movement with Laryngoscopy
- Cervical Spine Movement with Fiberoptic Intubation
- Cervical Spine Movement with Supraglottic Devices
- Extubation
- Guidelines for Airway Management in Trauma
- Further Reading

Introduction

Airway management for the patient with cervical spinal pathology is a core skill for the neuroanesthetist but can present a number of problems. Physical access to the airway may be limited by an external frame (HALO jacket) or hard collar. Direct laryngoscopy may prove difficult due to either an immobile fixed spine from chronic disease (ankylosing spondylitis), or fear that movement of the cervical spine may cause neurological deterioration (unstable cervical spine injury).

Acute Spinal Injury

Acute traumatic spinal cord injury occurs in 4% of trauma patients, and up to 5% of patients with head injury. Of these patients, 20% will have more than one cervical fracture, up to 75% are considered to have an unstable bony column, and many (30–70%) have an associated spinal cord injury. Although a significant number of fractures occur at C2 (24%), the vast majority of fractures occur in the lower cervical vertebrae (C6 > C7 > C5), as do fracture dislocations (C5/6 > C6/7 > C4/5) (Table 25.1). When there is significant disruption of the spinal column, the formation of a prevertebral hematoma should be considered. These can be large and occlude the airway.

Table 25.1 Incidence and Distribution of Cervical Fractures According to Cervical Level

Level	% Cervical Fractures	Level	% Fracture Dislocation
Occipital	1.7	A-O	2.2
C1	8.8	C1/2	10.0
C2	24.0	C2/3	9.1
C3	4.3	C3/4	10.0
C4	7.0	C4/5	16.5
C5	15.0	C5/6	25.1
C6	20.3	C6/7	23.4
C7	19.1	C7/T1	3.9

Chronic Cervical Spine Disease

Chronic disease affecting the cervical spine that is of greatest concern to the anesthetist relates to (1) excessive movement and instability of the OAA joint with the potential for spinal cord compression during intubation (e.g., rheumatoid arthritis, Down's syndrome) or (2) a rigid spinal column with no movement making direct laryngoscopy and tracheal access challenging (e.g., ankylosing spondylitis, previous spinal fixation).

Preoperative Assessment

Medical history and examination should include assessment of cardiorespiratory status and concomitant medication. Tolerance to awake procedures or increased sensitivity to sedative agents may influence the anesthetic technique.

Airway Assessment

Special attention should be paid to the following:

Mouth Opening

Reduced mouth opening can occur as a result of the rigid collar, reduced movement at the OAA joint or arthritis at the temporo-mandibular joint.

Reduced Neck Movement

Accessibility of trachea for trans-tracheal ventilation.

Soft Tissue Injury

This can result from arthritis of the cricoarytenoid joints, prevertebral hematoma, laryngeal injury and damage to the innervation (vagal nerve) of the laryngeal inlet with partial vocal cord paralysis. Patients with soft tissue injury present a potentially difficult airway at induction and extubation. Any soft tissue swelling should prompt a search for a bony injury. Swelling at C1 (nasopharyngeal space, normal <10 mm) precludes a nasal intubation, swelling between C2 and C4 (retropharyngeal space, normal <7 mm) can cause airway occlusion on induction of general anesthesia or may make navigation of the airway and visualization of the laryngeal inlet difficult during fiberoptic intubation. Swelling between C5 and T1 (retrotracheal space, normal <22 mm) can distort the tracheal anatomy.

Radiology

Airway assessment by plain radiographs (Figure 25.1) have been superseded by 3D-reconstruction CT or MRI. Box 25.1 highlights the features that point to potential difficulty in airway management or visualizing the larynx at intubation in cervical disease.

Airway Management Techniques

The key questions relate to (1) the potential for cervical spine movement with BMV or laryngoscopy, with consequent secondary neurological injury, (2) visualization of the laryngeal inlet, and (3) safety and timing of extubation.

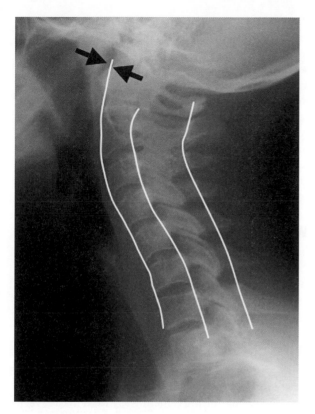

Figure 25.1 The cervical vertebral column "three lines" of alignment. These connect the anterior and posterior margins of the vertebral bodies, as well as the bases of the spinous processes. A further smooth curve can be traced between the tips of the spinous processes. The space between the odontoid peg and C1 should measure 3 mm or less in an adult (arrows).

BOX 25.1 Key Features on Cervical Imaging That Suggest a Difficult Intubation

Vertebral column	Check for alignment of the three vertebral columns. Misalignment of two or more vertebrae is considered an unstable injury
Unstable injuries	Facet joint dislocation Perched facets Subluxation Ligamentous injury
Atlantoaxial instability	Seen most commonly in Down's syndrome, rheumatoid arthritis or ligamentous injury
Soft tissue injury	Nasopharyngeal, retropharyngeal, and retrotracheal spaces should be inspected

High cervical fractures, fracture dislocations, and atlanto-occipital instability raise concern over the possibility of secondary neurological injury caused by movement of the cervical spine. Injury to the mid and lower cervical spine and fixed spine disease states may suggest difficulty visualizing the laryngeal inlet due to a prevertebral hematoma or difficulty accessing the valecula with the tip of the laryngoscope.

Not all cervical fractures are unstable injuries, but it can be assumed that fracture dislocation injuries are unstable placing the patient at risk of neurological deterioration with further cervical spine movement. The vast majority of fracture dislocation injuries occur at C4 or below. However, 10% occur at C1/2, and these patients present the greatest concern.

Patients with unstable spine injuries will be cared for in a hard collar or HALO jacket until the injury has been treated. A hard collar impedes mouth opening and visualization of the laryngeal inlet. Current best advice is to remove the anterior section of the hard collar and use MILS while securing the airway. This approach may not yield the best grade of view of the larynx (often Cormack and Lehane grade 3). A soft gum elastic bougie is a very useful adjunct and has been shown to reduce the time and increase the likelihood of successful intubation of the trachea. It is important to be aware that MILS reduces but does not stop all movement of the cervical spine.

Cervical Spine Movement with Bag Mask Ventilation

Some studies have shown that movement of the cervical spine during bag mask ventilation is far less than during direct laryngoscopy, yet others have shown the exact opposite. The safest choice is jaw thrust with an airway adjunct; a nasopharyngeal airway can be inserted with minimal OAA movement and is preferable in the absence of nasopharyngeal hematoma or skull base fracture.

Cervical Spine Movement with Cricoid Pressure

While many European countries do not use Sellick's maneuver during rapid sequence induction, it remains part of the protocol in UK practice. Measurements in anesthetized patients showed movement up to 5 mm, but negligible movement was found in cadaveric studies when cricoid pressure was applied. A two-handed technique for application of cricoid pressure in patients with cervical spine injury is sometimes used where the second hand is placed behind the neck to stabilize the spine and provide counter pressure.

Cervical Spine Movement with Laryngoscopy

Direct laryngoscopy causes the most OAA movement, and very little movement below C2. Many studies focus attention on movement at the level of the OAA area or C2 but few have looked at movement of the lower cervical spine where the majority of injuries occur. Flexion-extension views give information about movement of the atlanto-axial joint but not the atlanto-occipital joint. As most injuries occur below C2 it could be argued that quick successful placement of an endotracheal tube and restoration of adequate ventilation is safe and the greatest priority.

Studies have shown no difference in cervical movement or glottic views when comparing Macintosh and Miller laryngoscope blades. The McCoy blade produces the least movement and can improve the Cormack and Lehane view by at least 1 if not 2 grades. Videolaryngoscopy offers the advantage of direct laryngeal visualization from a camera at the tip of the laryngoscope blade with minimal cervical spine movement. In addition, studies have shown fewer failed intubations using videolaryngoscopes than when standard laryngoscope blades are used.

Cervical Spine Movement with Fiberoptic Intubation

Awake fiberoptic intubation is considered by many to be the gold standard for securing the airway in unstable cervical spine injuries as it permits neurological assessment immediately after intubation. However, significant movement can occur in poorly selected uncooperative patients and when practitioners are not well-practiced in the technique. The best advice is to select and prepare patients carefully and ensure the procedure is performed skillfully with trained assistance.

While an awake intubation affords the opportunity to perform an immediate neurological examination, it is not without risk and there are situations when it is not the method of choice. If there is significant concern that the laryngeal inlet cannot be visualized, the choices are awake intubation with a videolaryngoscope or fiberoptic scope, laryngeal mask insertion (if considered safe), or awake tracheostomy. Blood and secretions in the airway preclude the use of the fiberoptic scope, as does a large hematoma that completely occludes the airway. Asleep fiberoptic intubation is an alternative but movement at the OAA may occur if forceful jaw thrust is required to open the airway occluded by the soft tissues of the oropharynx.

Cervical Spine Movement with Supraglottic Devices

The movement of the cervical spine produced by the combitube and LMA is greater than with the McCoy laryngoscope. This may be irrelevant if the reason for difficulty is a fixed neck, as in ankylosing spondylitis, where an LMA may be a suitable rescue airway device in the "can't intubate, can't ventilate" scenario.

Extubation

Extubation after cervical spine surgery requires the same degree of planning and consideration as intubation. In addition to the presenting problems the patient may now have airway edema, secondary to prolonged prone or Trendelenburg positioning, and a fixed or fused cervical spine. The DAS guidelines for extubation in "at risk" patients, includes:

- Planning for emergency reintubation (should extubation fail)
- Optimization of cardiorespiratory systems
- Correction of metabolic derangements and temperature
- Assessment of whether extubation is safe

When attempting extubation the patient should be awake, able to follow commands and have normal airway reflexes.

Guidelines for Airway Management in Trauma

The ASA Closed Head Injury Algorithm, the ASA Cervical Spine Injury Algorithm, the ASA Difficult Airway Algorithm (modified for Trauma), and the Eastern Association for the Surgery of Trauma (EAST) Practice Management Guidelines, all recognize the importance of intubation and ventilation, but also the potential difficulty the anesthetist faces. In summary, the recommendations do not support one single correct method of intubation. Nonetheless, emphasis is placed on the need for adequate airway assessment,

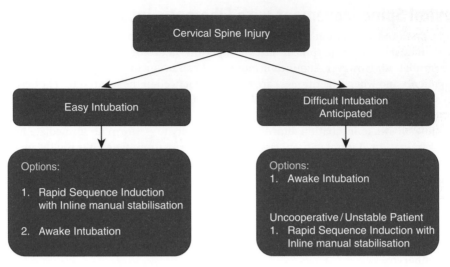

Figure 25.2 Airway management for cervical spine injury.

planning for a second airway management option if required and the maintenance of cervical spine immobilization (Figure 25.2).

Further Reading

Aziz, M.: Use of video-assisted intubation devices in the management of patients with trauma. *Anesthesiol Clin* 2013; **31**(1):157–166.

Crosby, E.T.: Airway management in adults after cervical spine trauma. *Anesthesiology* 2006;**104**(6):1293–1318.

Foulds, L.T., McGuire, B.E., Shippey, B.J.: A randomised cross-over trial comparing the McGrath((R)) Series 5 videolaryngoscope with the Macintosh laryngoscope in patients with cervical spine immobilisation. *Anaesthesia* 2016;**71**(4):437–442.

Suppan, L., Tramer, M.R., Niquille, M., Grosgurin, O., Marti, C.: Alternative intubation techniques vs Macintosh laryngoscopy in patients with cervical spine immobilization: Systematic review and meta-analysis of randomized controlled trials. *Br J Anaesth* 2016;**116**(1):27–36.

Popat, M., Mitchell, V., Dravid, R., et al: Difficult Airway Society Guidelines for the management of tracheal extubation. *Anaesthesia* 2012; **67**(3): 318–340.

Carotid Endarterectomy

Chapter 26

Jason Chui and Ian Herrick

Key Points

- The effectiveness and durability of CEA have been rigorously validated over the past three decades and it remains the gold standard surgical treatment for the secondary prevention of stroke in patients with advanced carotid atherosclerosis.
- Patients presenting for CEA frequently have a high burden of co-morbidities.
- Preoperative assessment should include: (1) risk stratification, (2) evaluation of the benefits and risks of revascularization, (3) optimization of pre-existing medical conditions, (4) identification of cardiac conditions and risk factors that merit management, and (5) formulation of an anesthetic plan.
- The main anesthetic goals are maintenance of hemodynamic stability with strict blood pressure control and preservation of cerebral perfusion throughout the perioperative period.
- CEA can be performed safely under regional or general anesthesia.
- Careful postoperative monitoring and vigilance is warranted to support timely recognition and intervention when complications arise (e.g., stroke, myocardial ischemia, hyperperfusion syndrome, neck hematoma).

Abbreviations

ACC	American College of Cardiology
ACT	Activated clotting time
AHA	American Heart Association
ASA	American Society of Anesthesiologists
CAS	Carotid angioplasty and stenting
CBF	Cerebral blood flow
CCA	Common carotid artery
CEA	Carotid endarterectomy
ECA	External carotid artery
ECG	Electrocardiograph
GA	General anesthesia
GALA	General anesthesia versus local anesthesia
ICA	Internal carotid artery
ICH	Intracranial hemorrhage
LA	Local anesthesia

NIBP   Non-invasive blood pressure
NIRS   Near infrared spectroscopy
RCR   Revised cardiac risk
SBP   Systolic Blood pressure
TCD   Transcranial doppler
TIA   Transient ischemic attack

Contents

- Introduction
- Indication for Surgery
- Preoperative Assessment
- Anesthetic Goals
- Mode of Anesthesia
  - General Anesthesia
  - Local Anesthesia
- Carotid Cross-Clamping
- Neurological Monitoring
- Postoperative Management
- Further Reading

Introduction

CEA involves the surgical removal of atherosclerotic plaque from the lumen of the extracranial portion of the carotid artery. Introduced in the early 1950s, CEA rapidly gained popularity as an intuitively appealing procedure directed at the surgical prevention of stroke. CEA has emerged, based on several large, international, randomized clinical trials as the "gold standard" surgical treatment, when combined with best medical therapy, for the prevention of stroke in patients with advanced extracranial carotid disease. Other cerebral revascularization procedures, specifically CAS, have been validated as alternative treatments in selected patients. CEA continues to represent a challenging procedure from an anesthesiologist's perspective as CBF is deliberately disturbed and many patients presenting for these procedures also have significant underlying cardiac disease and other comorbidities.

Indication for Surgery

Patients undergoing CEA may be symptomatic or asymptomatic with respect to their disease. Symptomatic patients present with a TIA or stroke. The primary aim of CEA is the secondary prevention of stroke in patients with advanced carotid atherosclerosis. Surgical intervention is indicated when the benefit of stroke risk reduction outweighs the surgical risk which is typically a 30-day risk of perioperative stroke or death. Recommendations from the AHA define complication rates that favor surgical benefit:

- In symptomatic patients with 70%–99% stenosis the surgical risk should be <6%.
- In asymptomatic patients with 60%–99% stenosis the surgical risk should be <3%.

Preoperative Assessment

The aims of preoperative assessment of patients presenting for CEA include: (1) risk stratification, (2) evaluation of the benefits and risks of revascularization, (3) optimization of pre-existing medical conditions, (4) identification of cardiac conditions or risk factors that warrant management, and (5) formulation of an anesthetic plan.

Preoperative assessment and optimization of symptomatic patients should be conducted expeditiously as the treatment benefit of CEA declines rapidly following the stroke event. Ischemic heart disease, a history of myocardial infarction or heart failure, and diabetes mellitus are prevalent among these patients. Considering that myocardial infarction is a major cause of perioperative mortality following CEA, cardiac evaluation represents an important part of preoperative assessment. There is no cardiac triage algorithm specific to patients presenting for CEA (e.g., indications for coronary angiography, etc.), as most studies that have focused on preoperative assessment and testing have traditionally excluded patients with severe carotid stenosis. Nevertheless, the approach to these patients generally follows the ACC/AHA guidelines for cardiac evaluation of patients undergoing non-cardiac surgery.

Neurological assessment should evaluate the risk of perioperative stroke. The risk of stroke is increased in patients with high-grade carotid stenosis, severe or unstable neurological symptoms (e.g., crescendo TIAs), inadequate collateral circulation or the presence of carotid ulceration/thrombus or an underlying hypercoagulable state. Other comorbidities such as hypertension, diabetes mellitus, chronic obstructive lung disease, and renal impairment which are common in patients presenting for CEA should be carefully evaluated and optimized. Several tools (e.g., Sundt, Halm, and Tu indices) have been devised to evaluate perioperative risk associated with CEA but the conventional risk stratification indices (i.e., the ASA Physical Status Classification and the Goldman, Detsky and RCR indices) are widely used and appear to perform similarly as predictors of postoperative cardiac and non-cardiac complications in patients presenting for CEA.

Antiplatelet medications, especially aspirin, should be continued throughout the perioperative period for prevention of postoperative carotid thrombosis. Continuation of thienopyridine agents such as clopidogrel (in addition to aspirin) may increase the bleeding risk and management of these drugs should be discussed with the surgical team. Other medications such as statins, anti-anginal, and anti-hypertensive medications including beta-blocking drugs should be continued preoperatively.

Anesthetic Goals

The primary anesthetic goals include: (1) maintenance of strict hemodynamic control to promote cerebral perfusion and CBF, (2) avoidance of secondary insults to the brain (e.g., hypoglycemia, hyperthermia, hypoxia), and (3) vigilance for potential perioperative complications, especially cardiac ischemia and neck hematoma.

SBP should be aggressively maintained at the patient's baseline level or slight hypertension (within 20% of baseline) prior to reperfusion (i.e., completion of the endarterectomy and re-establishment of cerebral circulation). Infusion of a vasoconstrictor such as phenylephrine or norepinephrine may be required to maintain cerebral perfusion pressure prior to reperfusion. The carbon dioxide reactivity of cerebral blood vessels is often impaired in patients undergoing CEA making the effects of hypocarbia or hypercarbia less predictable. Consequently, maintenance of normocarbia is recommended.

Mode of Anesthesia

The most appropriate choice of anesthetic technique, regional versus general anesthesia, has been the subject of intense debate and investigation for many years. The long-awaited GALA trial, a prospective, multi-center study involving 3526 patients in 24 countries, failed to demonstrate the superiority of either general or regional anesthesia for CEA based on the composite outcomes of stroke, myocardial infarction, and death. Some of the advantages and disadvantages of general and regional anesthesia are listed in Table 26.1. Given similar outcomes, the choice of technique should be based on patient factors, discussion with the surgeon, and familiarity and experience with the technique. The key stages associated with anesthetic management for CEA are outlined in Box 26.1.

General Anesthesia

General anesthesia remains the most popular anesthetic technique for CEA although there is limited evidence to support the use of any specific anesthetic drug or combination. Instead, the more important considerations include selection of a technique that promotes hemodynamic stability, smooth emergence, and facilitates early postoperative assessment. If intraoperative neurophysiologic monitoring is planned, anesthetic choices should avoid agents that compromise its reliability.

Local Anesthesia

Superficial cervical plexus block or local anesthetic infiltration by the surgeon are the most common techniques used for local/regional anesthesia. Deep cervical plexus block is not

Table 26.1 Advantages and Disadvantages of General and Regional Anesthesia for CEA

	Advantages	Disadvantages
General anesthesia	• Immobility • Suitable for anxious patients • Control of ventilation/CO_2 • Better suppression of autonomic reflexes • Facilitates management of complications such as stroke	• May result in significant hemodynamic changes during induction and emergence • Higher risk of complicating events such as difficult airway, delayed emergence, postoperative nausea, and vomiting • Requires surrogate monitor to assess carotid cross-clamping intolerance
Regional anesthesia	• Facilitates intraoperative neurological assessment with awake patient • Generally, less expensive • Potentially better neuro-cognitive performance in early postoperative period • Some reports of shorter length of hospital stay	• Less control of ventilation and CO_2 • Failure to tolerate prolonged procedure • May require conversion to GA for intraoperative complications (e.g., stroke, seizure, over-sedation, or agitation) • Complications related to cervical plexus block, if used (e.g., Horner's syndrome, phrenic nerve block, recurrent laryngeal nerve block, or LA toxicity)

BOX 26.1 Key Stages Associated with Anesthetic Management for CEA

1. Attach standard monitors (e.g., 5-lead ECG, SpO2, NIBP).
2. Arterial line insertion and preparation for neurophysiologic monitoring if planned (e.g., cerebral oximetry) and complete baseline assessment, if appropriate.
3. For general anesthesia

   a. Goal: Maintain cerebral perfusion (hemodynamic stability).
   b. Reinforced tracheal tube may avoid kinking or external compression during dissection.

4. For regional/local anesthesia

   a. Supplemental oxygen with CO_2 monitoring.
   b. Supplemental sedation (e.g., propofol or dexmedetomidine).
   c. Superficial cervical plexus block or subcutaneous infiltration.

5. Position: supine with neck slightly extended and rotated away from operative side.
6. Surgical Dissection

   a. Bradycardia, hypotension or hypertension may accompany manipulation of carotid sinus. Glycopyrrolate or atropine should be available. Local anesthetic infiltration of the carotid sinus during dissection may attenuate bradycardia and hypertension but can result in persistent hypotension.
   b. Hypertension may be due to visceral pain or signify cerebral ischemia – vigilance is warranted.
   c. Surgical retraction can cause cranial nerve dysfunction.

7. Heparinization: typically, 75–100 U/kg (target to double the baseline ACT) just prior to cross-clamping the carotid artery.
8. Carotid cross-clamping

   a. Cross-clamp sequence: distal ICA, proximal CCA and finally distal ECA (mnemonic ICE).
   b. Often associated with slight rise in BP because of loss of carotid sinus stretch (baroreflex).
   c. Modest induced hypertension (~20% above baseline BP) may be considered if evidence of cross-clamp intolerance (assessed by awake neurological evaluation when regional/local anesthesia used or neurophysiologic monitoring when surgery performed under general anesthesia).
   d. Consider shunt strategy: Routine, selective, or no shunt based on surgeon's preference and outcome of neurological assessment.

9. Arteriotomy and plaque removal.
10. Closure of arteriotomy: primary, patch arterioplasty, or eversion arterioplasty.
11. De-clamping (ECA, CCA, and then ICA) with reperfusion.
12. Meticulous wound hemostasis.
13. Management of anticoagulation. Consider reversal of heparin with protamine depending on the last dose of heparin, last ACT result, and surgeon's preference.
14. Skin closure.
15. Plan for smooth emergence with minimal strain on freshly repaired arteriotomy and transfer to recovery room (or high dependency unit) for observation.

popular for CEA since it is technically more difficult to perform and has been reported to have a higher risk of complications and conversion to general anesthesia. Supplemental sedation is usually used and common regimens include propofol or dexmedetomidine by infusion, with or without supplemental opioid (e.g., remifentanil or fentanyl). Access to the patient, particularly for airway support and monitoring of neurological status, is important when performing the procedure under regional or local anesthesia.

Carotid Cross-Clamping

Carotid cross-clamping isolates the extracranial portion of the diseased ICA allowing the surgeon to remove the atheromatous plaque. Occlusion of one ICA during CEA is associated with a risk of cerebral ischemia. Multiple factors contribute to the adequacy of cerebral perfusion during carotid cross-clamping including: (1) the adequacy of blood supply from collaterals, the contralateral carotid artery and the vertebrobasilar circulation, (2) the SBP and cardiac output, (3) the cerebral metabolic requirement, and (4) the duration of cross-clamping.

In practice, cross-clamp intolerance is managed by inducing a modest increase in SBP (typically to 20% above baseline) and/or insertion of an intra-carotid shunt that uses a specially designed silicone tube to bypass the arteriotomy to restore CBF. There are three strategies for shunt use: routine shunting (used for all patients), selective shunting (used in a subgroup of patients at high risk for cross-clamp intolerance) and no shunting.

The controversy surrounding the decision to deploy a shunt during CEA pertains to the fact that, despite the intent to restore brain perfusion, shunt use is also occasionally associated with complications that include cerebral embolism (atheromatous debris or air) and carotid artery dissection. Current evidence has failed to demonstrate an outcome benefit (30-day risk of stroke or death) associated with the routine or selective use of shunts. Despite longstanding controversy, a recent systematic review reported that few published studies met appropriate methodological criteria for inclusion and consequently available data was insufficient to identify a difference in outcome with selective or routine shunting. The choice of shunt strategy is therefore largely based on the preference of the surgeon.

Neurological Monitoring

The primary aim of neurological monitoring during CEA is to identify patients at risk of cross-clamping intolerance when a selective shunt strategy is used. Proponents of CEA performed under regional or local anesthesia cite the benefit of assessing cross-clamp tolerance in an awake patient. When general anesthesia is used for CEA, alternative monitoring techniques are often employed to evaluate the neurophysiologic response to cross-clamp application (e.g., electroencephalography, TCD, evoked potential monitoring, NIRS, carotid stump pressure measurement, etc.). However, the diagnostic test accuracies of all currently available neurophysiologic monitoring modalities are inadequate as sole confirmatory tests to identify cerebral ischemia. Despite these considerations, some form of neurophysiologic monitoring remains popular among surgeons who favor selective shunting.

Postoperative Management

Emergence and the early postoperative stage following CEA remain high risk periods. Emergence should be smooth with minimal strain to the freshly repaired arteriotomy site. Early awakening is preferred, in the absence of intraoperative complications, to facilitate postoperative assessment. Continuous monitoring of SBP, ECG, and oxygen saturation should be continued, and supplemental oxygen should be administered in the recovery room. Common complications arising in the postoperative period are summarized in Table 26.2.

Table 26.2 Summary of Perioperative Complications Associated with CEA

Complications	Mechanism	Notes
Myocardial infarction	• Unknown, may related to perioperative stress response • Some evidence linking increased risk to intraoperative use of vasopressor infusions	• Incidence ~ 2.3%* • 13%* of patients experience an asymptomatic postoperative increase in troponin • Incidence appears to be declining possibly because of more aggressive preoperative medical management
Stroke	Thromboembolic stroke	• Overall incidence 3.2%[#] (symptomatic patients); 1.4%[#] (asymptomatic patients) • Accounts for majority of strokes following CEA • Typically, embolic from endarterectomy site
	Acute Carotid thrombosis	• Technical error results in intimal flap and mural thrombus • Carotid artery dissection • Immediate reoperation to re-establish cerebral perfusion
	Intracerebral hemorrhage	• Often related to cerebral hyperperfusion syndrome or uncontrolled hypertension • Higher risk in patient with severe stenosis and poor collateral circulation
Hyper-perfusion syndrome	Dramatic increase in CBF following repair of stenotic vessel	• Pooled incidence 1.9%* • Ipsilateral headache, facial and eye pain, cerebral edema, seizure. and ICH • Relieved by upright posture • CBF usually exceeds 100% increase from baseline • Aggressive control of BP reduces risk

Table 26.2 (cont.)

Complications	Mechanism	Notes
Carotid hematoma	Surgical bleeding	• Incidence 7%* • Presents with hoarseness, neck swelling, dyspnea, dysphagia, and tracheal deviation, • Requires emergency intubation and surgical exploration • May produce challenging airway conditions for re-intubation
Cranial nerve palsy	Usually due to mechanical injury	• Overall incidence: 5%–12%* • Most common recurrent or superior laryngeal nerve palsy • Can present with hoarseness; usually temporary, rarely leads to airway obstruction • Other cranial nerves, hypoglossal nerve, vagus nerve, and branches of the facial nerve, can be injured

*From Herrick I. et al. (2016)
#From Brott T.G. et al. (2011)

Hemodynamic instability is common following CEA due to baroreceptor dysfunction following surgical manipulation. This may manifest as hypertension or hypotension. Other causes of hemodynamic instability after CEA should not be overlooked (e.g., myocardial ischemia, dysrhythmias, hypoxia, hypercarbia, pneumothorax, pain, confusion, stroke, and bladder distention).

Poorly controlled postoperative hypertension is a major risk factor for cerebral hyperperfusion syndrome. Risk is mitigated by maintaining systolic BP <140 mmHg. Neck circumference should be monitored and evidence of an expanding neck hematoma represents a surgical emergency for reintubation and urgent exploration.

Most patients will be admitted to a high-dependency (or step-down) unit for observation and monitoring. Patients should resume aspirin in the postoperative period to reduce the risk of postoperative acute carotid thrombosis.

Further Reading

Bouri, S., Thapar A., Shalhoub, J., et al: Hypertension and post-carotid endarterectomy cerebral hyperperfusion syndrome. *Eur J Vasc Endovasc Surg: The Official Journal of the European Society for Vascular Surgery* 2011; **41**(2):229–237.

Brott, T.G., Halperin, J.L., Abbara, S., et al (2013). 2011 ASA/ACCF/AHA/AANN/AANS/ ACR/ASNR/CNS/SAIP/SCAI/SIR/SNIS/SVM/ SVS guideline on the management of patients with extracranial carotid and vertebral artery disease: executive summary: A report of the American College of Cardiology Foundation/ American Heart Association Task Force on Practice Guidelines, and the American Stroke Association, American Association of Neuroscience Nurses, American Association of

Neurological Surgeons, American College of Radiology, American Society of Neuroradiology, Congress of Neurological Surgeons, Society of Atherosclerosis Imaging and Prevention, Society for Cardiovascular Angiography and Interventions, Society of Interventional Radiology, Society of NeuroInterventional Surgery, Society for Vascular Medicine, and Society for Vascular Surgery. Developed in collaboration with the American Academy of Neurology and Society of Cardiovascular Computed Tomography. Catheterization and Cardiovascular Interventions: Official Journal of the Society for Cardiac Angiography & Interventions, 81(1), E76–123.

Chongruksut, W., Vaniyapong, T., Rerkasem, K.: Routine or selective carotid artery shunting for carotid endarterectomy (and different methods of monitoring in selective shunting). *Cochrane Database Syst Rev* 2014; **6**:CD000190.

Guay, J., Kopp, S.: Cerebral monitors versus regional anesthesia to detect cerebral ischemia in patients undergoing carotid endarterectomy: A meta-analysis. *Can J Anaesth* 2013; **60**(3): 266–279.

Herrick, I., Chui, J., Higashida, R.T., et al: Chapter 16. Occlusive cerebrovascular disease: Anesthetic considerations. In Cottrell, J.E., Patel, P. (Eds.). *Neuroanesthesia*, 6th ed. NewYork, NY: Elsevier; 2016.

Lewis, S.C., Warlow, C.P., Bodenham, A.R., et al: General anaesthesia versus local anaesthesia for carotid surgery (GALA): A multicentre, randomised controlled trial. *Lancet* (London, England), 2008; **372**(9656):2132–2142.

Pandit, J.J., Satya-Krishna, R., Gration, P.: Superficial or deep cervical plexus block for carotid endarterectomy: A systematic review of complications. *Brit J Anaesth* 2007; **99**(2):159–169.

Shakespeare, W.A., Lanier, W.L., Perkins, W.J., Pasternak, J.J.: Airway management in patients who develop neck hematomas after carotid endarterectomy. *Anesth Analg* 2010; **110**(2):588–593.

Chapter 27

Anesthesia and Sedation for Neuroimaging

Tamsin Gregory

Key Points

- Neuroradiology plays an important part in neurological diagnosis and is an essential prerequisite to neurosurgical, neuroradiological, and neurointensive care interventions.
- Using a variety of imaging techniques, structural, and functional data relating to the brain and spinal cord can be obtained and interventional procedures can be performed.
- All individuals involved in the management of patients undergoing neuroradiological procedures must understand the principles of the techniques to ensure safety for patients and other healthcare personnel.
- The conduct of sedation and general anesthesia must reach the same standards as that available in the operating room.

Abbreviations

CBF	Cerebral blood flow
CBV	Cerebral blood volume
CI-AKI	Contrast-induced acute kidney injury
CT	Computed tomography
ECG	Electrocardiograph
fMRI	Functional magnetic resonance imaging
G	Gauss
MR	Magnetic resonance
MRI	Magnetic resonance imaging
T	Tesla

Contents

- Introduction
- Imaging Techniques

  - Computer Tomography
  - Magnetic Resonance Imaging
  - Interventional Neuroradiology

- Gamma Camera Imaging, Single-Photon Emission Computed Tomography, and Positron Emission Tomography
- Safety Concerns within the Imaging Environment
  - Radiation
  - MRI Safety
  - Contrast Agents
- Anesthesia and Sedation
- Further Reading

Introduction

Neuroradiology has seen the development of complex techniques and interventional procedures for patients with a variety of neurological disorders. These involve an increasing input from the neuroanesthetist and neuro-critical care physician who need to carefully manage prolonged procedures performed in sites remote from the operating theatre and on an aging population with multiple medical comorbidities.

Imaging Techniques

Computed Tomography

CT, using ionizing radiation, provides the ability to image in detail structures of the brain and spinal along with other organ systems. In addition, rapid sequential imaging before and after the administration of intravenous contrast allows CT angiography which can be used to calculate CBF and CBV. Imaging after the inhalation of 28% xenon can also be used to measure CBF. Stereotactic surgery which uses data from either CT or MRI modalities is used to improve surgical planning for minimally invasive excision of intracranial lesions or functional neurosurgery. In framed stereotaxy, a mechanical frame is attached to the patient's head, CT or MRI is performed, and a three-dimensional image of the patient's brain is computed. In frameless stereotaxy, the initial CT or MRI is stored onto a computer and fixed points on the skull are mapped onto the image with a sensor wand.

Magnetic Resonance Imaging

During MRI data acquisition, powerful static magnetic fields and intermittingly oscillating radiofrequency fields produce an image that is dependent on the distribution of hydrogen atoms in the body. Magnetic field strengths are measured in tesla (T) and gauss (G) where one tesla equals 10,000 G. The magnetic field strength of the earth is 0.5–1.5 G. Field strengths in clinical MRI range from 0.05 to 3 T. MRI which provides high-resolution structural images can also be adapted using different data acquisition protocols to provide functional activation information about various areas of the brain. This technique is known as functional MRI (fMRI). With the use of contrast agents, magnetic resonance angiography can demonstrate vascular patency while more rapid imaging can be used to generate data relating to cerebral perfusion. Evidence of cerebral ischemia and impending tissue necrosis can be determined with perfusion and diffusion-weighted imaging which can be very useful to the neuro-critical care physician. Magnetic resonance spectroscopy provides in vivo biochemical analysis of a variety of markers of cellular function including lactate and glutamate.

Intraoperative MRI involves scanning the patient during the surgical procedure. It allows the surgeon to avoid critical structures and ensure that surgical resection is complete. Surgery can either be continued during the procedure or halted to allow imaging to occur.

Interventional Neuroradiology

Flow-directed microcatheters are introduced into the blood vessels usually via the femoral artery under local or general anesthesia and manipulated through vertebral or carotid arteries to visualize the intracranial vessels. The venous circulation may also be imaged via the femoral or jugular veins. With the use of digital subtraction software, information relating to non-vascular structures can be removed from an image. After injection of a contrast agent, the resulting image of vascular anatomy can be saved as a "road map", and further fluoroscopic images can then be superimposed over this to aid manipulation and advancement of the microcatheter within the relevant cerebral vessel. This technique obviously requires the patient to remain immobile, although repeated injections can be used to update the road map image. Once the microcatheter is in the appropriate place, a variety of devices and drugs, including microcoils, stents, balloons, glue, thrombolytic drugs, sclerosing agents, and chemotherapeutic medicines can be introduced. Procedures that can be performed using this technique include diagnostic angiography, coiling of cerebral aneurysms, embolization of arteriovenous malformations, percutaneous transluminal angioplasty, and intravascular thrombolysis. Patients must remain immobile during these procedures to avoid complications including rupture or intimal tearing of vessels. Interventional neuroradiology is described in more detail in Chapter 28.

Gamma Camera Imaging, Single-Photon Emission Computed Tomography, and Positron Emission Tomography

Single-photon emission CT uses conventional γ-emitting nuclear medicine isotopes with multiple detectors to generate tomographic images of CBF that are nonquantitative. Positive emission tomography is a research technique in which isotopes such as ^{15}O and ^{18}F emit positrons. Annihilation of these positrons, resulting in gamma ray photons, can be localized in space by pairs of gamma detectors providing whole-brain quantitative imaging of many aspects of cerebral physiology including CBF, CBV, and oxidative and glucose metabolism.

Safety Concerns within the Imaging Environment

Radiation

All the previously described techniques, except MRI, involve exposure to ionizing radiation. To limit exposure to staff members, the maximum distance possible should be maintained from the X-ray source. Standard precautions including lead glass shields, lead aprons, thyroid shields, and protective glasses together with radiation exposure badges should be used by staff members in selected settings to limit the cumulative radiation burden. Female patients should have a negative pregnancy test before undergoing any procedure.

MRI Safety

Although exposure to magnetic fields is generally thought to be safe, unnecessary exposure to high strength fields should be minimized. Exposure can be reduced using custom-designed MRI monitoring equipment with slave patient monitors placed outside the MRI scanning room. No effects of MRI on the fetus have been documented but it is recommended pregnant women only undergo MRI if absolutely essential. The rapid alteration of magnetic fields during an MRI scan produces tapping or knocking noises which can be as loud as 140 dB so ear protection should be worn in the scanning room during the procedure.

Adverse incidents involving patients, equipment, and personal continue to occur within MRI scanners, thus underlining the importance of users understanding the MRI environment and ensuring that safe practice is observed. The magnetic field within the scanning environment is based on a cryogenic superconducting magnet that is maintained at −273°C by emersion in liquid helium. The helium can boil off ("quench") rapidly if the temperature rises. This has the potential to dilute room oxygen, and the cold vapor can cause frostbite and burns. Any loose ferromagnetic object can become a dangerous projectile and should not be taken into the MRI suite unless known to be safe. Even implanted ferromagnetic objects may move depending on their size and location (e.g., cochlear implants and aneurysm clips). Patients with an intracranial aneurysm clip should not undergo an MRI unless the clip has been documented not to be ferromagnetic. Nonferromagnetic implants can result in significant image distortion or cause local burns as their temperature is increased in the presence of radiofrequency currents. Deaths in patients with cardiac pacemakers have been reported as the magnetic field can cause the reed switch on pacemakers to stick and revert to a fixed-rate mode in which delivery of a pacing spike on the upstroke of a T wave can result in an R on T phenomenon and possibly trigger ventricular dysrhythmias. Therefore, MRI is usually contraindicated in patients with pacemakers and other implantable electronic devices unless they are known to function safely. However, MR compatible pacemakers are increasingly available for selected patients. If there is any doubt about the safety of implants, they should be checked against the manufacturers' specifications before the patient enters the MRI room. MRI units usually have a comprehensive checklist for patients and staff to complete to exclude the presence of implants. Devices are known as MRI *safe* when they do not pose a risk to the patient and MRI *compatible* when they continue to function in the MRI environment.

Although there are difficulties in the use of monitoring and anesthetic equipment within the MRI suite, integrated monitoring and anesthetic systems designed for use in the MRI environment are widely available and represent the standard of care. Many sensors are MRI safe but may not be MRI compatible and produce image artifacts. Leads from such devices present a particular risk because induced currents may result in burns. Electrocardiographic (ECG) monitoring within the MRI scanner is particularly problematic. Changes in T waves and ST segments can mimic hyperkalemia or pericarditis and radiofrequency produces ECG artefacts.

Contrast Agents

Patients can receive significant volumes of contrast agents during CT, angiographic, and MRI procedures and some are at risk of contrast-induced acute kidney injury (CI-AKI) as a result of the use of these agents. All patients should have their plasma creatinine levels and glomerular filtration rate checked prior to the procedure. Limiting the dose of contrast agents and maintaining good hydration pre- and post-procedure will lessen the risk of CI-AKI.

Anesthesia and Sedation

Anesthesia and sedation outside the operating theatre can be challenging as neuroradiological procedures have become more complex and prolonged. Additionally, many of these sites are not specifically designed for the delivery of anesthesia. Rooms may be darkened to provide optimal image viewing and access to the patient may be limited by radiological equipment. The risks associated with non-theater environment anesthesia and sedation can be minimized by proper planning and anesthetic provision. Most diagnostic procedures can be performed with sedation and local anesthesia. Midazolam, fentanyl, low-dose remifentanil, propofol, dexmedetomidine are all suitable. However, general anesthesia may be required for children, failed sedation, cases of claustrophobia and anxiety, and patients with movement disorders or learning disabilities. High-dose sedation may not be appropriate for those with concurrent medical disease or with raised intracranial pressure. General anesthesia may be required for prolonged and uncomfortable procedures and for critically ill patients requiring positive pressure ventilation. The anesthetic technique used should aim to maintain cerebral physiology by optimizing cerebral perfusion and controlling the intracranial pressure while providing the optimal conditions for the neuroradiolgist which should be determined by discussion before the case begins. Both volatile and intravenous anesthesia can be used and the specific choice depends on the circumstances.

Patients should be carefully positioned on the narrow scanning table. Consideration should be given to how the imagining equipment moves during the procedure and the subsequent risk of dislodgement of airway tubing, lines, and monitoring equipment. Patients should be adequately monitored while being transferred to and from the scanning room and throughout the procedure. The same standards of monitoring and general anesthesia should be available in remote locations as in the operating theater, including the routine use of capnography for all patients undergoing sedation. All personnel should be familiar with emergency protocols, and attention should be paid to any specific hazards of the environment.

Further Reading

Arlachov, Y., Ganatra, R.H.: Sedation/anaesthesia in paediatric radiology. *Br J radiol* 2012; **85**(1019):e1018–e1031.

Arthurs, O.J., Sury, M.: Anaesthesia or sedation for paediatric MRI: Advantages and disadvantages. *Curr opin Anaesthesiol* 2013; **26**(4):489–494.

Crute, D., Sebeo, J., Osborn, I.P.: Neuroimaging for the anesthesiologist. *Anesthesiol clin* 2012; **30**(2):149–173.

Henrichs, B., Walsh, R.P.: Intraoperative MRI for neurosurgical and general surgical interventions. *Curr opin anaesthesiol* 2014; **27**(4):448–452.

Landrigan-Ossar, M.: Common procedures and strategies for anaesthesia in interventional radiology. *Curr opin anaesthesiol* 2015; **28**(4):458–463.

Landrigan-Ossar, M., McClain, C.D.: Anesthesia for interventional radiology. *Paediatr anaesth* 2014; **24**(7):698–702.

Schulenburg, E., Matta, B.: Anaesthesia for interventional neuroradiology. *Curr opin anaesthesiol* 2011; **24**(4):426–432.

Tsai, L.L., Grant, A.K., Mortele, K.J., Kung, J.W., Smith, M.P.: A practical guide to MR imaging safety: What radiologists need to know. *Radiographics: A review publication of the radiological society of North America, Inc* 2015; **35**(6):1722–1737.

Chapter 28

Anesthesia for Interventional Neuroradiology

Chanhung Lee

Key Points

- Baseline blood pressure and cardiovascular reserve should be assessed carefully especially when blood pressure manipulation and perturbations are anticipated.
- Maintaining patient immobility during the procedure will facilitate imaging.
- Careful management of coagulation is required to prevent thromboembolic and hemorrhagic complications during and after the procedure.
- Complications during endovascular instrumentation of the cerebral vasculature can be rapid and life-threatening, and require multidisciplinary collaboration.
- Signs of hemodynamic instability or neurologic deterioration need to be monitored during the post-operative period.

Abbreviations

ACT   Activated clotting time
ARUBA   A randomized trial of unruptured brain arteriovenous malformations
BAVM   Brain arteriovenous malformation
CT   Computed tomography
ICU   Intensive care unit
INR   Interventional neuroradiology
ISAT   International subarachnoid aneurysm trial
MRI   Magnetic resonance imaging

Contents

- Introduction
- Pre-anesthetic Considerations
- Monitoring and Vascular Access
- Anesthetic Technique
  - Intravenous Sedation
  - General Anesthesia
- Anticoagulation
- Deliberate Hypotension

Introduction

This chapter focuses on anesthetic management for major INR procedures, including treatment of cerebral aneurysms, carotid stenosis, ischemic stroke, and BAVMs. INR may be broadly defined as treatment of central nervous system disease by endovascular access allowing delivery of therapeutic agents, including both drugs and devices. Because of rapid advances in INR, anesthesiologists are increasingly involved in this arena.

Pre-anesthetic Considerations

Baseline blood pressure and cardiovascular reserve should be carefully assessed especially when blood pressure manipulation and perturbations are anticipated. Pre-operative calcium channel blockers used in vasospasm treatment or prophylaxis can affect hemodynamic stability.

For cases managed with an unsecured airway, routine evaluation of the potential ease of laryngoscopy in an emergency situation, should take into account that direct access to the airway may be limited by table or room logistics. The possibility of pregnancy in female patients and a history of adverse reactions to radiographic contrast agents should be explored.

Monitoring and Vascular Access

Secure intravenous access should have adequate extensions to allow drug and fluid administration at maximal distance from the image intensifier. Access to intravenous or arterial catheters can be difficult when the patient is draped and the arms are restrained at the sides. Therefore, all connections should be secure. Infusions of anticoagulant, anesthetics or vasoactive agents, should be through proximal ports with minimal dead space.

In addition to standard monitors, a pulse oximeter probe can be placed on a toe of the leg with the femoral introducer sheath to provide early warning of femoral artery obstruction or distal thromboembolism. Since a significant volume of heparinized flush solution and radiographic contrast is often used, bladder catheters can assist in fluid management as well as patient comfort. Some intracranial procedures and post-operative care may benefit from beat-to-beat arterial pressure monitoring and blood sampling. A side port of the femoral artery introducer sheath can be used, but the sheath will be removed immediately after the procedure.

Anesthetic Technique

The choice of anesthetic technique varies among centers and there is no clear superior method. Rapid recovery from anesthesia is often preferred for neurological evaluation.

Intravenous Sedation

Many neuro-angiographic procedures, while not painful per se, can be psychologically stressful. Careful padding of pressure points and assisting the patient to obtain a comfortable position improves their ability to tolerate long periods lying supine and motionless, decreasing the requirement for medication.

Sedation techniques may facilitate early detection of neurological deficits, their causality and prompt management. A variety of sedation regimens can be used and specific choices are based on the experience of the practitioner and the goals of anesthetic management. Common to all intravenous sedation techniques is the potential for upper airway obstruction. Placement of nasopharyngeal airways may cause troublesome bleeding in anticoagulated patients and is generally avoided.

General Anesthesia

There is an increasing trend to utilize general anesthesia as it allows temporary periods of apnea and control of motion during imaging, especially in children and uncooperative adults. The specific choice of anesthesia is guided primarily by cardio- and cerebrovascular considerations plus clinician preference. Total intravenous anesthetic techniques or combinations of inhalational and intravenous methods may optimize rapid emergence.

Anticoagulation

Careful management of coagulation is required to prevent thromboembolic complications during and after the procedures. Generally, after obtaining a baseline ACT, intravenous heparin (70 units/kg) is given to a target prolongation of two to three times baseline. Then heparin can be given continuously or as an intermittent bolus with hourly monitoring of ACT. At the end of the procedure, heparin may be reversed with protamine.

Antiplatelet agents (aspirin, ticlopidine, and the glycoprotein IIb/IIIa receptor antagonists) are used for cerebrovascular disease management, as well as for rescue from thromboembolic complications. There is no simple monitoring technique. Because of the long effective duration of action, rapid reversal of antiplatelet activity can only be achieved through platelet transfusion. Concomitant heparin use may synergistically predispose to hemorrhage. In addition, the use of newer anticoagulants requires a good understanding of their mechanisms of action for appropriate perioperative therapeutic strategies.

Deliberate Hypotension

The two primary indications for induced hypotension are (1) to test cerebrovascular reserve in patients about to undergo permanent carotid occlusion; and (2) to slow the flow in a feeding artery of BAVMs before glue injection. The choice of agent should be determined by the experience of the practitioner, the patient's medical condition, and the specific goals of blood pressure reduction.

Deliberate Hypertension

During acute arterial occlusion or vasospasm, the only practical way to increase collateral blood flow may be an augmentation of the collateral perfusion pressure by raising the systemic blood pressure. The extent to which the blood pressure must be raised depends on the condition of the patient and the nature of the disease. Typically, the systemic blood pressure is raised by 30%–40% above the baseline or until ischemic symptoms resolve. Phenylephrine is commonly the first-line agent and is titrated to achieve the desired level of blood pressure. The risk of causing hemorrhage into the ischemic area must be weighed against the benefits of improving perfusion.

Management of Neurological and Procedural Crises

A well-thought-out plan, coupled with rapid and effective communication between the anesthesia and radiology teams, is critical for good outcomes.

The primary responsibility of the anesthesia team is to preserve gas exchange and if indicated, secure the airway. Simultaneous with airway management, the first branch in the decision-making algorithm is for the anesthesiologist to communicate with the INR team and determine whether the problem is hemorrhagic or occlusive. In the setting of vascular occlusion, the goal is to increase distal perfusion by blood pressure augmentation with or without direct thrombolysis.

If the problem is hemorrhagic, immediate cessation of heparin and reversal with protamine is indicated. As an emergency reversal dose, 1 mg protamine can be given for each 100 units of initial heparin dosage that resulted in therapeutic anticoagulation. The ACT can then be used to fine-tune the final protamine dose. Complications of protamine administration include hypotension, anaphylaxis and pulmonary hypertension. With the advent of newer long-acting direct thrombin inhibitors, new strategies for emergent reversal of anticoagulation will need to be developed.

Bleeding catastrophes are usually heralded by headache, nausea, vomiting, and vascular pain related to the area of perforation. Sudden loss of consciousness is not always due to intracranial hemorrhage. Seizures, as a result of contrast reaction or transient ischemia and the resulting post-ictal state, can also result in an obtunded patient. In the anesthetized patient, the sudden onset of bradycardia or the endovascular therapist's diagnosis of extravasation of contrast may be the only clues to developing hemorrhage.

Post-operative Management

Endovascular surgery patients spend the immediate post-operative period in a monitored or ICU setting so that signs of hemodynamic instability or neurologic deterioration can be detected. Blood pressure control, either induced hypotension or induced hypertension, may be continued into the post-operative period. Complicated cases may need CT or MRI and require critical care management during transport and imaging.

Procedures for Specific Cerebrovascular Diseases

Intracranial Aneurysm

The ISAT trial has made coil embolization the first-choice for many lesions, with proximal artery occlusion used occasionally. The aneurysmal sac is usually obliterated by using coils.

The anesthesiologist should be prepared for aneurysmal rupture occurring either spontaneously or from direct injury of the aneurysm wall by vascular manipulation.

Angioplasty may be used to treat symptomatic vasospasm refractory to maximal medical therapy. It is also possible to perform a "pharmacologic" angioplasty on more distal branches by direct intra-arterial vasodilator infusion. Treatment with papaverine, calcium channel blockers (nicardipine and verapamil), and milrinone are also being used. Significant, transient hypotension is common with these agents.

Carotid Stenosis

Carotid angioplasty has comparable overall outcomes comparted to endarterectomy but myocardial infarction rate is lower and stroke rate higher. Improved methods of embolic protection will likely result in further increases in endovascular treatment.

Carotid sinus distention may cause (severe) bradycardia. Intravenous atropine or glycopyrrolate may be used but occasionally transcutaneous pacing may be needed. As many patients also have coronary artery disease, caution is needed when increasing heart rate.

Potential complications include vessel occlusion, perforation, dissection, spasm, thromboemboli, transient ischemic episodes, and stroke. There is about a 5% risk of symptomatic cerebral hemorrhage and/or brain swelling after carotid angioplasty. This syndrome is associated with cerebral hyperperfusion, and may be related to poor post-operative blood pressure control and severe pre-procedural carotid stenosis.

Ischemic Stroke

The accessibility of radiological treatment for ischemic stroke is becoming more widespread with evidence of good outcome with early intervention. The anesthetic management of this condition is described in greater detail in Chapter 36.

Brain Arteriovenous Malformations

These are typically complex lesions made up of a tangle of abnormal vessels (called the nidus), frequently containing several discrete fistulae served by multiple feeding arteries and draining veins. The primary focus in brain AVM management is to prevent initial and recurrent rupture that can result in life-threatening intracranial hemorrhage. The goal of therapeutic endovascular embolization is to obliterate as many of the fistulae and their respective feeding arteries as possible. BAVM embolization is usually an adjunct for surgery or radiotherapy, although in rare cases, treatment results in total obliteration. While recent study results, including ARUBA, show superiority of medical management in unruptured AVMs compared with any intervention, there are ongoing debates about the applicability to all patients.

The cyanoacrylate glues offer relatively "permanent" closure of abnormal vessels. Passage of glue into a draining vein can result in acute hemorrhage and in smaller patients, pulmonary embolism of glue can be symptomatic. For these reasons, deliberate hypotension may increase safety of glue delivery.

Summary

This chapter has discussed the main anesthetic concerns for INR procedures, in addition to routine management of anesthetized patients. Anesthesia management should facilitate imaging and the procedures. Appropriate hemodynamic control is crucial for many procedures and good patient outcome. Prompt communication with neuroradiologists is essential in managing crises.

Further Reading

Degos, V., Westbroek, E.M., Lawton, M.T., et al: Perioperative management of coagulation in non-traumatic intracerebral hemorrhage. *Anesthesiology* 2013; **119**(1):218–227.

Lee, C.Z., Gelb, A.W.: Anesthesia management for endovascular treatment. *Curr Opin Anaesthesiol* 2014; **27**(5):484–488.

Mohr, J.P., Parides, M.K., Stapf, C., et al: Medical management with or without interventional therapy for unruptured brain arteriovenous malformations (ARUBA): A multicentre, non-blinded, randomised trial. *Lancet*(London, England) 2014; **383**(9917):614–621.

Molyneux, A.J., Birks, J., Clarke, A., Sneade, M., Kerr, R.S.C.: The durability of endovascular coiling versus neurosurgical clipping of ruptured cerebral aneurysms: 18-year follow-up of the UK cohort of the International Subarachnoid Aneurysm Trial (ISAT). *Lancet* (London, England) 2015; **385** (9969):691–697.

Pandey, A.S., Elias, A.E., Chaudhary, N., Thompson, B.G., Gemmete, J.J.: Endovascular treatment of cerebral vasospasm: Vasodilators and angioplasty. *Neuroimaging Clin N Am* 2013; **23**(4):593–604.

Chapter 29

Anesthesia for Neurosurgery in Infants and Children

Sulpicio G. Soriano and Craig D. McClain

Key Points

- Age-related factors, including blood pressure, heart rate, hematocrit, and fluid requirements, must be incorporated into the preoperative evaluation, intraoperative management, and postoperative care of infants and children.
- Newborns present specific challenges for anesthetic care because of their unique physiology associated with cardiorespiratory, renal, and hepatic immaturity.
- The effects of neurological injury/abnormalities, including vomiting, electrolyte derangements, increased ICP, and side effects of therapeutic agents (e.g., mannitol, diuretics, corticosteroids), must be meticulously evaluated in the perioperative setting.
- Induction of anesthesia is dictated by the patient's comorbidities and neurological status.
- Patient positioning requires careful preoperative planning to allow adequate access to the patient for both the neurosurgeon and anesthesiologist.
- Meticulous fluid and blood administration is essential in order to minimize hemodynamic instability.
- Heat loss may be significant during lengthy procedures in infants. Systems to prevent significant hypothermia must be incorporated into the intraoperative plan.
- The severity of the intraoperative course dictates the need for admission to an intensive care unit. Factors such as massive blood loss, hemodynamic instability, neurological deficits, seizures, and prolonged surgical time necessitate the need for continued observation.

Abbreviations

AVM	Arteriovenous malformation
CNS	Central nervous system
CSF	Cerebrospinal fluid
DI	Diabetes insipidus
ECG	Electrocardiogram
EEG	Electroencephalography
ECMO	Extracorporeal membrane oxygenation
ICP	Intracranial pressure

PICC   Peripherally inserted central catheters
VAE   Venous air embolism

Contents

- Introduction
- Preoperative Evaluation and Optimization
- Intraoperative Management
  - Induction of Anesthesia
  - Vascular Access and Positioning
  - Maintenance of Anesthesia
  - Management of Fluids and Blood Loss
- Anesthetic Management of Specific Neurosurgical Procedures
  - Myelomeningoceles and Encephaloceles
  - Hydrocephalus
  - Posterior Fossa Tumors
  - Supratentorial Tumors
  - Epilepsy
  - Cerebrovascular Disease
  - Minimally Invasive Neurosurgery
- Postoperative Care
- Further Reading

Introduction

Age has a significant impact on the management of pediatric patients undergoing neuro-surgical procedures. Various organ systems are in a state of flux as the neonate and infant matures and these changes alter the way drugs and techniques are utilized during the perioperative period. The CNS undergoes a tremendous amount of structural and physio-logical change during the first two years of life. Age-dependent differences in cranial bone development, cerebrovascular physiology, and neurological lesions distinguish neonates, infants, and children from their adult counterparts and has necessitated the emergence of subspeciality pediatric training in neurosurgery, anesthesiology and intensive care medi-cine. The goal of this chapter is to highlight the developmental differences that occur in the pediatric neurosurgical patient and how this impacts on anesthetic management.

Preoperative Evaluation and Optimization

Due to the relative immaturity of cardiopulmonary systems, neonates and infants have the highest risk for perioperative morbidity and mortality than any age group. Surgery and anesthesia produce non-physiological insults on this vulnerable group, which are magni-fied when combined with underlying congenital anomalies that increase the risk for adverse outcomes. It is essential to thoroughly review the patient's history to reveal conditions that may increase the risk of adverse reactions to anesthesia and identify patients who require more extensive preoperative evaluation or whose medical condition needs to be optimized prior to surgery (Table 29.1). If a cardiac defect is suspected (loud

Table 29.1 Coexisting Conditions that Influence Anesthetic Management

Condition	Anesthetic Implications
Congenital heart disease	Hypoxia Arrhythmias Cardiovascular instability Paradoxical air emboli
Prematurity	Postoperative apnea
Gastrointestinal reflux	Aspiration pneumonia
Upper respiratory tract infection	Laryngospasm, bronchospasm Hypoxia, pneumonia
Craniofacial abnormality	Difficult tracheal intubation
Denervation injuries	Hyperkalemia after succinylcholine, Resistance to non-depolarizing muscle relaxants Abnormal response to nerve stimulation
Epilepsy	Hepatic and hematological abnormalities Increased metabolism of anesthetic agents Ketogenic diet
AVM	Congestive heart failure
Neuromuscular disease	Malignant hyperthermia Respiratory failure Sudden cardiac death
Chiari malformation	Apnea Aspiration pneumonia
Hypothalamic/pituitary lesions	Diabetes insipidus Hypothyroidism Adrenal insufficiency

Table 29.2 Physiologic Effects of Patient Positioning

Position	Physiological Effect
Head-up/sitting	Increased cerebral venous drainage Decreased cerebral blood flow Increased venous pooling in lower extremities Postural hypotension
Head-down	Increased cerebral venous and intracranial pressure Decreased functional residual capacity (lung function) Decreased lung compliance
Prone	Venous congestion of face, tongue, and neck Decreased lung compliance Venocaval compression
Lateral decubitus	Decreased compliance of dependent lung

cardiac murmur, low room air oxygen saturation, cyanosis or respiratory distress), it is mandatory to obtain an echocardiography and an assessment by a pediatric cardiologist in order to optimize cardiac function prior to surgery. Neonatal and infants with large cerebrovascular malformations may develop high-output congestive heart failure requiring the administration of vasoactive drugs. Preoperative angiography and possible embolization of these high-flow lesions by interventional neuroradiologists should precede surgery.

Hemodynamic and metabolic derangements may influence neurological outcomes in anesthetized patients undergoing surgery or those sedated for painful procedures. Factors that have been implicated in causing poor outcomes include control of perioperative blood pressure, carbon dioxide tension, hyperoxia or hypoxia, temperature, and serum glucose levels. In infants and toddlers, prolonged fasting periods and vomiting may induce hypovolemia and hypoglycemia, which can exacerbate hemodynamic and metabolic instability under anesthesia. This is especially important during an inhalational induction where hypotension and bradycardia can occur in a hypovolemic patient breathing high concentrations of sevoflurane.

Intraoperative Management

Induction of Anesthesia

A smooth transition into the operating suite depends on the level of anxiety and the cognitive development and age of the child. Children between the ages of 9–12 months and 6 years may have separation anxiety. Midazolam, administered orally or intravenously, is effective in relieving anxiety and producing amnesia. Parental involvement during induction of anesthesia is common in pediatric operating rooms and requires full engagement of the surgical team. Obtunded and lethargic patients do not require premedication with sedatives and should have an anesthetic induction performed in an expeditious manner.

Induction of anesthesia is dictated by the patient's comorbidities and neurological status. If the patient does not have intravenous access, an inhalational induction with sevoflurane, nitrous oxide, and oxygen may be necessary. Intracranial hypertension is intensified with hypercarbia and hypoxia, which may occur if the airway becomes obstructed during induction but maintenance of a patent airway with mild hyperventilation will alleviate this problem. In patients with intravenous access, anesthesia can be induced with propofol. Some patients presenting for neurosurgical procedures may be at particular risk for aspiration of gastric contents, and a rapid-sequence induction of anesthesia with succinylcholine is required to expeditiously intubate the trachea. Contraindications to the use of succinylcholine include malignant hyperthermia susceptibility, muscular dystrophies, and recent denervation injuries.

Vascular Access and Positioning

Limited access to the patient during neurosurgical procedures requires secure intravenous access prior to the start of surgery. Large peripheral venous cannulae are sufficient for most craniotomies. If initial attempts fail, central venous cannulation may be necessary. However, the routine use of central venous catheters has shown to be unnecessary and given the small caliber of infant central venous catheters, its utility as a conduit for aspiration of a VAE is questionable. Placement of PICC under ultrasound guidance provide long-term central venous access without the complications associated with direct cannulation of the subclavian or jugular veins in infants and toddlers. Cannulation of the radial artery provides direct blood pressure monitoring and sampling for blood gas analysis. Other useful arterial sites in infants and children include the dorsalis pedis and posterior tibial arteries.

Patient positioning requires careful preoperative planning to allow adequate access to the patient for both the neurosurgeon and anesthesiologist. Infants and toddlers have thin skulls and are at risk for fractures and epidural hematomas with placement of head fixation devices such as the three-pin skull-clamp. Stabilizing the patient's head on a padded horseshoe headrest should be considered. Various surgical positions impact the physiologic status of the pediatric patient (Table 29.2). A large percentage of pediatric neurosurgical procedures are performed in the prone position. This can increase intra-abdominal pressure and lead to impaired ventilation, venocaval compression, and bleeding due to increased epidural venous pressure. Soft rolls are generally used to elevate and support the lateral chest wall and hips in order to minimize abdominal and thoracic pressure. Neurosurgical procedures are performed with the head slightly elevated to facilitate venous and CSF drainage from the surgical site. However, this increases the likelihood of a VAE. Significant rotation of the head can also impede venous return by compression of the jugular veins and can lead to impaired cerebral perfusion, increased ICP, and venous bleeding. Obese patients may be difficult to ventilate in the prone position and may benefit from the sitting position. In addition to the physiological sequelae of this position, a whole spectrum of neurovascular compression and stretch injuries can occur.

Maintenance of Anesthesia

The most frequently used technique during neurosurgery consists of an opioid (i.e., fentanyl, sufentanil, or remifentanil) and low-dose isoflurane or sevoflurane. Dexmedetomidine can be used as an adjunct and does not significantly affect most intraoperative neurophysiologic monitoring and reduces opioid requirements. Patients on chronic anticonvulsant therapy usually require a larger dose of neuromuscular blocking agents and opioids because of induced enzymatic metabolism of these agents. The maintenance of neuromuscular blocking agents should be discussed with the surgical and monitoring teams if assessment of motor function during seizure and spinal cord surgery is planned.

Management of Fluids and Blood Loss

In pediatric patients, meticulous fluid and blood administration is essential to minimize hemodynamic instability. Stroke volume is relatively fixed in the neonate and infant, so the patient should be kept normovolemic. Normal saline is generally chosen because it is mildly hyperosmolar and should minimize cerebral edema, but rapid infusion of more than 60 ml/kg may cause hyperchloremic acidosis. The routine administration of glucose-containing solutions is generally avoided during neurosurgical procedures, except in patients who are at risk for hypoglycemia. Premature and small new-born infants, patients with diabetes mellitus and those receiving total parental alimentation may require glucose-containing intravenous fluids.

Premature neonates have a circulating blood volume of approximately 100 ml/kg total body weight; full-term newborns have a volume of 90 ml/kg; infants have a blood volume of 80 ml/kg. Maximal allowable blood loss (MABL) can be estimated using a simple formula:

$$\text{MABL} = \text{Estimated circulating blood volume} * (\text{starting hematocrit} - \text{minimum acceptable hematocrit})/\text{starting hematocrit}.$$

Transfusion of 10 ml/kg of packed red blood cells increases hemoglobin concentration by approximately 2 g/dl. Pediatric patients are susceptible to dilutional thrombocytopenia in the setting of massive blood loss and multiple red blood cell transfusions. Administration of 5–10 ml/kg of platelets increases the platelet count by 50,000–100,000/mm^3. Routine use of the anti-fibrinolytic agent tranexamic acid has been shown to decrease blood loss in pediatric patients during surgical procedures where the risk of excessive bleeding exists.

Infants and children are at risk for hemodynamic collapse due to massive blood loss or VAE during major craniotomy surgery. Large-bore intravenous access and invasive arterial blood pressure monitoring are therefore essential for these procedures. Massive blood loss should be aggressively treated with crystalloid, blood replacement and vasopressor therapy (e.g., dopamine, epinephrine, norepinephrine). The relatively large head of infants and toddlers places them at risk for a VAE. Maintaining normovolemia minimizes this risk. Early detection of a VAE with continuous precordial doppler ultrasound may allow treatment to be instituted before large amounts of air are entrained. Neonates and young infants are at risk for sudden death because right-to-left cardiac mixing lesions can result in paradoxical emboli. In the case of severe cardiovascular collapse, some pediatric centers have rapid response ECMO teams that can provide cardiopulmonary support when the crisis is refractory to standard cardiopulmonary resuscitation measures.

Anesthetic Management of Specific Neurosurgical Procedures

Myelomeningoceles and Encephaloceles

Repair of myelomeningoceles and encephaloceles are urgent surgical procedures because of the risk of rupture and infection. Depending on the size and location of the defect, tracheal intubation of a neonate with these lesions can be challenging. Securing the airway can be accomplished in the supine position with the lesion being supported without direct pressure, in a hollowed-out soft head ring. Alternatively, the patient's trachea can be intubated in the left lateral decubitus position. Blood and fluid loss depend upon the size of the lesion and the amount of tissue dissection required to repair the defect. Twenty percent of these patients have hydrocephalus at birth, but eventually 80% of patients with a meningomyelocele will require ventricular shunting for hydrocephalus.

Hydrocephalus

Surgical management of hydrocephalus is the most common neurosurgical intervention in pediatric patients. The anesthetic technique depends on the patient's symptoms. In a patient with an intact mental status or one in whom intravenous access cannot be established, an inhalation induction with sevoflurane and gentle cricoid pressure may be used. If the patient is obtunded, at risk for cerebral herniation, or has a full stomach, intravenous access should be established in order to perform a rapid sequence induction followed by tracheal intubation. A VAE may occur during placement of the distal end of a ventriculo-atrial shunt if the operative site is above the heart. Acute obstruction of a ventricular shunt requires urgent treatment because an acute increase in ICP in the relatively small cranial vault of the infant and child can have devastating consequences.

Posterior Fossa Tumors

Posterior fossa tumors may impinge upon brain stem structures vital to the control of respiration, heart rate, and blood pressure, complicating the intraoperative management of these patients. Respiratory control centers can be damaged during surgical dissection. Stimulation of the nucleus of cranial nerve V can cause hypertension and tachycardia. Irritation of the nucleus of the vagus nerve may result in bradycardia or postoperative vocal cord paralysis. Continuous observation of the blood pressure and electrocardiogram (ECG) are essential to detect encroachment upon these vital structures. Inadvertent entry into the straight and transverse venous sinuses can precipitate a massive VAE.

Supratentorial Tumors

Craniopharyngiomas may be associated with hypothalamic and pituitary dysfunction. Steroid replacement therapy with either dexamethasone or hydrocortisone may be required because the integrity of the hypothalamic-pituitary-adrenal axis is uncertain. Perioperative DI can lead to electrolyte and hemodynamic derangements. Laboratory studies should therefore include serum electrolytes and osmolality, urine-specific gravity, and urine output. DI is marked by a sudden polyuria (>4 ml/kg/h), hypernatremia and hyperosmolarity. Initial management consists of infusion of aqueous vasopressin (1–10 mU/kg/h) and judicious fluid administration that matches urine output and estimated insensible losses.

Epilepsy

Epilepsy surgery poses several anesthetic management issues. Should non-invasive surface EEG fail to localize the source of the seizures (Phase I), a seizure map is generated by implantation of cortical (grids and strips) and depth electrodes (Phase II) followed by monitoring over several days. The second stage of the procedure occurs when the patient returns to the operating room for definitive resection. Nitrous oxide can precipitate pneumocephalus after a recent craniotomy (three weeks) and should be avoided until after the dura is opened. General anesthetics can compromise the effectiveness of intraoperative neurophysiological monitors that guide the detection and resection of the epileptogenic focus. High levels of volatile anesthetics may suppress cortical stimulation.

A variety of techniques have been advocated to facilitate intraoperative assessment of motor-sensory function and speech. In the 'sleep-awake-asleep' technique the patient undergoes general anesthesia for the surgical exposure. The patient is then awakened for functional testing and general anesthesia is reinstituted when patient cooperation is no longer needed. Most cooperative patients will tolerate sedation with propofol or dexmedetomidine. Propofol does not interfere with the electrocorticography if it is discontinued 20 minutes before monitoring in children undergoing an awake craniotomy. Supplemental opioids are administered to provide analgesia. It is, however, imperative that candidates for craniotomy under local anesthesia or sedation be mature and psychologically prepared to participate in this procedure.

Cerebrovascular Disease

The primary goal of the anesthesiologist during cerebrovascular surgery is to optimize cerebral perfusion while minimizing the risk of bleeding. Large AVM in neonates may be associated with high-output congestive heart failure requiring vasoactive support. Hypertensive crisis after embolization or surgical resection of the AVM should be rapidly treated with vasodilators.

The goal of anesthetic management of patients with Moyamoya syndrome is to optimize cerebral perfusion with aggressive preoperative hydration and maintaining normotension or mild hypertension during surgery and the postoperative period. Intraoperative normocapnia is essential, because both hyper- and hypocapnia can lead to steal phenomenon from the ischemic region. Intraoperative EEG monitoring may utilize during surgery to detect cerebral ischemia, but it has low specificity. Optimization of cerebral perfusion should be extended into the postoperative period where euvolemia should be maintained. Sedatives and/or opioids may need to be used to prevent hyperventilation induced by pain and crying.

Minimally Invasive Neurosurgery

Minimally invasive pediatric neurosurgical techniques include endoscopy and stereotactic guided insertion of intracranial devices. Given the relatively small size of the cranial vault in pediatric patients, life-threatening intracranial hypertension can occur insidiously.

Neuroendoscopic techniques have been utilized for treatment of hydrocephalus and tumor biopsies. Infants with hydrocephalus can be treated with the creation of a ventriculostomy on the floor of the third ventricle followed by cauterization of the choroid plexus to attenuate excessive production of CSF. Precise insertion of ventricular shunt catheters can be facilitated with endoscopy as well. Despite the relative safety of this procedure, hypertension, arrhythmias, and neurogenic pulmonary edema have been reported in conjunction with acute intracranial hypertension due to lack of egress of irrigation fluids and/or manipulation of the floor of the third ventricle.

Innovations in stereotactic surgery have been implemented in the management of deep brain lesions in pediatric patients. Patients with dystonia have been traditionally managed by placement of deep brain stimulator electrodes in the awake state with minimal sedation. However, most pediatric patients cannot tolerate these lengthy procedures. Skull-mount aiming devices guided by MRI-derived software have been successfully utilized to implant electrodes in pediatric patients under general anesthesia. Similar techniques have also been applied in placement of depth electrodes for detection of deep seated seizure foci. Magnetic resonance guided laser interstitial thermal therapy is another minimally invasive technique that has been used to ablate tumors and seizure foci in pediatric patients. Since these techniques are associated with negligible blood loss and fluid shifts, placement of arterial catheters is not indicated. However, vascular injuries can occur and post procedural imaging (MRI or CT) should be performed to rule-out any evolving processes. Despite the relatively minimally invasive nature of these procedures, malignant cerebral edema, hemorrhages, and onset of new neurological deficits have been reported.

Postoperative Care

The severity of the intraoperative course dictates the need for admission to an intensive care unit. Factors such as massive blood loss, hemodynamic instability, neurological deficits, seizures, and prolonged surgical time necessitate the need for continued observation. The intensive care setting is essential for early detection and treatment of evolving postoperative events which include bleeding, seizures, neurological deficits, electrolyte abnormalities, respiratory distress, and fluid shifts. The immediate availability of a MRI or CT scanner is mandatory in order to assess evolving neurological deficits. The incidence of perioperative seizures in pediatric neurosurgical patients is 7.4% with 4.4% of the whole cohort receiving prophylactic anticonvulsant drugs. Independent factors associated with perioperative seizures include supratentorial tumor, age <2 years, and hyponatremia. Given the equivocal impact of prophylactic anticonvulsants, its routine use needs further investigation.

Postoperative neurosurgical patients should be comfortable, awake, and cooperative to complete serial neurological examinations. In pediatrics, these goals can be difficult to achieve due to the cognitive level of the patient. The mainstay of sedation in the pediatric intensive care unit remains a combination of opioid and benzodiazepine. Opioids such as morphine and fentanyl should be carefully titrated to minimize post-craniotomy pain while maintaining consciousness. The use of propofol infusions over extended periods in small children on the pediatric intensive care unit is limited. This is due to its association with a fatal syndrome of bradycardia, rhabdomyolysis, metabolic acidosis, and multiple organ failure which is known as propofol infusion syndrome. Dexmedetomidine has analgesic properties and is a useful agent for reversible sedation.

Further Reading

Bray, R.J.: Propofol infusion syndrome in children. *Paediatr Anuesth* 1998; **8**:491–499.

McCann, M.E., Soriano, S.G.: Perioperative central nervous system injury in neonates. *Br J Anaesth* 2012; **109**(Suppl 1):i60–i67.

Faraoni, D., Goobie, S.M.: The efficacy of antifibrinolytic drugs in children undergoing noncardiac surgery: A systematic review of the literature. *Anesth Analge* 2014; **118**:628–636.

Hardesty, D.A., Sanborn, M.R., Parker, W.E., Storm, P.B.: Perioperative seizure incidence and risk factors in 223 paediatric brain tumor patients without prior seizures. *J Neurosurg Pediatr* 2011; **7**:609–615.

Limbrick, D.D., Jr., Baird, L.C., Klimo, P., Jr., Riva-Cambrin, J., Flannery, A.M.: Paediatric hydrocephalus systematic R, evidence-based guidelines task F: Paediatric hydrocephalus: Systematic literature review and evidence-based guidelines. Part 4: Cerebrospinal fluid shunt or endoscopic third ventriculostomy for the treatment of hydrocephalus in children. *J Neurosurg Pediatr* 2014; **14**(Suppl 1):30–34.

Meier, P.M., Guzman, R., Erb, T.O.: Endoscopic paediatric neurosurgery: Implications for anesthesia. *Paediatr Anaesth* 2014; **24**:668–677.

Soriano, S.G., Martyn, J.A.J.: Antiepileptic-induced resistance to neuromuscular blockers: Mechanisms and clinical significance. *Clin Pharmacokinet* 2004; **43**:71–81.

Soriano, S.G., Sethna, N.F., Scott, R.M.: Anesthetic management of children with moyamoya syndrome. *Anesth Analg* 1993; **77**:1066–1070.

Stricker, P.A., Lin, E.E., Fiadjoe, J.E., et al: Evaluation of central venous pressure monitoring in children undergoing craniofacial reconstruction surgery. *Anesth Analg* 2013; **116**:411–419.

Tovar-Spinoza, Z., Choi, H.: Magnetic resonance-guided laser interstitial thermal therapy: Report of a series of paediatric brain tumors. *J Neurosurg Pediatr* 2016; **17**:723–733.

Chapter 30

Anesthetic Considerations for Pediatric Neurotrauma

Monica S. Vavilala and Randall Chesnut*

Key Points

- Traumatic brain injury is the leading cause of death in children >1 year of age.
- Fifty percent of children with spinal cord injury have an associated traumatic brain injury.
- Diffuse brain injury and cerebral edema are the most common findings on computed tomography.
- Children with a Glasgow Coma Scale score <9 need tracheal intubation for airway protection and management of increased intracranial pressure.
- The cervical spine must be immobilized in all cases of suspected injury.
- General anesthesia consisting of an intravenous or volatile anesthetic agents (<1 minimum alveolar concentration), opioid boluses and muscle relaxants is considered suitable for children with neurotrauma.
- Hypotension after head injury should be treated firstly by restoring euvolemia and thereafter with vasopressors.
- Hyperventilation ($PaCO_2 < 30$ mmHg)(< 4 kPa) should be avoided unless evidence of brain herniation is present.
- Intracranial hypertension may need treatment with hyperosmolar therapy.
- Secondary brain injury caused by hyperglycemia, hyperthermia, hypoxia, and/or coagulopathy should be prevented or aggressively treated.

Abbreviations

CBF	Cerebral blood flow
CMR_{glu}	Cerebral metabolic rate for glucose
$CMRO_2$	Cerebral metabolic rate for oxygen
CPP	Cerebral perfusion pressure
CT	Computed tomography
DAI	Diffuse axonal injury
GCS	Glasgow Coma Scale
ICP	Intracranial pressure

* Funding was provided by NIH grant # 1R01NS072308-06 (MSV)

iTBI	Inflicted traumatic brain injury
LLA	Lower limit of autoregulation
MAC	Minimum alveolar concentration
SBP	Systolic blood pressure
SCI	Spinal cord injury
SCIWORA	Spinal cord injury without radiological abnormalities
TBI	Traumatic brain injury

Contents

Introduction

Pediatric neurotrauma (TBI and SCI) is the leading cause of death in children over one year of age. Significant disability following pediatric neurotrauma is frequent and often has profound impact on functional long-term outcomes.

Traumatic Brain Injury

Epidemiology

TBI should be considered in all children following trauma, particularly those with a suspicious mechanism of injury, loss of consciousness, multiple episodes of emesis, and extracranial injuries. Most children with multiple trauma have TBI and most trauma deaths are associated with TBI. Motor vehicle related crash (blunt trauma) and falls are the most common causes of TBI. However, in infants and young children <4 years of age, inflicted TBI (iTBI) is a common cause. Ten to fifteen percent of TBI in children is classified as severe with an associated mortality rate of 50%. After TBI, mortality is lower in children compared to adults (10.4% vs. 2.5%), but certain factors predict worse outcomes (Box 30.1). Sports related concussion may also be associated with long-term sequelae and cerebrovascular derangements which affect cerebral physiology after injury.

Patterns of Injury

Children are more susceptible to TBI because they have a larger head to body size ratio, thinner cranial bones providing less protection to the intracranial contents, less myelinated neural tissue which makes them more vulnerable to damage and a greater incidence of diffuse injury and cerebral edema compared to adults. Children have a higher incidence of increased ICP following TBI than adults (80% vs. 50%). Diffuse TBI is the most common type of injury seen causing concussion to DAI and permanent disability.

Diagnosis

The diagnosis of TBI is primarily made by CT which may be initially normal in those with DAI despite significant neurological findings and increased ICP. Repeat imaging often shows secondary injury due to cerebral edema. In view of growing concerns about cumulative radiation exposure during CT scans, recent guidelines have been updated to discourage routine imaging in favor of follow-up scans only when there is neurological decline.

BOX 30.1 Predictors of Poor Outcome after Pediatric TBI

Age < 4 years
Cardiopulmonary resuscitation
Multiple trauma
Hypoxia (PaO2 < 60 mmHg) (<8 kPa)
Hyperventilation (PaCO2 < 30 mmHg)(< 4 kPa)
Hyperglycemia (glucose > 250 mg/dl)(> 5.5 mmol/L)
Hyperthermia (Temperature > 38°C)
Hypotension (SBP < 5th percentile for age)
Intracranial hypertension (ICP > 20 mmHg)
Poor rehabilitation

Physiology and Pathophysiology

Cerebral Hemodynamics

Global $CMRO_2$ and CMR_{Glu} is higher in children than in adults (oxygen: 5.8 vs. 3.5 ml/100 g /min, glucose: 6.8 vs. 5.5 ml/100 g min). Unlike adults, CBF changes with age and may be higher in girls compared to boys. Following TBI, CBF and $CMRO_2$ may not be matched, resulting in either cerebral ischemia or hyperemia. Recent work demonstrates that the incidence of cerebral hyperemia is only between 6% and 10% and $CMRO_2$ may be normal, low or high after TBI. Data suggest that healthy infants may autoregulate CBF as well as older children during low dose sevoflurane anesthesia. However, the long-held assumption that the LLA is lower in young than in older children may not be valid (same LLA range for younger and older children 46–76 mmHg). Since blood pressure increases with age, young children may be at increased risk of cerebral ischemia due to lower blood pressure reserve (mean arterial pressure – LLA). Like adults, the incidence of impaired cerebral autoregulation in children is higher following severe versus mild TBI and can lead to poor outcomes. One potential explanation for this association may be hypotension, which is common after pediatric TBI and may lead to cerebral ischemia.

Intracranial Pressure

In adults, normal ICP is between 5 mmHg and 15 mmHg compared to 2–4 mmHg in young children. Unlike the adult with relatively poor cranial compliance, the infant with open fontanels may be able to accommodate slow and small increases in intracranial volume by expansion of the skull. However, rapid expansion of intracranial volume, may lead to rapid deterioration in infants following TBI. The indications for ICP monitoring and treatment threshold for increased ICP are given in Table 30.2.

Inflicted Traumatic Brain Injury

Most inflicted injury deaths involve TBI. Children with iTBI commonly present with altered consciousness, coma, seizures, vomiting, or irritability. Histories are often lacking and injuries out of proportion to history or developmental milestone should alert clinicians to consider this diagnosis. Types of injuries include subdural hematoma, subarachnoid hemorrhage, skull fractures or DAI with or without cerebral edema. Outcome is poor after iTBI.

Cervical Spine and Spinal Cord Injury

Children with an unknown mechanism of injury, multisystem trauma, TBI or injury above the clavicle should be suspected of having cervical spine injury. The incidence of SCI is low (1%) because of greater flexibility of their tissues compared to adults. A motor vehicle crash is the most common cause although sports injuries are a second common mechanism in adolescents. Half of all children with SCI die at the scene of the injury. Approximately 50% of children with cervical spine injury have concomitant TBI and the presence of TBI increases the risk of spine injury. The role of high dose steroids in pediatric SCI is unclear and its use is therefore not routine.

Sixty to seventy percent of cervical spine injuries occur in children >12 years of age. Young patients have injuries to the upper cervical spine and this is related to the fulcrum of

Table 30.1 Glasgow Coma Scale and Modification for Young Children

Glasgow Coma Scale	Pediatric Coma Scale	Infant Coma Scale	Score
Eyes	Eyes	Eyes	
Open spontaneously	Open spontaneously	Open Spontaneously	4
Verbal command	React to speech	React to speech	3
Pain	React to pain	React to pain	2
No response	No response	No response	1
Best verbal response	Best verbal response	Best verbal response	5
Oriented and converses	Smiles, oriented, interacts	Coos, babbles, interacts	4
Disoriented and converses	Interacts inappropriately	Irritable	3
Inappropriate words	Moaning	Cries to pain	2
Incomprehensible sounds	Irritable, inconsolable	Moans to pain	1
No response	No Response	No response	
Best motor response	Best motor response	Best motor response	6
Obeys verbal command	Spontaneous or obeys verbal command	Normal spontaneous movements	5
Localizes pain	Localizes pain	Withdraws to touch	4
Withdraws to pain	Withdraws to pain	Withdraws to pain	3
Abnormal flexion	Abnormal flexion	Abnormal flexion	2
Extension posturing	Extension posturing	Extension posturing	1
No response	No response	No response	

cervical motion (C1–C3). In children >12 years of age, the fulcrum moves down to C5–C6. Complete plain radiographic assessment of the cervical spine includes an antero-posterior image, lateral views of the cervico-thoracic junction and odontoid views. Due to the increased proportion of upper cervical injuries in young children, adding cuts through C3 to the initial head CT should be considered. The spine cannot be 'cleared' by radiographic examination alone. A child with normal cervical spine radiographs should be maintained with cervical spine immobilization until she/he can be thoroughly examined.

In children, cervical spine fractures can occur without neurological deficit and visa versa. A neurological deficit without a fracture has been termed spinal cord injury without radiological abnormalities (SCIWORA). SCIWORA was a diagnosis made in the pre-MRI era and, nowadays, most children have an MRI within a week after TBI. SCIWORA can occur in the cervical or thoracic spine and the onset of neurological deficit is delayed in about 25% of children. Symptoms include brief sensory or motor deficits initially with later onset of more severe signs. Most SCIWORA injuries appear to be due to flexion or hyperextension and are caused by ligamentous stretching or disruption without bony injury. Children with these injuries need to be treated with spine immobilization because recurrent injury can occur. Neurogenic shock can occur and early use of vasopressor therapy to maintain spinal cord perfusion is important.

Table 30.2 Select 2012 Brain Trauma Foundation Guidelines for the Management of Severe Brain Injury

Physiological Parameter	Recommendations
Blood glucose	Avoid dextrose containing solutions Keep blood glucose <200–250 mg/dl (4.4–5.5 mmol/L)
Temperature	Avoid hyperthermia: cool patients to 36–37° C Hypothermia (32–34 C) may be considered for refractory ICP
CBF and P_aCO_2	Avoid mild/prophylactic hyperventilation (P_aCO_2 < 30 mmHg) (<4 kPa) Mild hyperventilation if acute brain stem herniation exists Mild hyperventilation may be considered for refractory ICP
SBP	Hypovolemia should be corrected ASAP SBP should be maintained at least >5th percentile for age. May be beneficial to maintain SBP in normal range (>50th percentile)
CPP	Keep CPP >40 mmHg CPP 40–65 mmHg may represent an age-related continuum for best treatment
ICP	Monitor if Glasgow Coma Scale score <9 Treat intracranial pressure >20 mmHg Ventriculostomy or intraparenchymal catheter
Hypertonic solutions	3% Saline 0.1–1.0 ml/kg/h Mannitol 0.25–1.0 g/kg

Adapted from Adelson PD, Bratton SL, Carney NA, et al. "Guidelines for the acute medical management of severe traumatic brain injury in infants, children and adolescents." *Pediatric Critical Care Medicine* Vol 4, No 3 Suppl. 2012

Clinical Management

The original 2003 TBI Guidelines for the management of severe pediatric TBI were revised in 2012, with the addition of some new recommendations.

Initial Assessment

The initial approach to the traumatized child involves a primary and secondary survey followed by definitive care of all injuries in a timely fashion (Table 30.2). The GCS score (modified for children) is the most commonly used neurological assessment (Table 30.1). Discussed below are relevant issues specific to the different components of the anesthetic management for children with neurotrauma.

Cervical Spine Immobilization

In infants <6 months of age, the head and cervical spine should be immediately immobilized using a spine board with tape across the forehead and blankets or towels around the neck. In infants >6 months of age, the head should be immobilized either in the manner described above or by using a small rigid cervical collar. Children >8 years of age require a medium-sized cervical collar. The use of rigid cervical collars is essential as it prevents cervical distraction during laryngoscopy. Since children under 7 years have a prominent occiput, a pad placed under the thoracic spine provides neutral alignment of the spine and avoids excessive flexion that may occur in the supine position. These two maneuvers are paramount in avoiding iatrogenic cervical spine injury.

Airway Management

During the primary survey, it is essential to establish an adequate airway. The lucid and hemodynamically stable child can be managed conservatively but if the child has altered mental status, attempts should be made to establish the airway by suctioning the pharynx, chin-lift and jaw thrust maneuvers, or insertion of an oral airway. Children with a GCS score <9 require tracheal intubation for airway protection and management of increased ICP. However, recent studies demonstrate no survival or functional advantage of pre-hospital tracheal intubation compared to pre-hospital bag-valve-mask ventilation in pediatric TBI. The most common approach to airway management involves induction of anesthesia, manual in-line stabilization, cricoid pressure, direct laryngoscopy, oral intubation, and ventilation with high oxygen concentrations. Naso-tracheal intubations are contraindicated in patients with basal skull fractures. The 2012 Guidelines recommend avoidance of prophylactic severe hyperventilation to a P_aCO_2 less than 30 mmHg (<4 kPa) within the first 48 hours after injury. If hyperventilation is used in the management of severe intracranial hypertension, evidence suggests that advanced neuromonitoring for evaluation of cerebral ischemia should be used concurrently.

Anesthetic Technique

Most recommendations regarding choice of anesthetic technique and monitoring are extrapolated from data in adults and anesthesiologists should be aware of the hemodynamic and physiological recommendations given in Box 30.2. The 2012 Guidelines highlight that choice and dosing of analgesics, sedatives, and neuromuscular-blocking agents are left to the discretion of the treating physician.

Intravenous Agents

All intravenous sedative-hypnotic induction agents, including barbiturates, etomidate, and propofol, that are used to facilitate tracheal intubation are potent cerebral vasoconstrictors, cause coupled reduction in CBF and $CMRO_2$, and can decrease ICP. Opioids and benzodiazepines can be safely used to facilitate tracheal intubation but should be used in small doses. Ketamine may be safe in pediatric TBI as a recent study has shown an association with a reduction in ICP in TBI. Lidocaine is commonly used as an anesthetic adjunct to prevent increases in ICP induced by laryngoscopy and tracheal intubation in patients whose hemodynamic instability precludes use of large doses of sedative hypnotic agents. Dexmedetomidine has favorable profiles in TBI, including preservation of cerebral autoregulation and the ability to facilitate a neurological examination. The 2012 Guidelines recommend barbiturate therapy in hemodynamically stable patients when maximal medical and surgical therapy has failed to control ICP.

Volatile Agents

All inhalational agents are cerebral vasodilators but <1 MAC of sevoflurane does not increase CBF velocities compared to other agents. Consequently, sevoflurane may be the preferred volatile agent in comparison to isoflurane, desflurane, or halothane in pediatric TBI. Nitrous oxide can increase ICP.

Muscle Relaxants

Muscle relaxants have little effect on the cerebral circulation. Succinylcholine can be safely administered without causing an increase in ICP with or without a defasiculation dose of a nondepolarizing muscle relaxant. Succinylcholine is a better choice than rocuronium when airway management is anticipated to be difficult.

Intravenous Access

Obtaining vascular access in the traumatized child can be very challenging. A functioning 20-gauge or larger peripheral intravenous catheter will suffice for induction of anesthesia. Saphenous veins are commonly used. A second intravenous line should be started once the child is anesthetized. In emergency cases, if peripheral access is unsuccessful after two attempts, an interosseous line should be placed. Central venous catheters should be inserted by experienced personnel.

Intravenous Fluids

Unlike adults, children can become hypovolemic from scalp injuries and isolated TBI. Isotonic crystalloid solutions are commonly used during anesthesia and for cerebral resuscitation. Hypotonic crystalloids should be avoided and the role of colloids is controversial. The use of hydroxyethyl starch is discouraged because of its role in exacerbating coagulopathy. Hypertonic saline 3% may be used to lower ICP and improved CPP and is recommended by 2012 Guidelines.

Glucose

Retrospective studies suggest that hyperglycemia (glucose 200–250 mg/100 ml) (4.4–5.5 mmol/L) is associated with poor outcome. Provision of nutrition is associated with better outcomes and hence, early provision of enteral or parenteral nutrition should be initiated after TBI.

Monitoring

Standard monitoring (e.g., electrocardiograph, oximetry, end-tidal CO_2) and invasive arterial blood pressure measurement is recommended in TBI. Central venous pressure monitoring can be useful. An internal jugular catheter may be safely placed and used without increasing ICP. Retrograde jugular venous saturation monitoring can be useful to guide the degree of hyperventilation in patients with TBI but is not standard of care. ICP monitoring is useful during intrahospital transfer and during surgery involving extracranial injuries since CPP can be calculated but any pre-existing coagulopathy must be treated prior to monitor placement. Urine output must be monitored. The 2012

Guidelines recommend that if hypothermia is employed, it should be continued for >24 hours, and rewarming should be carried out at a pace slower than 0.5°C per hour. Regular assessment of arterial blood gases and coagulation is essential. ICP monitoring should be used to guide blood pressure management in children with TBI undergoing non-neurosurgical procedures.

Cerebral Hemodynamics

While SBP <5th percentile defines hypotension, in the absence of ICP monitoring and suspected increased ICP, supranormal SBP may be needed to maintain CPP. At a minimum, MAP should not be allowed to decrease below values normal for age and the use of vasopressors may be required. Intravenous phenylephrine or norepinephrine infusions are commonly used to treat hypotension and maintain CPP using age appropriate thresholds. Although the exact optimal CPP in the pediatric patient is unknown, CPP <40 mmHg should be avoided and CPP of 50–60 mmHg should be maintained in older children. The 2012 Guidelines recommend maintaining brain tissue oxygenation ($PbtO_2$) greater than 10 mmHg, based on level III evidence.

Indications for Surgery

Evidence-based practice guidelines have recently been published for surgical management of TBI in general and more specifically for the surgical management of ICP in pediatric TBI. Nevertheless, the indications remain controversial for many procedures. The major goal of surgery for TBI is to optimize the recovery of viable brain. Most operations deal with the removal of mass lesions to prevent herniation, intracranial hypertension, or alterations in CBF. In general, unless small and deemed likely venous, epidural hematomas should be evacuated in patients with coma. Subdural hematomas that are associated with herniation are greater than 10 mm thick, or produce a midline shift of >5 mm should be evacuated. Indications for surgical treatment of intraparenchymal mass lesions include progressive neurological deterioration referable to the lesion, signs of mass effect on CT, or refractory intracranial hypertension. Penetrating injuries can often be managed with local debridement and watertight closure if not extensive and there is minimal intracranial mass effect (as defined above). The 2012 Guidelines recommend consideration of craniectomy in pediatric patients who are showing early signs of neurologic deterioration or herniation, or are developing intracranial hypertension refractory to medical management. A generous decompressive craniectomy with duraplasty can be considered when intracranial hypertension reaches or approaches medical refractoriness in salvageable patients where the ICP elevation and its effects are felt to be the major threat to recovery. Unilateral craniectomy is appropriate for lateralized swelling; bifrontal decompression is selected for diffuse disease. However, studies suggest no benefit and potential harm with decompressive craniectomy for TBI.

In general, surgical removal of mass lesions in comatose patients should be performed as early as safely feasible. As this often involves incompletely resuscitated patients, close collaboration between surgery and anesthesia is critical. Bidirectional communication should be maintained regarding issues such as the stage of the procedure, anticipated and ongoing blood loss, systemic stability, and unanticipated events so that the procedure can be altered or even terminated if necessary.

Summary

Pediatric TBI results in large societal costs. Therefore, efforts to improve outcome are extremely important. Although many general principles of managing pediatric TBI are similar to adults, there are unique anatomic, physiological, and patho-physiological features of children with TBI worth recognizing.

Further Reading

Bullock, M.R.1, Chesnut, R., Ghajar, J., et al: Surgical management of acute epidural hematomas. *Neurosurgery* 2006; **58**(Suppl 3): S7–S15.

Bullock, M.R.1, Chesnut, R., Ghajar, J., et al: Surgical management of acute subdural hematomas. *Neurosurgery* 2006; **58**(Suppl 3): S16–S24.

Chaiwat, O., Sharma, D., Udomphorn, Y., Armstead, W.M., Vavilala, M.S.: Cerebral hemodynamic predictors of poor 6-month Glasgow outcome score in severe pediatric traumatic brain injury. *J Neurotrauma* 2009 May; **26**(5):657–663. doi: 10.1089/neu.2008.0770.

Crosby, E.T.: Airway management in adults after cervical spine trauma. *Anesthesiology* 2006; **104**(6):1293–1318.

Gausche, M., Lewis, R.J., Stratton, S.J., et al: Effect of out-of-hospital pediatric endotracheal intubation on survival and neurological outcome: A controlled clinical trial. *JAMA* 2000; **283**:783–790.

Kochanek, P.M., Carney, N., Adelson, P.D., et al: Guidelines for the acute medical management of severe traumatic brain injury in infants, children, and adolescents–second edition. *Pediatr Crit Care Med* 2012 January; **13**(Suppl 1):S1–S82.

Pediatric Trauma in Advanced Trauma Life Support Course for Physicians. USA, American College of Surgeons, 1993 pp 261–281.

Skippen, P1., Seear, M., Poskitt, K., Kestle, J., Cochrane, D., Annich, G., Handel, J.: Effect of Hyperventilation on regional blood flow in head injured children. *Crit Care Med* 1997; **25**:1402–1409.

Vavilala, M.S., Kernic, M.A., Wang, J., et al: Pediatric guideline adherence and outcomes study. Acute care clinical indicators associated with discharge outcomes in children with severe traumatic brain injury. *Crit Care Med* 2014 October; **42**(10):2258–2266.

Chapter

31

Post-Anesthesia Care Unit

Veena Sheshadri and Pirjo H. Manninen

Key Points

- Continuous postoperative monitoring and careful management of airway, oxygenation and hemodynamics are important to avoid neurological adverse events.
- The potential for rapid neurological deterioration requires regular and frequent neurological monitoring.
- Pharmacological and physiological causes for neurological deterioration should be ruled out first before considering imaging and surgical consultation.
- When used carefully, potent opioids (morphine, hydromorphone) are appropriate for pain management.
- 5HT3 antagonists are suitable antiemetics but multiple agents may be needed.
- Discharge from the post-anesthesia care unit to a suitable location occurs when all discharge criteria have been met.

Abbreviations

COX-2	Cyclooxygenase-2
CT	Computed tomography
GCS	Glasgow Coma Scale
ICP	Intracranial pressure
ICU	Intensive care unit
MRI	Magnetic resonance imaging
NSAIDs	Non-steroidal anti-inflammatory drugs
OSA	Obstructive sleep apnea
PACU	Post-anesthesia care unit
PCA	Patient controlled analgesia
PONV	Postoperative nausea and vomiting

Contents

- Introduction
- General Considerations
    - Monitoring
    - Airway and Ventilation

Introduction

Postoperative recovery of patients is a critical phase after neurosurgical procedures encompassing continued patient care and monitoring with the primary goal of timely recognition and treatment of complications. The immediate recovery may take place in a PACU or an ICU depending on institutional resources, individual patient factors, and the surgical procedure. Not all patients require ICU care after elective neurosurgery. Early postoperative complications usually occur within the first 2 hours. Close monitoring is focused on the detection of neurological deterioration and the optimization of physiological parameters that influence neurological outcome.

General Considerations

Monitoring

On arrival in the recovery location, the airway, oxygenation, and hemodynamics should be assessed immediately, along with a neurological examination. Following this, there should be regular and frequent (every 15 minutes) assessment of:

- Respiratory Function (oxygen saturation, respiratory rate, and pattern) Cardiovascular Function (heart rate, rhythm, blood pressure – invasive/non-invasive)
- Neurological Function (GCS, pupil size and symmetry, sensory and motor function of upper and lower extremities, new onset neurological deficits, and seizures)
- Temperature
- Fluid balance and urine output
- Pain scores (verbal or visual)
- Presence of PONV

BOX 31.1 Indications for Postoperative Ventilation

Airway concerns	Likelihood of upper airway obstruction (airway edema, macroglossia)
	Failure to regain conscious state or return of airway reflexes
Oxygenation concerns	Concurrent severe respiratory disease
Cardiovascular instability	Poor cardiac function, hypovolemia, major blood loss
Neurological concerns	Decreased level of consciousness
	Neurological deficit
	Raised ICP
	Brainstem injury or cranial nerve dysfunction (lack of gag reflex)
Physiological disturbances	Hypothermia, acid-base abnormities

Additional neurological monitoring includes ICP especially for patients with a deteriorating level of consciousness, traumatic brain injury, or hydrocephalus. Advanced monitoring techniques such as electroencephalography, transcranial doppler, jugular bulb venous oximetry, and near infrared spectroscopy may aid in early detection of secondary adverse events but are not routine.

Airway and Ventilation

Extubation of an awake patient is appropriate for most patients prior to arriving in the PACU. Early extubation is generally preferred over elective postoperative ventilation to facilitate early neurological examination, avoidance of unnecessary diagnostic and/or therapeutic interventions as well as stress-induced increases in catecholamines and other ventilator-associated challenges. Assessment of the gag reflex is warranted after posterior fossa surgery as brainstem and cranial nerve function may be altered. Airway edema may occur after prolonged prone position surgeries, cervical spine surgery, carotid endarterectomy, and procedures involving large fluid shifts. Postoperative ventilation may be required for some patients. The indications are shown in Box 31.1.

Fluids and Electrolytes

The perioperative fluid goals for neurosurgical patients should be to maintain normovolemia and to avoid reduction in serum osmolality, hyperglycemia, and hyponatremia. This is discussed in more detail in Chapters 40 and 41.

Laboratory Parameters

Correction of changes in plasma biochemistry and rheology may need to be commenced in the PACU. Laboratory parameters are obtained as indicated by each patient's needs. Management of sodium disorders is reviewed in Chapter 41.

Hyperglycemia may be attributed to stress, insulin resistance, and/or steroid administration and can lead to poor wound healing, infection, and a worse neurological outcome. Blood glucose levels should be maintained in the range of 140–180 mg/dl (7.8–10 mmol/L).

The available clinical data does not support tight glucose control in this subgroup of patients.

Position

A head up position, approximately 30 degree, is used to improve ventilation; reduce face, neck, and airway edema; and facilitate cerebral venous and cerebrospinal fluid drainage. Patients should lay flat following evacuation of a chronic subdural hematoma and endovascular procedures requiring femoral artery cannulation.

Temperature

Maintain normothermia using warming blankets if necessary.

Imaging

A chest X-ray should be performed to check central line placement. Advanced imaging (CT, MRI, and angiography) may be required after major surgery or following any deterioration in neurological function. Patient should be transported from the radiology suite with appropriate monitoring and supplemental oxygen.

Complications

Airway and Respiratory

Deterioration in the level of consciousness (GCS ≤ 8) and lower cranial nerve dysfunction are indications for re-intubation as these patients are at risk of airway obstruction, aspiration and are vulnerable to hypoxia and hypercarbia. A nasopharyngeal airway may be considered for airway obstruction due to over-sedation. It is also important to rule out any residual neuromuscular blockade leading to respiratory distress. Following neck surgery (carotid endarterectomy, cervical spine procedures), monitoring of the airway is required because of possible edema and hematoma formation. Measuring neck circumference may be helpful.

Macroglossia is a potentially serious cause of airway obstruction. Risk factors include prone positioning, severe flexion of the neck, venous or lymphatic engorgement from oropharyngeal airway, or from tongue protrusion. Patients with OSA are at higher risk of airway obstruction or hypoxemia postoperatively. Whenever required, continuous positive airway pressure should be considered unless contraindicated by the surgical procedure.

Cardiovascular

Maintenance of stable hemodynamics and cerebral perfusion pressure is important. Both hypertension and hypotension may independently lead to adverse neurological outcomes. The planned postoperative target blood pressure should be agreed upon. A compromise may be needed between a high blood pressure (for cerebral perfusion) and a lower blood pressure (to avoid bleeding). Following surgery for arterio-venous malformations, avoidance of hypertension may be critical to prevent postoperative bleeding or hyperperfusion syndrome. Pharmacological control of blood pressure is often required.

Neurological causes of cardiovascular instability include cerebral ischemia, raised ICP, brainstem injury, involvement of T1–T4 sympathetic nerves, spinal shock, and autonomic hyper-reflexia after spinal injury. Cardiac dysfunction and neurogenic pulmonary edema may be secondary to sympathetic activation following subarachnoid hemorrhage. Cardiac and respiratory support with inotropes, invasive hemodynamic monitoring, and ventilation may be indicated.

Neurological

Any deterioration in the neurological state requires immediate attention to the airway, oxygenation, and ventilation. Optimization of hemodynamic parameters and cerebral perfusion pressure, followed in most cases by prompt diagnosis via imaging (CT, MRI) will determine if surgical intervention is warranted. The possibility of pharmacological causes (opioids or sedative agents) and physiological abnormalities (airway, oxygenation, hemodynamics, temperature, acid-base status, electrolytes, and blood glucose) should be considered. (See Chapters 5, 34, 35, 42 for management of increased ICP, seizures, and vasospasm.)

Pain

Pain should be assessed with a scoring system (verbal or visual) to help guide treatment. Post-craniotomy pain may be moderate or severe but treatment remains inadequate, challenging, and controversial. Management should balance adequate analgesia and avoidance of excessive sedation that masks new neurological deficits.

A scalp block may be associated with significant short-term reduction of postoperative pain. Parenteral opioids (fentanyl, morphine, and hydromorphone) are the cornerstone of management. Although intermittent administration is most commonly used, PCA may also be used. Codeine (intramuscular) should not be used as it is not effective. Side effects include nausea, vomiting, pruritus, over sedation, and respiratory depression. Tramadol has less respiratory depression and sedation compared with opioids, but has a higher incidence of nausea and vomiting.

Acetaminophen orally or intravenously alone is inadequate but should be used as an adjunct. The use of NSAIDs is controversial in view of possible platelet dysfunction, hematoma formation, and renal failure. There is limited evidence of the benefit of selective COX-2 inhibitors.

Postoperative pain after spinal surgery is proportional to the number of levels of vertebrae operated upon. There is no significant difference in the severity of pain between cervical, thoracic, and lumbar spine surgeries. Superior analgesia is obtained with PCA. Multidrug regimens allow for opioid sparing and fewer side effects. Intrathecal or epidural opioids can also be used. Other adjuvants used are NSAIDs, COX-2 inhibitors, acetaminophen, steroids, ketamine, and gabapentin.

Postoperative Nausea and Vomiting

The incidence of PONV is high following both craniotomy and spine surgery. Antiemetic prophylaxis with 5-HT3 antagonists is effective in decreasing PONV after both

Table 31.1 Antiemetic Treatment Options

Class of Drug	Examples (IV Doses)	Important Side Effects
5HT3 antagonists	Ondansetron (4 mg), Tropisetron (2 mg), Granisetron (1 mg), Dolasetron (12.5 mg), Palanosetron (0.25 mg)	Headaches
Antihistamines	Dimenhydrinate (25 mg), Promethazine (12.5 mg)	Drowsiness
Anticholinergics	Scopolamine (transdermal patch)	Drowsiness, mydriasis
Antidopaminergics	Droperidol (1 mg), Metoclopramide (20 mg)	Extrapyramidal symptoms
Steroids	Dexamethasone (8 mg)	Hyperglycemia

supratentorial and infratentorial surgery. Multiple antiemetics may be used when indicated. Suppression of hypothalamo-pituitary axis may occur with use of dexamethasone for PONV. Options for treatment are shown in Table 31.1.

Shivering

Treatment of shivering is by rewarming and pharmacological agents including intravenous meperidine (12.5–25 mg), clonidine (75 µg), ketanserin (10 mg), or magnesium sulfate (30 mg/kg).

Urinary Retention

Postoperative urinary retention is common (up to 39%) following neurosurgical spine procedures and these patients may require bladder catheterization.

Emergence Agitation

Risk factors for agitation during emergence include male sex, use of antidepressants or benzodiazepines, frontal craniotomy, and long duration of anesthesia. Initial management is to protect the patient, and rule out and treat hypoxemia, metabolic, or neurological disorders. Treatment with sedatives or analgesics may be required.

Thromboembolism

The frequency of deep vein thrombosis is high after neurosurgical procedures (cranial 3.4%, spinal 1.1%). Pneumatic compression stockings are recommended but not always practical. Heparinization requires individual risk assessment.

Other Complications

Some procedures are associated with specific postoperative concerns such as endoscopic transsphenoidal hypophysectomy (aspiration of blood in pharynx), neuroendoscopy (delayed arousal, hyperkalemia, diabetes insipidus, and hypothalamic dysfunction) and deep brain stimulation (movement disorder symptoms).

Discharge Criteria

Disposition of neurosurgical patients from PACU may be to an ICU, an intermediate care unit, the ward and in some cases home. Ambulatory day surgery is feasible for procedures like lumbar microdiscectomy and awake craniotomy for tumor. The American Society of Anesthesiologists practice guidelines do not recommend any mandatory minimum stay in PACU before discharge. Criteria used for general PACU patients (modified Aldrete score) do not sufficiently address the postoperative risks specific to the neurosurgical population in whom rapid neurological deterioration may occur. A longer stay in PACU or earlier discharge to an intermediate care unit equipped for frequent neurological assessments may be appropriate.

In general, the following principles apply prior to the discharge from PACU:

* No airway or respiratory problems
* Stable hemodynamics
* No major neurological problems (awake/alert/orientated, no new major sensory or motor deficits)
* Other physiological parameters within normal range (temperature, acid-base status, and blood sugar level)
* Adequate pain control and minimal PONV

Further Reading

Alsaidi, M., Guanio, J., Basheer, A., et al: The incidence and risk factors for postoperative urinary retention in neurosurgical patients. *Surg Neurol Int* 2013; **4**:61.

Apfelbaum, J.L., Silverstein, J.H., Chung, F.F., et al: Practice guidelines for post anesthetic care: An updated report by the American Society of Anesthesiologists task force on post anesthetic care. *Anesthesiology* 2013; **118**:291–307.

Ayrian, E1., Kaye, A.D2., Varner, C.L1., et al: Effects of anesthetic management on early postoperative recovery, hemodynamics and pain after supratentorial craniotomy. *J Clin Med Res* 2015; **7**:731–741.

Flexman, A.M., Ng, J.L., Gelb, A.W.: Acute and chronic pain following craniotomy. *Curr Opin Anaesthiol* 2010; **23**(5):551–557.

Godoy, D.A., Di Napoli, M., Biestro, A., Lenhardt, R.: Perioperative glucose control in neurosurgical patients. *Anesthesiol Res Pract* 2012; **2012**:690362.

Gross, J.B., Apfelbaum, J.L., Connis, R.T., Nickinovich, D.G. for American Society of Anesthesiologists Task Force on Perioperative Management of patients with obstructive sleep apnea et al.: Practice guidelines for perioperative management of obstructive sleep apnea. *Anesthesiology* 2014; **120**:268–286.

Jian, M., Li, X., Wang, A., et al: Flurbiprofen and hypertension but not hydroxyethyl starch are associated with post-craniotomy intracranial haematoma requiring surgery. *Br J Anaesth* 2014; **113**(5):832–839.

Kirkman, M.A., Smith, M.: Multimodal intracranial monitoring: Implications for clinical practice. *Anesthesiol Clin* 2012; **30**:269–287.

Lai, L.T., Ortiz-Cardona, J.R., Bendo, A.A.: Perioperative pain management in the neurosurgical patient. *Anesthesiol Clin* 2012; **30**:347–367.

Latz, B., Mordhorst, C., Kerz, T., et al: Postoperative nausea and vomiting after craniotomy: Incidence and risk factors. *J Neurosurg* 2011; **114**:491–496.

Rhondali, O1., Genty, C., Halle, C., et al: Do patients still require admission to an intensive care unit after elective craniotomy for brain surgery? *J Neurosurg Anesthesiol* 2011; **23**:118–123.

Siegemund, M., Steiner, L.A.: Postoperative care of neurosurgical patient. *Curr Opin Anesthesiol* 2015; **28**:487–493.

Chapter

32

Spinal Cord Injury

Mark Plummer and Ronan O' Leary

Key Points

- Survival following spinal cord injury (SCI) is common but is associated with significant morbidity arising from both the primary and secondary insults.
- The so called "secondary injury", is a poorly understood vascular and inflammatory response which commences immediately after injury and persists for several weeks.
- Intensive care management involving maintenance of spinal cord perfusion and oxygenation is required to prevent exacerbation of secondary injury.
- In tetraplegic patients, acute and long-term respiratory complications commonly cause further disability and death.
- A mean arterial pressure of 85–90 mmHg should be maintained for at least the first week following injury.
- Spinal protection can reliably be removed from an obtunded trauma patient after a negative whole-spine computed tomography (CT) scan is reported by an experienced radiologist.
- All patients with a SCI should have their neurology regularly graded using the American Spinal Injury Association (ASIA) system.

Abbreviations

ASIA   American Spinal Injury Association
CT   Computed Tomography
ICU   Intensive Care Unit
NMDA   N-Methyl D-Aspartate
SCI   Spinal Cord Injury

Learning Objectives

- To understand the pathophysiological processes causing primary and secondary spinal cord injury (SCI) following trauma and other causes of acute SCI.
- To develop strategies for preventing the common, life threatening complications of SCI within the critical care environment.
- To understand and describe the essential aspects of critical care management for patients with SCI.
- To establish a safe algorithm to allow removal of spinal protection from obtunded trauma patients.

Contents

Introduction

Spinal cord injury (SCI) is a devastating event and care needs to be focused on aggressive prevention of further injury and optimization for early rehabilitation. The estimated annual global incidence of SCI is 40–80 cases per million, the vast majority of which are secondary to trauma (90%) and occur in previously healthy young men (80%). SCI may be thought of as progressing from a primary injury, which is the damage to the cord at the time of insult, to a secondary injury where high-quality intensive care medicine may improve the prognosis. This chapter will discuss SCI due to traumatic and vascular injures but other conditions such as inflammatory, infective, autoimmune, and neoplastic may also cause damage to the spinal cord. Improved outcomes for these patients require a multi-disciplinary approach involving critical care units experienced in the management of SCI and its complications.

Classification

The American Spinal Injury Association (ASIA) scoring system is frequently used to assess and classify SCI but it requires a clinical examination on a conscious and co-operative patient. The level of neurological injury is described as the lowest spinal level with normal motor and sensory function. The lesion is described as complete if there is no sensory or motor function in the anal and perineal region representing the lowest sacral cord (S4–S5) and "incomplete" if some function is preserved (Table 32.1). In practice, many ICU patients suffer from high, complete lesions. The ASIA score at 72-hours post injury is currently the most sensitive tool to determine longer term prognosis and it is imperative that the score is

Table 32.1 ASIA Assessment

Category	Description	Frequency
A = Complete	No motor or sensory function is preserved in the sacral segments S4–S5	49%
B = Incomplete	Sensory but not motor function is preserved below the neurological level and includes the sacral segments S4-S5	13%
C = Incomplete	Motor function is preserved below the neurological level, and more than half of key muscles below the neurological level have a muscle grade <3	16%
D = Incomplete	Motor function is preserved below the neurological level, and at least half of the key muscles below the neurological level have a muscle grade ≥3	22%
E = Normal	Motor and sensory function are normal	-

documented regularly throughout the intensive care admission to help guide rehabilitation. It is especially important to distinguish between complete lesions (ASIA-A) and lesions with preserved sacral sensory function (ASIA-B), as a substantially greater proportion of the latter will eventually regain some motor function at one year (8% vs 39%).

Pathophysiology

In the context of trauma, the primary injury occurs due to direct neuronal disruption at the time of the incident. This acute physical damage initiates a complex cascade of secondary molecular and vascular mechanisms culminating in vasospasm, thrombosis, loss of micro-circulatory autoregulation, lipid peroxidation, edema, apoptosis, and ultimately glial cell death. This secondary injury worsens neurological status and the functional cord level may ascend within the first 48 hours. Eventually, the processes driving the secondary injury subside leaving glial scar tissue around a central cord cavity thereby obstructing cord regeneration.

In patients with traumatic or sudden vascular SCI, there is an immediate period of "spinal shock" which results in flaccid paralysis below the level of the injury which may last many months. This is then followed by a period or spastic paralysis when chest wall rigidity can lead to an improvement in respiratory mechanics assuming diaphragmatic function is maintained.

The overwhelming majority of the acute management issues after the first 72 hours are respiratory. These are compounded by the degree of systemic traumatic injures (measured by injury severity score), age of the patient and co-existing pathologies. Respiratory function and therefore ventilator weaning, correlates with the level of injury. High cervical injuries (C1–C4) are more likely to develop pneumonia while atelectasis occurs more often in lower cervical injuries.

Initial Management

Evaluation and Imaging

SCI rarely occurs in isolation and, as with all trauma patients, the acute management should follow an ABC approach. The spine should be immobilized and the patient kept flat, but a reverse Trendelenburg position of up to 30 degree may improve comfort in conscious patients and ventilation in all groups.

All trauma patients with neck pain, neurologic compromise, and/or a suggestive mechanism of injury should undergo computed tomography (CT) imaging of the entire spine. Fractures of cervical transverse foramina raise concern for a vertebral artery injury. This will require a CT angiogram for confirmation and multi-disciplinary consultation to discuss the merits of anti-coagulation, antiplatelet therapy, or procedural intervention.

All vertebral fractures need early discussion with neuro-spinal surgeons to discuss the merits of early (first 24 hours) decompression and definitive fixation. In many cases, spinal surgery is not possible due to other traumatic injuries and in these cases, conservative management of the spinal fracture while allowing some amount of sitting up for respiratory care must be agreed upon.

Clearing the Cervical Spine in the Obtunded Trauma Patient

The spine should be assessed and cleared as early as is practical, with guidelines supporting the safety of removing spinal precautions following a negative CT scan reported by an experienced radiologist (see Chapter 12). While this practice fails to detect isolated ligamentous injury, these lesions are of questionable clinical significance and extremely unlikely to result in permanent neurological deficit. Importantly, spinal immobilization has the potential to cause harm and is associated with pressure sores, raised intracranial pressure, ventilator associated pneumonia and difficult central venous access.

Subsequent Management

The presence of SCI compromises multiple organ systems and following resuscitation the goal of management should be physiological optimization to prevent exacerbation of secondary injury and to aid early rehabilitation.

Respiratory

The trauma patient with SCI presents unique difficulties for induction of anesthesia and intubation. Inadequacy of ventilation may be due to pain, rib fractures, pneumo/hemothoraces, traumatic brain injury, or the level of the SCI (Table 32.2). Respiratory function is further compromised by a lack of sympathetic outflow predisposing to bronchospasm and hypersecretion.

Patients with complete injuries at C4 and above will frequently fail to maintain respiratory effort in the acute phase and may benefit from early tracheostomy judged on the extent of injuries and pre-existing diseases. Injuries at C5 and below may not require intubation in the acute setting and respiratory function should be monitored closely with a low threshold for early intubation. For patients with cervical SCI requiring mechanical ventilation, a complete lesion (ASIA-A) is the greatest predictor for requirement of a tracheostomy.

Early and on-going physiotherapy is essential. Hypersecretion should be managed with the routine use of nebulized mucolytics. Flaccid abdominal musculature contributes to decreased vital capacity and an impaired cough. This can be improved with the use of abdominal binders and lying flat during spontaneous ventilation.

Table 32.2 Respiratory Function at SCI Lesion Level

SCI level	Effect on Respiration	Consequence
C1-3	Complete paralysis of all respiratory muscles	Apnea requiring mechanical ventilation. Absent cough. Consider early tracheostomy.
C4-5	Variable impairment of diaphragm and accessory muscles.	Ventilation often necessary acutely but there is potential to wean from mechanical ventilation. Weak cough.
C6-T1	Diaphragm and accessory muscles intact. Intercostal and abdominal muscles paralyzed.	Passive expiration. Decreased vital capacity. Weak cough.
T2-T11	Abdominal muscles paralyzed.	Rarely requires ventilation in isolated SCI. Weak cough. May benefit from abdominal binder.

Cardiovascular

Systemic hypotension may be due to hypovolemia secondary to hemorrhage, cardiac dysfunction, vasoplegia due to the spinal trauma, or a combination of these. It is essential to identify the causes of hypotension and treat each aggressively.

The penumbra surrounding the injured cord is also particularly susceptible to hypotensive ischemia due to a loss of vascular auto-regulation. Accordingly, maintaining adequate perfusion is paramount with guidelines recommending mean arterial pressure thresholds of 85–90 mmHg up to seven days. Sympathetic cardiac afferents exit the spinal cords in the ventral roots of T1–T5 and injury at or above this level disrupts sympathetic outflow culminating in vasodilatation, venous pooling, and bradycardia.

All SCI patients should be managed with invasive arterial pressure monitoring. Hypotension in an isolated SCI should be managed with cautious crystalloid fluid resuscitation. However, for active hemorrhage control in the acute trauma setting, blood products should be administered as per local protocols and vasoactive drugs may be required to maintain an adequate spinal cord perfusion pressure. The oral α-agonist midodrine should be considered early following admission, once hemorrhage has been excluded. This allows weaning from intravenous vasoactive medications and can reduce the risk of catheter-related sepsis.

Vagal hypersensitivity also predisposes to acute bradydysrhythmias, which may be triggered by routine suctioning and turning. If these episodes result in hemodynamic compromise management should be with anti-cholinergic agents such as glycopyrrolate or atropine.

Neurogenic Shock

Resolution of neurogenic shock is associated with the return of deep tendon reflexes and usually occurs after 4–6 weeks but may occur as early as 4 days. While patients with lesions above T6 commonly develop resting and orthostatic hypotension, the majority also experience autonomic dysreflexia. This is an inappropriate autonomic response to stimuli below the level of injury resulting in episodes of malignant hypertension accompanied by headache, sweating, flushing, and pallor above the level of the lesion. Common precipitants in the intensive care unit include constipation, urinary tract infections, and pressure sores. Management is directed at eliminating the stimulus and if needed, the use of a short-acting vasodilator.

Genitourinary Care

All patients should be catheterized on admission to avoid bladder distension and to aid fluid management. In time, the in-dwelling catheter can be removed and four hourly intermittent catheterization commenced.

Gastrointestinal and Nutrition

Paralytic ileus and constipation are almost ubiquitous in this patient group and should be anticipated and managed early.

Hypermetabolism and marked nitrogen depletion frequently occur early resulting in loss of lean muscle mass, contributing to both short and long-term morbidity. Early feeding by any available route is currently preferred, ideally via the enteral route. Unopposed gastric vagal activity predisposes to gastroparesis and may require the use of prokinetics. Maintenance of caloric delivery is key, which may be achieved via the post-pyloric or parenteral routes. It is imperative to assess swallowing function prior to commencing oral feeding.

The parasympathetic dominance coupled with the stress response to trauma also predisposes this population to stress ulceration warranting routine stress ulcer prophylaxis. The stress response also predisposes to dysglycemia and both hyper and hypoglycemia exacerbate secondary cord injury. Intravenous insulin infusion protocols should target blood glucose between 6 and 10 mmol/L (110–180 mg/dl).

Thermoregulation

Altered autonomic signaling results in impaired thermoregulatory capacity and regular monitoring of body temperature is vital. Vasodilation below the cord lesion predisposes to hypothermia whereas an inability to sweat impairs heat dissipation, which can lead to fatal hyperthermia. Therapeutic hypothermia in acute SCI remains experimental and maintenance of normothermia is encouraged.

Prevention of Thromboembolic Complications

The immobile SCI patient is at considerable risk of deep venous thrombosis. All patients should have compression stockings and pneumatic compression devices from admission. Pharmacological prophylaxis with low molecular weight heparin should be commenced as soon as possible and continued for a minimum of three months. Inferior vena cava filters should only be considered for patients with a significant bleeding risk that is likely to persist for >72 hours.

Skin Ulceration

Immobility and impaired sensation predispose to pressure ulcers, with a reported incidence as high as 30%. Pressure ulcers markedly impair rehabilitation and nursing care with a focus on preserving tissue viability is paramount. Patients should be managed on a pressure-reducing mattress, repositioned frequently and hard collars should be removed once daily to assess underlying skin integrity.

Pain

Pain following SCI may be secondary to spinal nerve damage at the level of the injury, concomitant injuries at or above the level of injury and/or deafferentation of the cord. Deafferentiation frequently occurs following incomplete injuries and results in allodynia whereby severe cutaneous pain is evoked by non-noxious stimuli.

Psychological Support

SCI is a devastating event for a patient and their family. Patients frequently experience feelings of despair, uncertainty, and loss, and it is difficult to distinguish grief from pathological depression in the acute setting. It is important for the treating health-care team to proactively manage the psychosocial health of the patient by offering professional counseling, promoting effective coping strategies, fostering independence and outlining realistic expectations while maintaining realistic hope.

Pharmacological Neuroprotective Agents

Despite promising in vitro and pre-clinical data, the neuroprotective properties of a number of agents, including corticosteroids, GM-1 gangliosides, NMDA receptor antagonists and naloxone, have failed to translate to clinical benefit in human trials. The use of methyl-prednisolone is no longer recommended for the treatment of acute SCI and high dose steroids have been associated with harm including sepsis, gastrointestinal bleeding, delirium, and impaired wound healing. At present, no pharmacotherapies are recommended for the management of acute SCI.

Summary

Primary SCI is an acute, frequently irreversible insult, usually occurring in a young and previously healthy population. The pathophysiological response contributes to neuronal loss and persists for several weeks. Preservation of neurological function begins with avoidance of hypoxemia and hypotension, spinal immobilization with early surgical decompression and stabilization. Secondary complications of bowel and bladder dysmotility, pressure ulcers, venous thrombosis, and pain should be anticipated and preventative measures initiated early. Identification of a neuroprotective or neuroregenerative agent that translates to meaningful clinical improvement is a priority for future research.

Further Reading

Abranowicz, A., Bustillo, M.: Anesthesia for cervical spinal cord injury. In: Scher, C. (Ed.). *Anesthesia for Trauma*. New York: Springer; 2014: 167–192.

Berney, S., Bragge, P., Granger, C., Opdam, H., Denehy, L.: The acute respiratory management of cervical spinal cord injury in the first 6 weeks after injury: A systematic review. *Spinal Cord* 2011; **49**(1):17–29.

Ryken, T.C., Hurlbert, R.J., Hadley, M.N., et al: The acute cardiopulmonary management of patients with cervical spinal cord injuries. *Neurosurgery* 2013; 72(Suppl 2):84–92.

Walters, B.C., Hadley, M.N., Hurlbert, R.J., et al: Guidelines for the management of acute cervical spine and spinal cord injuries: 2013 update. *Neurosurgery* 2013; 60(Suppl 1):82–91.

Chapter 33

Head Injury: Initial Resuscitation and Transfer

Joanna L. C. White and Jane E. Risdall

Key Points

- Hypoxia and hypotension are the two major contributors to secondary brain injury.
- Assume that the cervical spine is unstable and maintain appropriate immobilization until no injury has been demonstrated.
- Resuscitate and stabilize a head-injured patient before transfer.
- Communicate early with the receiving neurosurgical center.
- Ensure that appropriate personnel, monitoring equipment, and records accompany the patient when transferred.

Abbreviations

$CMRO_2$	Cerebral metabolic rate for oxygen
CPP	Cerebral perfusion pressure
CSF	Cerebrospinal fluid
CVP	Central venous pressure
EEG	Electro-encephalographic
ETT	Endotracheal tube
FiO_2	Inspired oxygen fraction
GCS	Glasgow coma scale
ICP	Intracranial pressure
MAP	Mean arterial pressure
PEEP	Positive end-expiratory pressure
PTS	Post-traumatic seizures
TBI	Traumatic brain injury
TCDB	Traumatic Coma Data Bank
VQ	Ventilation-perfusion

Contents

- Introduction
- Initial Resuscitation and Stabilization
  - Airway and Breathing
  - Circulation and Fluid Resuscitation

- Neurological Protection
    - Seizure Control
    - Temperature Control
    - Glycemic Control
- Transfer of the Head-Injured Patient
- Further Reading

Introduction

Head injuries can be divided into direct injuries to the structures of the external cranium and injuries to the cranial contents (brain tissue, intra-cranial blood vessels, and structures that control CSF mechanics). Traumatic injuries to the cranial contents result from flexion, extension, or shearing forces as the brain moves within the cranium, as well as from the direct effects of the injury mechanism.

> *Primary injury*: Describes damage that occurs at the time of the initial brain insult. The resulting damage is not usually reversible, and the magnitude of the primary injury is the principal factor differentiating a survivable from a non-survivable injury.

> *Secondary injury*: Is the subsequent insult(s) resulting from derangement of normal physiology following the primary injury. Neuro-protective strategies should be used to prevent and limit secondary injury.

With increasing centralization of neurosurgical services, safe and timely transfer of brain-injured patients to tertiary neurosurgical centers is required. The management and maintenance of neuro-protective physiology during this critical time is paramount.

Initial Resuscitation and Stabilization

The focus of initial resuscitation and stabilization of the brain-injured patient is to limit the primary insult and prevent secondary brain injury. Meticulous attention to the maintenance of normal physiology is imperative (Box 33.1).

Airway and Breathing

Adequate levels of oxygenation and ventilation are required to avoid secondary brain injury. Endotracheal intubation is indicated whenever there is concern about the patient's

---

BOX 33.1 Physiological Targets for Resuscitation and Maintenance of the Brain-Injured Patient

Physiological Targets

PaO_2	≥11 kPa
$PaCO_2$	>80 mmHg
pH	34–37 mmHg
MAP	≥70 mHg
CVP	6–10 cmH_2O
Glucose	4–10 mmol/L (70–180 mg/dl)
Core Temperature	≤37°C

BOX 33.2 Indication for Intubation and Controlled Ventilation in Brain Injured Patients

Indications for Intubation and Controlled Ventilation

Immediate	Loss of protective airway reflexes Inadequate ventilation (poor effort, respiratory pattern, or chest movement) Deteriorating gas exchange (PaO$_2$ < 11 kPa (80 mmHg), PaCO$_2$ > 5.0 kPa or < 4.0 kPa (>37 or <30 mmHg), pH > 7.45 or < 7.35) Uncontrolled seizures
Pre-transfer	Deteriorating level of consciousness or falling Glasgow Coma Score Facial, mouth, or airway injuries Seizures

---

ability to maintain a patent airway or where inadequate gas exchange requires ventilatory support. Emergency intubation can be avoided by early recognition of the "at risk" patient (Box 33.2).

Endotracheal intubation of obtunded patients assumes a full stomach and requires a rapid sequence induction. Severe head injuries are often associated with cervical spine injuries, mandating in-line cervical immobilization at intubation. This may make intubating conditions more difficult and equipment for difficult airway management should be available.

Pre-oxygenation should precede cautious administration of intravenous anesthetic agents. While the use of ketamine and succinylcholine in the presence of raised ICP is debatable, any transient rise in ICP associated with these agents is outweighed by the benefit of rapid control of ventilation and avoidance of hypotension. Prospective data from the TCDB showed that episodes of hypoxemia (SpO$_2$ < 90% or PaO$_2$ < 8 kPa) (< 60 mmHg) were associated with increased morbidity and mortality. Although not reproduced during in-hospital trials, clinical experience suggests that correcting hypoxia improves outcomes.

Controlled ventilation is indicated in patients with severe brain injuries to optimize arterial oxygen (PaO$_2$) and carbon dioxide (PaCO$_2$). The FiO$_2$ is important but prolonged periods at high oxygen levels should be minimized to reduce the risk posed by oxygen free radicals. PEEP can mitigate VQ mismatch but should be used judiciously as it increases intra-thoracic pressure and impedes cerebral venous drainage. Peak inspiratory ventilator pressures should be limited to reduce the risk of pulmonary barotrauma and to minimize intra-thoracic pressure. Excessive hyperventilation (PaCO$_2$ < 4 kPa)(<30 mmHg) should be avoided because it is associated with worsening of cerebral ischemia secondary to cerebral vasoconstriction. The only exception is in the emergency management of raised ICP, when brief periods of controlled hyperventilation can reduce ICP pending definitive intervention.

Circulation and Fluid Resuscitation

Maintenance of an adequate MAP is key in preventing secondary brain injury. Hypotension should always prompt examination for hemorrhage which may require urgent surgical intervention. TCDB data show that systolic hypotension is one of five major predictors of poor outcome from TBI. An isolated episode of hypotension below 90 mmHg increases morbidity and doubles mortality compared to matched patients and is statistically independent of other predictors (age, admission GCS, admission motor score, intracranial diagnosis, and pupillary status). While these results have not yet been mirrored in hospital-based trials, there is compelling evidence that episodes of hypotension are associated with worse outcome.

ICP and CPP are commonly measured in specialist neurosurgical units. Since CPP is determined by MAP and ICP, MAP is sometimes used as a temporary surrogate target to maintain adequate cerebral perfusion until ICP monitoring is instituted. Maintaining a CPP target of 50–70 mmHg is usually achieved with a MAP ≥ 70 mmHg. However, the MAP target may be increased if elevated ICP is suspected. Systolic hypertension can be tolerated in TBI, as it may be the only means of maintaining CPP in the presence of intracranial hypertension. However, MAP above 130 mmHg should always be controlled with short-acting intravenous antihypertensive agents (e.g., labetalol or hydralazine).

Patients with acutely raised ICP, mass lesions (subdural/extradural hematomas), or subarachnoid hemorrhage may have intense sympathetic activity causing increased systemic vascular resistance. This may mask inadequate circulating blood volume. CVP and urine output monitoring can guide intravenous fluid resuscitation. However, the massive diuresis following the administration of hyperosmolar agents such as mannitol or hypertonic saline for acutely raised ICP renders urine output ineffective in monitoring intravascular status.

Brain injury can occur following myocardial injury (e.g., cardiac arrest and hypoxic brain injury), or myocardial injury can occur as a result of primary brain injury (e.g., myocardial ischemia secondary to subarachnoid hemorrhage). Either invasive (e.g., pulmonary artery catheter) or non-invasive cardiac output monitors may assist with assessment of intravascular fluid status, systemic vascular resistance, and cardiac output in these circumstances. Intravenous fluid therapy and/or vasopressor agents can be used to augment MAP. Current opinion favors Hartmann's solution or 0.9% saline since maintenance of serum sodium concentration is important in the prevention of seizures and brain edema. Colloids and human albumin solutions are now used less often.

Boluses of hyperosmolar solutions (20% mannitol or 5% saline) are administered to treat acutely raised ICP. Mannitol has been used for the last three decades replacing most other osmotic diuretics. Its beneficial effects on ICP, CPP, cerebral blood flow and brain metabolism are the result of immediate plasma expansion and reduction in blood viscosity which increases cerebral blood flow and oxygen delivery. While benefiting brain edema, mannitol's diuretic effect can cause profound intravascular volume depletion, hypotension, and acute electrolyte disturbances. Hypertonic saline acts by osmotic mobilization of water across the blood-brain barrier, a reduction in cerebral water content, and a dehydration effect on endothelial cells. All of these effects can improve brain microcirculation. However, the agent can dramatically increase serum sodium concentrations risking central pontine myelinolysis particularly in patients with pre-existing chronic hyponatremia.

Coagulopathy should be corrected aggressively as further intra-cerebral bleeding will exacerbate secondary brain injury. Mechanical deep venous thrombosis prophylaxis should be instituted immediately but chemical prophylaxis withheld pending neurosurgical opinion.

Neurological Protection

Maintaining adequate oxygenation and perfusion of the brain is essential in limiting secondary brain damage and improving outcome. An optimal balance in brain oxygen requirement can be achieved by (1) moderating brain oxygen consumption by adequate sedation and the prevention and treatment of fever and seizures and (2) optimizing brain oxygen delivery by managing MAP, CVP, ICP, avoiding hypocapnia, and hypoxia and ensuring an adequate hemoglobin.

Neurological status is monitored by frequent assessment of a patient's GCS and pupillary light responses which must be documented prior to the use of sedation and muscle relaxants since these confound the assessment of GCS.

Seizure Control

Seizure activity is associated with an increased $CMRO_2$ and should always be controlled. Treatment of seizures with boluses of intravenous benzodiazepine should be followed by anticonvulsant drugs such as levetiracetam or phenytoin. If this fails to control the seizures, consider using an intravenous anesthetic agent, commonly propofol, until effective anticonvulsant therapy can be established. Patients in status epilepticus require intubation and controlled ventilation for airway protection. The use of muscle relaxants will mask seizure activity and only EEG monitoring can confirm cessation.

PTS are those occurring within seven days of TBI. The risk factors for PTS are:

- GCS < 10
- Cortical contusion
- Depressed skull fracture
- Subdural, epidural, or intra-cerebral hematoma
- Penetrating head wound
- Seizures within 24 hours of injury

The incidence of PTS in patients with penetrating brain injuries is 50% and for other high-risk patients the incidence is reported as 4%–25%. Prophylactic anticonvulsants are recommended in high-risk TBI patients but do not improve outcomes.

Temperature Control

Pyrexia in acute brain injury is associated with adverse clinical outcomes. Patients who are hyperthermia should be cooled to normothermia. Trials following resuscitation from cardiac hyperthermic showed that reducing temperature to 33°C conferred no benefit over 36°C but was associated with increased complications. Multi-center trials and meta-analyses of induced hypothermia in TBI have shown that temperatures of 32–35°C in patients with ICP > 20 mmHg are effective in reducing ICP but increase overall complications without conferring a better outcome over standard treatment.

Glycemic control

Glucose is the preferred substrate for brain metabolism. However, hyperglycemia lowers the ischemic neuronal threshold in the presence of neurological injury. Studies have shown that complications arise in critical care patients with poor glycemic control (hypo and hyperglycemia). Recent studies have undertaken subgroup analysis looking at intensive

(4.6–6.0 mmol/L) (82–108 mg/dl) versus conventional (<10 mmol/L) (<180 mg/dl) glycemic control and have shown no outcome benefit with tight control. Despite an increase in hypoglycemic episodes in the tight control group, there was no increase in morbidity or mortality.

Transfer of the Head-Injured Patient

Transferring critically ill patients is complex, and even transient derangement of physiology in brain-injured patients can have catastrophic short and long-term consequences. The same strategies and transfer protocols should apply to both intra-hospital and inter-hospital transfers of brain-injured patients.

Optimal transfer of head-injured patients demands the maintenance of normal physiology (Box 33.1). All brain-injured patients should be managed with the following goals in mind:

- Optimize brain oxygen delivery – achieve adequate MAP, hemoglobin, and FiO_2.
- Minimize brain oxygen demand with sedation, normothermia and seizure control.
- Reduce ICP by: (1) optimizing central venous drainage (head-up 30 degree or reverse Trendelenburg if cervical spine injury), (2) avoiding constrictive ETT ties and cervical collars, (3) keeping the head in a midline position, and (4) reducing intra-thoracic pressure by controlling PEEP.

All patients with severe brain injuries should be referred to regional neurosurgical services in accordance with local protocols, to discuss treatment strategies and expedite transfer.

Successful and safe transfer involves:

- Good communication
- Adequate patient resuscitation and stabilization
- Appropriate monitoring and resuscitation
- Escorts (medical and nursing) with appropriate training, skills, and experience
- Comprehensive patient handover to the receiving team including:
  - Verbal handover to medical and nursing staff
  - Written clinical records
  - Radiology investigations and written reports
  - Relevant laboratory results

Inter-hospital transfers are usually undertaken by road or air. Vehicles fitted with specialist transfer equipment are preferred. Monitoring cables, intravascular infusion lines, ETT tubes, and all other drains should be well secured and positioned so that escorts can access them from a seat-belted position. Journey times, the amount of drugs needed, oxygen usage, and battery requirements must be estimated allowing some provision for delays and deteriorations. Escorts should carry a mobile phone to allow communication with senior staff at both the referring and receiving units.

Further Reading

Andrews, P.J., Sinclair, H.L., Rodriguez, A., et al; Eurotherm3235 Trial Collaborators.: Hypothermia for intracranial hypertension after traumatic brain injury. *N Eng J Med* 2015; **373**:2403–2412.

Association of Anaesthetists of Great Britain and Ireland. Inter-Hospital Transfer. Online (2009).

Brain Trauma Foundation: Guidelines for the Management of Severe Traumatic Brain Injury (4th Edition). https://braintrauma.org/guide lines/guidelines-for-the-management-of-sever e-tbi-4th-ed#/.

Stocchetti, N., Taccone, F.S., Citerio, G., et al: Neuro-Protection in acute brain injury: An up-to-date review. *Crit Care* 2015; **19**:186.

Chapter 34

Intensive Care Management of Acute Head Injury

Susan Stevenson and Ari Ercole

Key Points

- Hypotension and hypoxia are consistent predictors of mortality and poor outcome after severe TBI. Prompt control of hemodynamics and ventilation are crucial.
- A complex inflammatory cascade leads to the development of cerebral edema in the hours after TBI. The disease is highly heterogeneous in its evolution.
- Cerebral perfusion can be maintained by measures to achieve an adequate blood pressure and a reduction in ICP.
- Treatments to manage raised ICP may be medical or surgical and potentially harmful treatments are reserved as rescue therapies.
- Systemic physiological derangements are common after TBI and may impact on outcome.

Abbreviations

ARDS   Acute respiratory distress syndrome
CBF   Cerebral blood flow
CBV   Cerebral blood volume
CMR   Cerebral metabolic rate
CPP   Cerebral perfusion pressure
CSF   Cerebrospinal fluid
GCS   Glasgow Coma Score
HTS   Hypertonic saline
ICP   Intracranial pressure
$PbtO_2$ Brain tissue oxygen tension
TBI   Traumatic brain injury

Contents

- Cerebral Monitoring
  - Intracranial Pressure Monitoring
  - Brain Tissue Oxygenation
  - Other Modalities
- Controlling Intracranial Pressure
  - Osmotherapy
  - Hyperventilation
  - Cerebrospinal fluid Drainage
- Rescue Therapies for Refractory Intracranial Hypertension
  - Temperature Control
  - Barbiturates
  - Decompressive Craniectomy
- Other Issues
  - Systemic Effects
  - General Issues Relating to Intensive Care Management
- Further Reading

Introduction

TBI is a major global public health problem with an increasing incidence. In Europe there are 2.5 million cases per year (500 per 100,000 of the population) resulting in 1 million hospitalizations (250 per 100,000) and 75,000 deaths (9 per 100,000). . The economic burden of acute and chronic medical care, long-term disability, and loss of work is considerable. The annual costs in most western countries amount to billions of dollars.

The median age of those affected by this condition has increased from 27 years in the 1980s to 51 years in 2015. Road traffic collisions remain the leading cause of TBI in the young where mortality is decreasing, however, mortality in the elderly is increasing with falls being the predominant mechanism. The increased incidence within the elderly population is multifactorial and includes an ageing population, better mobility, higher alcohol consumption, and polypharmacy. Additionally, increasing use of antiplatelet and anticoagulant medications are resulting in a greater severity of TBI. It is important to remember that age itself is a predictor of a poorer outcome in all grades of TBI.

TBI severity is classified according to initial GCS as mild (13–15), moderate (9–12) or severe (≤8) although this is increasingly recognized as an imperfect definition. Subsequent disease evolution is heterogeneous and sustained by an inflammatory response. Very soon after a TBI, some patients will go on to develop cerebral edema due to cellular energetic failure (cytotoxic edema) and/or increased capillary permeability (vasogenic edema), which can lead to a rise in ICP. Contusions, hematomas, and disordered CSF circulation may further increase this pressure and the resulting cerebral circulatory compromise will alter oxygen delivery and cause secondary injury to the brain. It is the goal of critical care to monitor cerebral physiological parameters and institute treatment in an attempt to mitigate against this injury.

Initial Measures

Cerebral edema develops over hours and the dominant pathology is usually local hypoperfusion of the injured brain rather than raised ICP except in those patients with a space occupying lesion or particularly severe trauma. Initial measures initiated in the pre-hospital setting or during resuscitation in the emergency department aim to prevent hypoxia (by intubation and mechanical ventilation) and hypotension (by aggressive hemorrhage control), both of which have been repeatedly shown to negatively influence outcome. Early CT scanning on arrival to hospital is essential to determine the extent of intra and extracranial injuries. Systematic targets of care and their rationale are outlined in Table 34.1. Large hematomas causing significant mass effect must be evacuated quickly.

Cerebral Monitoring

Since it is not possible to assess cerebral function clinically in unconscious patients, alternative monitoring methods are needed to assess and diagnose a deterioration in neurological function. Many neurocritical care units now employ multimodality monitoring with protocol-driven therapy to more fully characterize cerebral physiology and facilitate prompt intervention.

Intracranial Pressure Monitoring

ICP monitoring is frequently instituted in the neurocritical care setting and allows the calculation of CPP as a surrogate for perfusion adequacy (see Chapters 3 and 5). Monitoring must be coupled to effective treatments to be useful, including prompt access to neurosurgical intervention. Invasive ICP monitoring should be considered in any patient at risk of intracranial hypertension (Table 34.2). Mortality increases with ICP > 20 mmHg and sustained rises above this level should initiate prompt intervention. There are multiple methods available for ICP measurement but intraventricular and intraparenchymal devices are most commonly employed (see Chapter 45).

The pathobiology of TBI is complex and the dominant contributors to cellular failure may vary between patients and over time thus ICP alone does not provide a complete picture. Many processes in addition to intracranial hypertension may lead to secondary injury which has led to some debate on the effectiveness of ICP-directed therapy for TBI.

Brain Tissue Oxygenation

Measurement of cerebral venous oxygen saturation (jugular bulb oximetry) can reveal critical levels of oxygen extraction and has been used as a guide to the adequacy of cerebral perfusion. $PbtO_2$ can now be measured directly with miniature intraparenchymal probes and this has largely replaced jugular bulb oximetry. Several devices based on miniature electrochemical or optical technologies are now available and may be combined with other measurement modalities. It is difficult to define a "normal" range for $PbtO_2$. However, observationally, oxygen tensions of less than 15 mmHg correlate with a poor outcome and should precipitate intervention (see Chapter 47).

Table 34.1 Initial Physiological Targets

System	Target(s)	Rational
	Intubation (full stomach precautions, manual in-line stabilization).	Secure airway, facilitate ventilation, avoid aspiration.
	Avoid Hypoxia: • SpO_2: >94%	Avoids cellular injury
	Maintain normocapnia: • $PaCO_2$: 4.5–5.0 kPa (34–38mmHg)	CBF proportional to $PaCO_2$. Hypercapnia associated with increased CBV and ICP. Hypocapnia associated with cerebral ischaemia.
	Paralyze using neuromuscular blocking drugs	Ensures better gas exchange, prevents coughing/straining.
Cardiovascular	Initially maintain normotension. Once ICP monitoring established, maintain CPP 50–70 mmHg:	CPP is determined by MAP-ICP. Hypotonic solutions worsen cerebral edema;
	• Correct fluid losses or hypovolaemia (avoid hypotonic solutions and albumin)	Albumin harmful after TBI.
	• Vasopressors to maintain MAP > 90 mmHg	
Brain	Sedation and analgesia (e.g., propofol/fentanyl infusions)	Provides tolerance to intubation and invasive monitoring. Lowers CMR.
	Osmotic therapy if evidence of raised ICP (e.g., blown pupil). Hypertonic saline or mannitol.	No evidence for routine administration.
	Maintain plasma glucose of: 6.0–10.0 mmol/L(110- 180mg/dl	
	Anti-epileptic drugs relative indications if: • Witnessed seizure • High risk, for example, open depressed skull fracture, temporal lobe injuries • Seizure demonstrated on EEG monitoring	Seizures significantly increase CMR and therefore CBF and CBV. Non-convulsion seizures are common following TBI
External	Temperature:	Temperature directly affects CMR.
	Position: • Head-up 30° (unless contraindicated)	Ensure adequate cerebral venous return

Table 34.2 Possible Indications for ICP Monitoring (after Brain Trauma Foundation)

TBI	AND
Severe TBI	Abnormal CT: • Hematomas • Contusion • Swelling • Herniation • Compressed Basal Cisterns
OR	
Severe TBI	Normal CT. But 2 or more of the following: • Age > 40 years • Uni- or bilateral motor posturing • Systolic BP < 90 mmHg

Other Modalities

A number of other neuromonitoring strategies have been employed. Cerebral microdialysis is used in some centers to measure extracellular concentrations of small molecules such as lactate, pyruvate, and glucose. Elevations of the lactate/pyruvate ratio are thought to indicate failure of aerobic cerebral metabolism and are associated with poor outcome. Low cerebral tissue glucose concentrations are also harmful and may be associated with energetic crisis through a variety of mechanisms (see Chapter 48).

Near infrared spectroscopy (NIRS) is another technology for assessing cerebral oxygenation and has the advantage of being non-invasive (see Chapter 47). The signal is largely a reflection of cerebral venous oxygen saturation (i.e., oxygen extraction) but may be contaminated by absorption from extracranial or venous sinus blood.

Controlling Intracranial Pressure

Neuromonitoring is of little use unless coupled to interventions and treatment that can be escalated quickly. An example of a typical protocol is shown in Figure 34.1. Progression between stages of care is prompted by a sudden or unexpected deterioration in the patient's clinical condition or deviation from monitored targets. Prior to commencement of the next treatment stage urgent imaging should always be considered to exclude a surgically amenable lesion.

It is important to realize that, although numerous therapies exist for controlling intracranial hypertension and optimizing oxygen delivery, all of these therapies carry risks. For that reason, it is usual to escalate treatment in a stepwise manner with the most potentially harmful therapies being reserved as rescue strategies for refractory pathology.

Osmotherapy

Interventions for neurological deterioration include osmotherapy, CO_2 control, and CSF drainage. Osmotherapy is the administration of hyperosmotic agents such as HTS or mannitol. These increase plasma osmolality (and extracellular osmolality in the case of

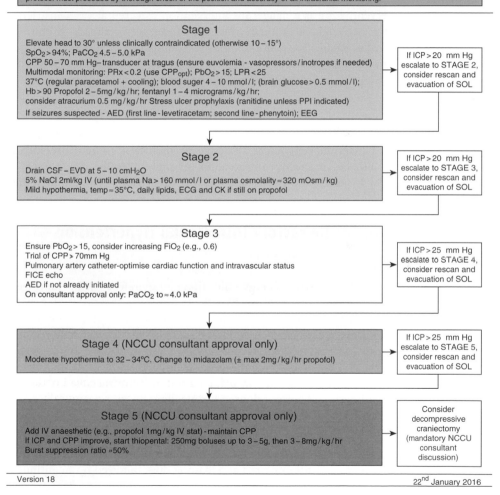

Neurosciences and Trauma Critical Care Unit
Addenbrooke's Hospital, Cambridge, UK

Cambridge University Hospitals
NHS Foundation Trust

Traumatic Brain Injury ICP/CPP Algorithm

Patients with traumatic brain injury admitted to NCCU must be managed according to this protocol.
All patients with or, at risk of developing, intracranial hypertension must have the following within 4h of admission to NCCU:

1) Invasive arterial (transducer at tragus) and central venous monitoring
2) ICP monitoring
3) Cerebral microdialysis catheter and PbO_2 probe
4) ICM+
5) Selected patients: Early MRI ± clinical PET

Initial target CPP 70 mmHg (CPP > 60 mm Hg is acceptable in most patients). Autoregulation parameters and brain biochemistry should be used to individualise targets. Stage 4 and 5 treatments only after approval by NCCU consultant. Evacuate significant space occupying lesions (SOL) and drain CSF (surgical referral for EVD) before escalating medical treatment. Each step of the protocol must preceded by thorough check of the position and accuracy of all intracranial monitoring.

Stage 1

Elevate head to 30° unless clinically contraindicated (otherwise 10 – 15°)
$SpO_2 > 94\%$; $PaCO_2$ 4.5 – 5.0 kPa
CPP 50 – 70 mm Hg – transducer at tragus (ensure euvolemia - vasopressors/inotropes if needed)
Multimodal monitoring: PRx < 0.2 (use CPP_{opt}); $PbO_2 > 15$; LPR < 25
37°C (regular paracetamol + cooling); blood suger 4 – 10 mmol/l; (brain glucose > 0.5 mmol/l);
Hb > 90 Propofol 2 – 5mg/kg/hr; fentanyl 1 – 4 micrograms/kg/hr;
consider atracurium 0.5 mg/kg/hr Stress ulcer prophylaxis (ranitidine unless PPI indicated)
If seizures suspected - AED (first line - levetiracetam; second line - phenytoin); EEG

If ICP > 20 mm Hg escalate to STAGE 2, consider rescan and evacuation of SOL

Stage 2

Drain CSF – EVD at 5 – 10 cmH_2O
5% NaCl 2ml/kg IV (until plasma Na > 160 mmol/l or plasma osmolality ≈ 320 mOsm/kg)
Mild hypothermia, temp ≈ 35°C, daily lipids, ECG and CK if still on propofol

If ICP > 20 mm Hg escalate to STAGE 3, consider rescan and evacuation of SOL

Stage 3

Ensure $PbO_2 > 15$, consider increasing FiO_2 (e.g., 0.6)
Trial of CPP > 70mm Hg
Pulmonary artery catheter-optimise cardiac function and intravascular status
FICE echo
AED if not already initiated
On consultant approval only: $PaCO_2$ to ≈ 4.0 kPa

If ICP > 25 mm Hg escalate to STAGE 4, consider rescan and evacuation of SOL

Stage 4 (NCCU consultant approval only)

Moderate hypothermia to 32 – 34°C. Change to midazolam (± max 2mg/kg/hr propofol)

If ICP > 25 mm Hg escalate to STAGE 5, consider rescan and evacuation of SOL

Stage 5 (NCCU consultant approval only)

Add IV anaesthetic (e.g., propofol 1mg/kg IV stat) - maintain CPP
If ICP and CPP improve, start thiopental: 250mg boluses up to 3 – 5g, then 3 – 8mg/kg/hr
Burst suppression ratio ≈ 50%

Consider decompressive craniectomy (mandatory NCCU consultant discussion)

Version 18

22nd January 2016

Figure 34.1 Example of an ICP and CPP targeted treatment algorithm (Addenbrooke's neurosciences and trauma critical care unit).

HTS), drawing fluid out of edematous brain parenchyma. Additionally, a similar effect on red cells improves rheology and flow through the cerebral microcirculation. HTS has several advantages over mannitol in that it appears to be more effective and leads to intravascular expansion. Mannitol administration on the other hand is associated with a diuresis that can cause hypovolemia and hypotension, which is more undesirable.

Hyperventilation

Arterial CO_2 tension has a potent influence on CBV. Therefore, normal $PaCO_2$ should be carefully maintained in patients with poor intracranial compliance because even if the absolute CBV reduction is small, the effect on ICP can be significant. Hyperventilation or hypocapnia to $PaCO_2$ 4.5–5 kPa (34–38mmHg) is effective in reducing dangerously raised ICP. However, hyperventilation is a dangerous intervention as cerebral vasoconstriction may worsen cerebral ischaemia at a time when blood supply is already precarious. Furthermore, the effect is transient as CSF chemistry will compensate and rebound hyperemia may then occur. For these reasons, hypocapnia below $PaCO_2 < 4.5$ kPa (<34mmHg) should only be considered in extremis as a holding measure until further definitive treatment.

Cerebrospinal Fluid Drainage

CSF drainage via an external ventricular drainage to maintain an ICP pressure of 10–15 cmH_2O may also be an effective intervention for preventing the development of dangerous intracranial hypertension. Even small reductions in CSF volume may reduce ICP significantly.

Rescue Therapies for Refractory Intracranial Hypertension

Temperature Control

Induced hypothermia reduces cerebral energy utilization and therefore CMR. Conversely, pyrexia is well recognized as being harmful in TBI patients. However, these possible benefits must be balanced against harmful side effects such as myocardial depression, immunoparesis, hypotension, hypokalaemia, coagulopathy, increased blood viscosity, and altered drug pharmacokinetics (such as sedative agent accumulation). Despite positive animal model data, use as a primary treatment has recently been associated with harm in humans. However, it is effective as a rescue-therapy in reducing otherwise intractable intracranial hypertension. Re-warming should be very slow and controlled.

Barbiturates

Thiopentone (sodium thiopental) is also an effective medical rescue strategy for refractory intracranial hypertension and is administered as a loading dose followed by a continuous infusion. Barbiturates cause a profound reduction in the CMR and therefore CBF, CBV, and ICP. The exact dose is titrated until electroencephalographic burst suppression is achieved. However, resultant hemodynamic instability can offset its beneficial effects on ICP unless carefully managed. Additionally, at the doses given, the pharmacokinetics of thiopentone become zero-order and recovery time proportional to duration of therapy. Therefore, length of critical care stay becomes prolonged with resultant difficulty in neurological assessment, particularly if plasm thiopentone levels are not measured. Thiopentone infusions are also complicated by hypokalemia, respiratory and infectious complications, and sometimes, hepatic and renal dysfunction, all of which must be carefully managed.

Decompressive Craniectomy

Decompressive craniectomy (DC) involves surgical removal of part of the skull to allow for expansion of the underlying edematous brain. Although effective in reducing ICP, studies have failed to demonstrate benefits of DC as a primary intervention. Its use as a rescue strategy is also controversial. Recent data (RESCUE-ICP Trial) has shown that at 6 months, DC in patients with TBI and refractory intracranial hypertension resulted in lower mortality and higher rates of vegetative state, lower severe disability, and upper severe disability than medical care.

Other Issues

In addition to the optimization of cerebral physiology, TBI care includes management of other associated traumatic injuries, systemic non-trauma effects of TBI, and issues relating to general critical care patients.

Systemic Effects

Cardiovascular Effects

The inflammatory cascade associated with trauma can have multisystem effects. Myocardial impairment can arise due to multiple mechanisms including direct cardiac contusion. Neurogenic catecholamine release from brainstem or medullary injury can place significant demands on the myocardium and potentially leading to a neurogenic stress cardiomyopathy. Additionally, inotropic/vasoactive support to maintain CPP may further worsen myocardial demands.

Respiratory Effects

Respiratory complications are also common following trauma. Intubation, ventilation and paralysis predispose to potential infective consequences. Cardiomyopathy may cause pulmonary edema. Finally, the management of TBI is particularly difficult in the presence of severe thoracic trauma, and it can be particularly difficult to balance the need for tight CO_2 control with the need for permissive and gentle ventilation in ARDS patients.

Metabolic Effects

Significant metabolic disturbances can arise in TBI patients. Both hyperglycemia and hypoglycemia are harmful after acute brain injury and must be avoided. Disturbances in sodium homeostasis are particularly prevalent. Serum sodium is the main control of intracellular volume and a degree of hypernatremia is common and probably inevitable as a result of TBI treatment. Hyponatremia ($Na^+ < 135$ mmol/L) may, however, occur as a result of cerebral salt wasting syndrome (CSWS) or syndrome of inappropriate antidiuretic hormone (SIADH). The former is thought to be due to increased renal sodium loss and is treated with sodium and volume replacement. Conversely, SIADH is due to excessive ADH and renal water retention with resultant plasma sodium dilution requiring fluid restriction although this may be inappropriate in a patient whose circulation is being supported.

Hyponatremia or sudden falls in serum sodium are highly undesirable as they will worsen cerebral edema and should be treated aggressively in the acute phase (e.g., with HTS – See Chapter 41).

A degree of hypernatremia ($Na^+ > 155$ mmol/L) is most commonly iatrogenic from the effects of osmotherapy and may be, to an extent, inevitable and perhaps even desirable. However, central diabetes insipidus (DI) can occur because of pituitary dysfunction; inadequate ADH release results in large quantities of dilute urine being passed. Mild DI may be treated with meticulous fluid replacement. However, if severe, DI can lead to very rapid rises in sodium and dangerous hypovolemia and may require administration of desmopressin.

General Issues Relating to Intensive Care Management

Like all critically unwell patients, specific caution must be made to prevent additional complications associated with critical illness. All patients should receive stress ulcer and deep vein thrombosis prophylaxis. Early enteral feeding reduces the catabolic effects associated with the exaggerated inflammatory response of TBI and improves outcome. Hypotonic fluids and fluids containing glucose should be avoided because of the potential to worsen cerebral edema, excepting for the specific purpose of treating hypoglycemia. The use of albumin as a resuscitation fluid is associated with a worse outcome after TBI.

Anemia is common in all ICU and trauma patients and there is some debate over the ideal hemoglobin target and whether a truly permissive approach is appropriate after TBI. Permissive transfusion thresholds are believed to reduce infectious and ischemic complications in general ICU patients. However, this must not be at the expense of a precarious cerebral oxygen delivery situation that may exist after TBI. Consensus is lacking but a hemoglobin target of 8.0 or 9.0 g/dL is usually accepted.

Disordered coagulation is common after trauma and may occur even after isolated TBI. Coagulopathy is associated with increased contusion evolution and must be avoided. Anticoagulant use is associated with poorer outcome after TBI and therapeutic anticoagulation should be reversed. Pharmacological venous thromboembolism prophylaxis is usually not appropriate in the acute setting but mechanical prevention is important.

Further Reading

Andrews, P.J., Sinclair, H.L., Rodriguez, A., et al: Eurotherm3235 trial collaborators. Hypothermia for intracranial hypertension after traumatic brain injury. N Engl J Med 2015; 373 (25):2403–2412.

Brain Trauma Foundation: Guidelines for the Management of Severe Traumatic Brain Injury (4th Edition). https://braintrauma.org/guide lines/guidelines-for-the-management-of-severe -tbi-4th-ed#/.

Chesnut, R.M., Temkin, N., Carney, N., et al: A trial of intracranial-pressure monitoring in traumatic brain injury. N Engl J Med 2012; 367 (26):2471–2481.

Cooper, D.J., Rosenfeld, J.V., Murray, L., et al: Decompressive craniectomy in diffuse traumatic brain injury. N Engl J Med 2011; 364(16):1493–1502.

Hutchinson, P.J., Kolias, A.G., Timofeev, I.S., et al: Trial of decompressive craniectomy for traumatic intracranial hypertension. N Engl J Med 2016; 375(12):1119–1130.

Chapter

35

Intracranial Hemorrhage: ICU Management

Erika Brinson and Anne L. Donovan

Key Points

- Patients are at high risk of developing complications after subarachnoid hemorrhage.
- Initial management should focus on evaluation and treatment of neurologic and cardiac dysfunction, hemodynamic control, airway and ventilation management, pain control, and sedation.
- Pain should be treated first and sedation minimized when possible to allow frequent neurological examinations.
- Aneurysms are definitively treated with either coil embolization or microsurgical clip ligation which should be performed early when clinically possible.
- Cerebral vasospasm may occur from 3 to 14 days post-bleed and is treated with a combination of medical and interventional therapies.

Abbreviations

CSF	Cerebrospinal fluid
CSW	Cerebral salt wasting
CT	Computed tomography
DCI	Delayed cerebral ischemia
DND	Delayed neurologic deterioration
DVT	Deep venous thrombosis
EEG	Electroencephalography
EVD	External Ventricular Drain
ICP	Intracranial pressure
ICU	Intensive care unit
SAH	Subarachnoid hemorrhage
SIADH	Syndrome of inappropriate antidiuretic hormone

Contents

- Introduction
- Clinical Findings and Diagnosis

- Initial Management
  - Elevated Intracranial Pressure
  - Hemodynamic Control
  - Volume Status
  - Neurocardiogenic Injury
  - Airway and Ventilation Management
  - Pain and Sedation Management
- Definitive Treatment of Subarachnoid Hemorrhage
- Treatment of Complications
  - Delayed Neurologic Deterioration
  - Delayed Cerebral Ischemia
  - Cerebral Vasospasm
  - Other Critical Care Issues
- Timeline for Recovery
- Further Reading

Introduction

Intracranial hemorrhage refers to the rupture of a vessel inside the cranial cavity. Intracerebral hemorrhage refers specifically to bleeding into the brain parenchyma caused most frequently by hypertension, amyloid disease, anticoagulation, tumor, drug abuse, or arteriovenous malformation. Bleeding into the subarachnoid space and CSF is called SAH and is usually caused by rupture of a cerebral aneurysm.

This chapter will focus on the ICU management of acute SAH, which is associated with significant morbidity and up to 50% mortality. Patients surviving the initial event often have a prolonged course and ultimately only one third of survivors achieve a good functional outcome.

Clinical Findings and Diagnosis

SAH most commonly presents with a sudden severe headache. A sentinel bleed may precede a larger hemorrhage by days to weeks. Patients often have a history of hypertension, smoking or drug, and alcohol abuse. Examination findings include focal neurological deficits, meningismus, and retinal hemorrhages. A non-contrast head CT scan is the initial imaging modality of choice. If the head CT is negative but suspicion for SAH is still high, a lumbar puncture may reveal elevated CSF red blood cell count and xanthochromia (see Chapter 16).

Initial Management

Patients with significant intracranial hemorrhages are admitted to the ICU for management. Patients treated at a high volume center with a neurointensive care unit after initial stabilization have significantly improved outcomes. Common management considerations are discussed below.

Elevated Intracranial Pressure

Elevated ICP, which may be caused by hematoma, edema, hydrocephalus, impaired auto-regulation, or infarction, may present with somnolence, headache, nausea, vomiting, and papilledema. Decreased cerebral perfusion pressure may lead to ischemia. Interventions to decrease ICP include elevating the head of the bed, optimizing pain control and sedation, and administering intravenous osmotic agents. ICP may increase due to impaired CSF drainage caused by the hemorrhage necessitating insertion of an external ventricular drain (EVD). Hemicraniectomy may be performed when medical management fails to control ICP. Temporary hyperventilation to a $PaCO_2$ no lower than 30 mmHg can be used if brain herniation is imminent.

Hemodynamic Control

The incidence of re-bleeding, a common and devastating event, is highest within the initial 72 hours after aneurysm rupture. Early repair of the ruptured aneurysm significantly reduces the risk for re-rupture. A short course of antifibrinolytic therapy is sometimes used prior to securing the aneurysm, but may increase the risk of DVT.

To prevent re-bleeding prior to securing the aneurysm, blood pressure targets include mean arterial pressure <110 mmHg and systolic blood pressure <160 mmHg. Initial antihypertensive agents of choice include intravenous labetalol or hydralazine, while infusions of nicardipine or labetalol may be used for refractory cases. Hypotension is less common but requires prompt treatment since it can lead to decreased cerebral perfusion and ischemia.

Volume Status

Hypovolemia is associated with cerebral infarction and poor outcomes. Clinical assessment of volume status with strict measurement of input and output is the best guide. In most patients, use of central venous pressure or a pulmonary artery catheter does not add significant benefit. Isotonic crystalloids are generally the resuscitation fluid of choice.

Neurocardiogenic Injury

Blood levels of epinephrine and norepinephrine spike within minutes of aneurysm rupture and fall back to normal levels within two hours. This catecholamine response can have many physiologic sequelae, including myocardial and pulmonary vascular injury. So-called "neurogenic stress cardiomyopathy," which bears many similarities to Takotsubo cardiomyopathy, is associated with DCI and worsening outcomes. Patients may complain of chest pain, or have dyspnea, hypoxemia, elevated cardiac biomarkers, and develop cardiogenic shock. Common electrocardiographic abnormalities include QT-segment prolongation, ST-segment changes, and dysrhythmias. Wall motion abnormalities unrelated to coronary artery territories and apical ballooning may be visible on echocardiography. Myocardial dysfunction appears early after the bleed and generally resolves within a week. Treatment is supportive and follows the same guidelines as those used to manage patients without neurological injury.

Airway and Ventilation Management

Pulmonary complications, including pneumonia, pulmonary edema, and acute respiratory distress syndrome are a major cause of mortality following SAH. Up to 80% of patients will have impaired oxygenation which can be due to neurogenic pulmonary edema, cardiac failure, and fluid overload. Patients may require intubation for airway protection or respiratory distress. Special care must be taken to avoid large blood pressure changes during laryngoscopy. Ventilation goals include tidal volumes of 6–8 ml/kg of ideal body weight, $PaCO_2$ 30–40 mmHg, (4–5.3 kPa) and oxygen saturation >94%. Permissive hypercapnia should be used cautiously. Spontaneously breathing patients often have a respiratory alkalosis, which should only be treated if it is causes excessive work of breathing or signs of cerebral ischemia.

Pain and Sedation Management

Headaches and other pain can be treated with acetaminophen (paracetamol) or opioids, but avoidance of over-sedation is key. Sedation choice must weigh the ability to perform an accurate neurological examination with the potential benefits of reduced ICP and cerebral oxygen consumption, improved tolerance of mechanical ventilation, reduced sympathetic activity, anxiolysis, and comfort. It is important to minimize sedation as much as safely possible while ensuring adequate pain control. Standard delirium precautions including frequent reorientation should also be employed. During the use of common sedative agents such as propofol and dexmedetomidine, attention must be paid to maintaining adequate cerebral perfusion pressure while avoiding excessive increases in $PaCO_2$ which increases ICP. The favorable hemodynamic profile of benzodiazepines may be outweighed by their long half-life and association with delirium when used as an infusion. Neuromuscular blockers should be avoided unless their use is necessary.

Definitive Treatment of Subarachnoid Hemorrhage

Aneurysmal SAH is definitively treated with either coil embolization or microsurgical clip ligation, which should be performed as early as possible to decrease re-bleeding risk. For more information on these procedures, see Chapters 16 and 28.

Treatment of Complications

Common complications associated with SAH are discussed below. In addition, patients are also at risk for medical complications affecting the general ICU population.

Delayed Neurologic Deterioration

DND describes clinically significant worsening of a patient's neurological status not caused by further bleeding. There are many causes including; vasospasm, cerebral edema, hydrocephalus, seizures, fever, and metabolic disturbances.

Delayed Cerebral Ischemia

Worsening neurologic status related to cerebral ischemia after SAH is referred to as DCI, a complex and incompletely understood phenomenon. It occurs in 30%–40% of patients and is the major cause of morbidity after the bleed itself.

Cerebral arterial vasospasm is one of the most recognized and potentially treatable causes of DCI. Other proposed causes include disruption of the blood-brain barrier, apoptosis, oxidative stress, microvascular spasm, impaired cerebral autoregulation, and microthrombosis.

Cerebral Vasospasm

Vasospasm can lead to stroke or death. It is seen as early as 3 days after aneurysm rupture, but the highest risk occurs 5–14 days after the bleed. Risk increases with larger hemorrhages and with poorer clinical grades. Vasospasm is likely driven by accumulation of blood degradation products in the subarachnoid space.

There are many available techniques to aid in early diagnosis of vasospasm, including frequent neurological examination, daily transcranial Doppler ultrasound studies, EEG, CT perfusion scanning, and near-infrared spectroscopy. If suspicion for vasospasm exists, further imaging and/or empiric treatment should occur.

Vasospasm can be treated with medical and interventional therapies. "Triple-H" therapy refers to the combination of hypertension, hypervolemia, and hemodilution. Induced hypertension has been shown to increase cerebral blood flow and improve the patient's neurology. In particular, after securing the aneurysm, patients with evidence of clinical deterioration should have their blood pressure augmented to target a goal at which neurological status improves. Phenylephrine or norepinephrine are considered the vasopressor of choice. CT perfusion is a useful imaging modality to help target MAP (see Chapter 51). The use of hypervolemia for blood pressure augmentation increases the risk of cardiopulmonary complications without additional benefits. Hemodilution increases cerebral blood flow, but oxygen delivery does not improve since the oxygen carrying capacity of the blood is decreased. The latter two interventions are therefore not considered especially important in treatment.

Nimodipine, a calcium channel blocker, is the only intervention shown to improve outcomes in prospective randomized controlled trials. Nimodipine is thought to prevent vasospasm by inhibiting the adverse effects of certain substances on the cerebral vasculature and by increasing fibrinolytic activity. However, it does not actually treat established vasospasm. All patients should receive oral nimodipine for 21 days following SAH unless it causes problematic hypotension.

Endovascular treatment of vasospasm involves local injection of vasodilators and/or angioplasty. The risks of the procedure include hypotension and vessel rupture.

Other Critical Care Issues

Blood glucose

Maintain blood glucose between 80 and 200 mg/dl and avoid hypoglycemia. Glucose levels >220 mg/dl are associated with infection and worsening outcomes.

Anemia

Anemia occurs in approximately 50% of patients after SAH and the average hemoglobin drop is 3 g/dl. It is important to maintain hemoglobin above 7 g/dl but to avoid unnecessary transfusions which can alter cerebral hemodynamics unfavorably.

DVT Prophylaxis

DVTs can occur in up to 18% of SAH patients due to a prothrombotic state and limited mobility. Sequential compression devices should be used in all patients where possible. Subcutaneous unfractionated heparin 5000 units 2–3 times daily once is usually allowed once the aneurysm is secure. However, it is often held for 24 hours before and after invasive procedures.

Stress Ulcer Prophylaxis

Patients with a high-grade SAH or those intubated but not fed enterally are at risk of stress ulcers. The use of either an H_2-blocker or proton pump inhibitor is recommended.

Seizure Prophylaxis

Seizures occur in up to 20% of patients and may be a sign of aneurysm re-rupture. Consider a non-phenytoin anticonvulsant in high-risk patients and continuous EEG if there is evidence of neurological deterioration. Phenytoin is associated with a worse outcome following SAH.

Temperature Management

Pyrexia in SAH patients is often due to a non-infectious systemic inflammatory reaction or centrally driven due to blood within the ventricular system. However, infective causes must be ruled-out particularly in patients with an EVD in-situ (see Chapter 37). Every attempt should be made to diagnose the source of infection but treatment is often started when there is a strong clinical suspicion. Normothermia should be maintained by using pharmacological agents or surface/invasive cooling methods.

Electrolyte Management

Electrolyte abnormalities are not uncommon in SAH patients. Hypernatremia due to hypovolemia, osmotic agents, or neurogenic diabetes insipidus along with hyponatremia due to the SIADH or CSW can occur in these patients. These electrolyte problems are discussed in detail in Chapter 41.

Timeline for Recovery

The ICU stay can range from days to weeks depending on the patient's clinical course and complications. Physical and occupational therapy should be started as soon as possible. Tracheotomy and gastrostomy or jejunostomy tube placement may be appropriate for some patients. Recovery is often prolonged and many, particularly young patients, continue to improve for more than a year.

Further Reading

Budohoski, K.P., Guilfoyle, M., Helmy, A., et al: The pathophysiology and treatment of delayed cerebral ischaemia following subarachnoid hemorrhage. *J Neurol Neurosurg Psychiatry* 2014; **84**:1343–1353.

Claassen, J., Bernardino, G.L., Kreiter, K., et al: Effect of cisternal and ventricular blood on risk of delayed cerebral ischemia after subarachnoid hemorrhage: The fisher scale revisited. *Stroke* 2001; **32**:2012–2020.

Diringer, M.N., Bleck, T.P., Hemphill, C., et al: Critical care management of patients following aneurysm subarachnoid hemorrhage: Recommendations from the neurocritical care society's multidisciplinary consensus conference. *Neurocrit Care* 2011; **15**:211–249.

Elkind, M.S.V., Sacco, R.L.: Chapter 37: Pathogenesis, classification, and epidemiology of cerebrovascular disease. In: Rowland, L.P., Pedley, T.A. (Eds.) *Merritt's Neurology*, 12th ed. Philadelphia: Lippencott Williams, & Wilkins;2010: 258.

Green, D.M., Burns, J.D., DeFusco, C.M.: ICU management of aneurysmal subarachnoid hemorrhage. *J Intensive Care Med* 2013; **28**:341–354.

Hunt, W., Hess, R.: Surgical risk as related to time of intervention in the repair of intracranial aneurysms. *J Neurosurg* 1968; **28**:14–20.

Salem, R., Vallée, F., Dépret, F., et al: Subarachnoid hemorrhage induces an early and reversible cardiac injury associated with catecholamine release: One-week follow-up study. *Crit Care* 2014; **18**:558–568.

Seder, D.B., Jagoda, A., Riggs, B.: Emergency neurological life support: Airway, ventilation, and sedation. *Neurocrit Care* 2015; **23**:S5–S22.

Wilson, D.A., Nakaji, P., Albuquerque, F.C., et al: Time course of recovery following poor-grade SAH: The incidence of delayed improvement and implications for SAH outcome study design. *J Neurosurg* 2013; **119**:606–612.

Zoerle, T., Lombardo, A., Colombo, A., et al: Intracranial pressure after subarachnoid hemorrhage. *Criti Care Med* 2015; **43**:168–176.

Management of Acute Stroke

Philip E. Bickler

Key Points

- Acute stroke is a medical emergency that requires quick action to preserve neurological function.
- Recent studies show a clear benefit of endovascular clot retrieval for treatment of acute anterior circulation stroke compared to chemical thrombolysis alone.
- Mean arterial blood pressure should be maintained >85 mmHg, with a systolic pressure between 140 and 180 mmHg.
- Blood glucose concentration should be maintained in the range of 70–140 mg/dl. (3.8–7.8 mmol/L)
- During interventional radiology procedures for clot retrieval, the choice of general anesthesia versus sedation/monitored care must be made based on the patient's ability to cooperate and to protect their airway.
- Emerging evidence suggests better neurological outcomes following clot retrieval under sedation than general anesthesia.

Abbreviations

CT   Computed tomography
DALYs   Disability adjusted life years
ICU   Intensive care unit
r-tPA   Recombinant tissue plasminogen activator
SNACC   Society of Neuroanesthesia and Critical Care

Contents

- Overview of Acute Stroke
    - Urgency of Treating Acute Stroke
    - Stroke Outcomes and Epidemiology
    - Perioperative Stroke Risk
    - Current Stroke Management

- Management of Patients for Clot Retrieval
  - Blood Pressure
  - Airway Management
  - Temperature Management
  - Glucose Management
  - Monitoring
  - Anticoagulation
- Anesthetic Management for Endovascular Stroke Treatment

Overview of Acute Stroke

Urgency of Treating Acute Stroke

An acute stroke is a true medical emergency. Complete occlusion of a large cerebral artery kills 1.9 million neurons every minute. An hour of ischemia is equivalent to the cell death that occurs during 3.6 years of normal brain aging. Therefore, the speed of restoring cerebral circulation is critically important for improving neurological outcome. Every institution that cares for stroke patients should have policies and procedures in place that ensure timely care of these patients.

Stroke Outcomes and Epidemiology

Cerebrovascular disease causes significant morbidity and mortality. The long-term mortality following a significant cerebrovascular event is high. Death rates in the 10-year period following a stroke are increased 30% over those of age-matched controls. Stroke survivors require expensive health care and experience significant loss of DALYs. Ischemic cerebrovascular disease is the fourth leading cause of death in the USA and the fifth leading cause of healthcare expenditure. Ischemic cerebrovascular disease is the sixth leading cause of death worldwide, and was responsible for the loss of 50 million DALYs in 2014. The incidence of stroke is increasing in the developing world, with more than 90% of the global burden of ischemic cerebrovascular disease now occurring in low and middle-income countries.

Perioperative Stroke Risk

Patients undergoing low-risk surgery have a slightly increased stroke risk, with a perioperative risk of approximately 0.1% in non-neurosurgical, non-cardiovascular procedures. However, patients who suffer a stroke following these low risk procedures experience longer hospital stays and up to an eight-fold increase in hospital death. Higher rates of stroke (0.1–4%) and similar rates of mortality apply to neurological and cardiovascular surgery, depending on patient co-morbidities and the type of surgery.

Current Stroke Management

Neurological assessment and brain imaging are the foundations of stroke diagnosis. Typically, a CT scan is used to determine the likelihood of the occurrence of an ischemic or hemorrhagic stroke. For those diagnosed with an ischemic stroke, two main treatment options are available: thrombolysis with chemical agents and endovascular (mechanical)

BOX 36.1 Contraindications to Recombinant Tissue Plasminogen Activator (r-tPA)

Contraindications to r-tPA

Sustained hypertension above 180/110 mm Hg
Symptoms suggestive of subarachnoid hemorrhage
Previous history of intracranial hemorrhage
ST elevation myocardial infarction within the previous 3 months
Seizure at onset with suspected postictal deficits
Minor or rapidly improving neurological deficits
Major head trauma or stroke within the previous 3 months
Major surgery within the previous 14 days
Gastrointestinal or urinary tract hemorrhage within the previous 21 days
Arterial puncture at a non-compressible site within the previous 7 days
Active bleeding or acute traumatic fracture on examination
Head CT showing hemorrhage or multilobar infarction
Oral anticoagulation with INR > 1. 7
Heparin within previous 48 hours
Platelet count <100,000 per mm^3
Blood glucose level <50 mg/dl

---

clot retrieval. Thrombolytic drugs such as r-tPa remain the mainstay of early treatment of acute ischemic stroke. Intravenous thrombolytic treatment is given to patients without CT imaging evidence of hemorrhage, and who have presented within 4.5 hours of the onset of stroke symptoms. For contraindications to this therapy see Box 36.1. The incidence of hemorrhagic conversion increases with time from stroke symptom onset, so there is a relatively limited time window for thrombolysis therapy.

Endovascular stroke therapy is now the standard of care for some types of stroke. Three randomized trials for endovascular stroke therapy published in 2015 demonstrated a clear benefit of endovascular clot removal (plus intravenous tPa) compared to standard therapy with intravenous thrombolysis alone. The recently released American Heart Association/American Stroke Association guidelines (2015) recommend endovascular treatment of acute ischemic stroke in patients with a large vessel anterior circulation occlusion, independent pre-stroke functional status and favorable imaging. These trials and guidelines will change clinical practice and have significant ramifications for anesthesia care providers.

Management of Patients for Clot Retrieval

The management of acute stroke patients must be based on specific targets for blood pressure, blood glucose, assessment of airway or breathing compromise, and the ability of the patient to co-operate with the procedure. In addition, in the event of peri-procedural complications, the anesthesiologist should be immediately available to reverse heparin with protamine, manage blood pressure, and convert to general anesthesia. There are several fundamental management issues in addition to the choice of anesthetic.

Blood Pressure

Patients who present with acute ischemic stroke have decreased perfusion to at least one brain region, and may have multiple areas of the cerebral or spinal cord that is threatened with ischemia due to underlying ischemic vascular disease, chronic hypertension, and other medical co-morbidities. Therefore, a goal of a MAP >85 mmHg is recommended, but no outcomes studies have investigated this. The systolic blood pressure should be maintained >140 mmHg and <180 mmHg with fluids and vasopressors, as indicated. In a recent American Heart Association review of stroke therapy, it was concluded that for most patients a systolic blood pressure in the 140–150 mmHg range was associated with the best outcomes. The diastolic blood pressure should be maintained at <105 mmHg. Causes of hypotension, such as volume depletion, myocardial infarction, cardiac arrhythmia, blood loss, retroperitoneal hemorrhage, and aortic dissection from endovascular complications should be identified and treated. These recommendations also apply to patients who are being treated with intravenous thrombolytic agents. Following thrombolysis and successful recanalization of occluded vessel(s), blood pressure targets may be adjusted (lowered) in communication with the neuro-interventional radiologists and neurologists because the reperfused brain often lacks autoregulation leading to a risk of hyperperfusion causing hemorrhage.

Airway Management

Tracheal intubation is not required if (1) adequate oxygenation can be maintained without high levels of supplemental oxygen; (2) adequate ventilation exists to achieve normocapnia or only mild hypercapnia; and (3) adequate cooperation can be expected when there is a need for remaining motionless or for breath holding during critical neuro-imaging. Of course, patients with decreased consciousness, signs of brainstem dysfunction with compromised protective airway reflexes, and those with active nausea or vomiting require intubation of the trachea. Intubation may also be required for patients who develop agitation or inability to communicate and those who develop airway obstruction under sedation.

Temperature Management

It is good practice to maintain body temperature between 35°C and 37°C during endovascular treatment. Antipyretics and cooling devices are indicated if the patient is febrile. Shivering should be treated with a forced air warming blanket and only when necessary should intravenous meperidine be administered.

Glucose Management

The blood glucose should be measured in patients arriving for endovascular treatment and repeated at least once every hour. Hyperglycemia is an independent predictor of poor outcome following ischemic and hemorrhagic stroke. Blood glucose should be maintained in the range of 70–140 mg/dl(3.8 – 7.8 mmol/L). Insulin should be given for glucose values of >140 mg/dl(>7.8 mmol/L), using a protocol-driven intravenous insulin infusion. Fluids containing dextrose should be avoided during endovascular treatment unless hypoglycemia is present. The goal of treatment of hypoglycemia should be to achieve glucose levels of >70 mg/dl(>3.8 mmol/L).

Monitoring

Hemodynamic monitoring and management should commence as soon as the diagnosis of acute ischemic stroke has been made. At a minimum, the standard American Society of Anesthesiologists recommendations for patient monitoring during general anesthesia or sedation should be followed. The continuously measured parameters include heart rate and rhythm, blood pressure, expired CO_2, body temperature, and respiratory rate. Close monitoring and control of arterial pressure is a requirement in all acute stroke cases, and invasive blood pressure monitoring is recommended for this. An arterial line also facilitates care in the ICU or stroke unit and is used for blood samples for blood gas analysis. Arterial pressure can easily be obtained from the femoral artery catheter allowing the procedure to progress while a radial catheter is inserted. There are no trials that demonstrate superior outcomes with EEG and/or cerebral oximeters.

Anticoagulation

The optimal level of anticoagulation during endovascular treatment of stroke has not been established. Heparin is frequently administered as requested by the interventional team. Anesthesiologists must be prepared to administer protamine (typically 50 mg IV) immediately to a heparinized patient who is experiencing an acute intracerebral hemorrhage.

Anesthetic Management for Endovascular Stroke Treatment

A consensus statement from the SNACC states that the optimal anesthetic care for stroke treatment remains controversial. The use of general anesthesia may be associated with an increased risk of adverse outcome when compared to monitored anesthesia care. However, these data are likely confounded by selection bias, based on the presumption that sicker patients tend to receive general anesthesia for airway protection or because they are comatose. The choice of anesthetic technique and pharmacological agents should be individualized based on the patient's medical condition in communication with the neurointerventional radiologist. If monitored anesthesia care/sedation is used, minimal doses of agents like fentanyl are recommended to preserve patient cooperation and maintain adequate breathing and oxygenation. Even if it is ultimately shown that outcomes are better with MAC compared to GA, the decision over anesthetic choice will rarely be at equipoise; other factors such as patient ability to cooperate, and the need for airway protection will continue to determine the choice. Anesthesia assessment and care should be done quickly to avoid delay in endovascular treatment.

General anesthesia is preferable in uncooperative or agitated patients and for patients who cannot protect their airway, e.g., those patients with posterior circulation stroke who experience brainstem/bulbar dysfunction, depressed level of consciousness or respiratory compromise. Local anesthesia with sedation is an option for patients with anterior circulation strokes who can protect their airway and are cooperative. In all patients receiving local anesthesia with sedation, the anesthesia provider should be prepared to rapidly change to a general anesthetic with an endotracheal tube, if needed. With general anesthesia, early post-procedural neurological assessment and extubation should be the goal when selecting types and doses of anesthetic agents.

Further Reading

Saver, J.L.: Time is brain – quantified. *Stroke* 2006; **237**:263–266.

Mozaffarian, D., Benjamin, E.J., Go, A.S., *et al.* American Heart Association Statistics Committee and Stroke Statistics Subcommittee.: Heart disease and stroke statistics–2015 update: A report from the American Heart Association. *Circulation* 2015; **131**:e29–e322.

Berkhemer, O.A., Fransen, P.S., Beumer, D., *et al.* MR CLEAN Investigators.: A randomized trial of intraarterial treatment for acute ischemic stroke. *N Engl J Med* 2015; **372**:11–20.

Campbell, B.C., Mitchell, P.J., Kleinig, T.J., *et al.* EXTEND-IA Investigators. Endovascular therapy for ischemic stroke with perfusion-imaging selection. *N Engl J Med* 2015; **372**:1009–1018.

Goyal, M., Demchuk, A.M., Menon, B.K., *et al.* ESCAPE Trial Investigators.: Randomized assessment of rapid endovascular treatment of ischemic stroke. *N Engl J Med* 2015; **372**:1019–1030.

2015 American Heart Association/American Stroke Association Focused Update of the 2013 Guidelines for the Early Management of Patients With Acute Ischemic Stroke Regarding Endovascular Treatment: A Guideline for Healthcare Professionals From the American Heart Association/American Stroke Association.: AHA/ASA focused update of the 2013 guidelines for the early management of patients with acute ischemic stroke regarding endovascular treatment: A guideline for healthcare professionals from the American Heart association/American Stroke association. *Stroke* 2015; **46**(10):3020–3035.

Talke, P.O., Sharma, D., Heyer, E.J., *et al.* Republished: Society for neuroscience in anesthesiology and critical care expert consensus statement: Anesthetic management of endovascular treatment for acute ischemic stroke. *Stroke* 2014; **45**(8): e138–e150.

Chapter 37

Central Nervous System Infections

Kelsey Innes and Mypinder Sekhon

Key Points

- Central nervous system infections are common in neuro-critically ill patients and can be associated with long-term neurological sequelae.
- Prompt diagnosis and management with antimicrobials is of paramount importance to improve outcome.
- Cerebrospinal fluid examination is essential for the diagnosis of bacterial meningitis and other central nervous system infections.
- Neuroimaging may assist in delineating the etiology of various forms of encephalitis, immunocompromised infections, and bacterial cerebral abscesses.

Abbreviations

BM   Bacterial meningitis
CA   Cerebral abscess
CNS   Central nervous system
CSF   Cerebrospinal fluid
EVD   External ventricular drain
HIV   Human immunodeficiency virus

Learning Objectives

- Describe the risk factors, clinical manifestations, diagnosis, and management of bacterial meningitis.
- Describe the etiology, diagnosis, and management of encephalitis.
- Describe the etiology, pathophysiology, diagnosis, and management of bacterial cerebral abscess.
- Describe the causes, diagnosis, and management of immunocompromised central nervous system infections.

Contents

- Introduction
- Bacterial Meningitis

- Encephalitis
- Ventriculitis
- Infections in Immunocompromised Patients
  - Cryptococcus
  - Toxoplasmosis
  - Mycobacterium Tuberculosis
- Cerebral Abscess
- Further Reading

Introduction

CNS infections including meningitis, encephalitis, ventriculitis, and CAs can result in devastating outcomes. The clinical index of suspicion should be high for a CNS infection in the acutely obtunded patient with signs of infection or meningeal irritation. Prompt diagnosis including physical examination, CSF analysis and neuroimaging is required to delineate the underlying etiology. Simultaneously, antimicrobial therapy with a broad spectrum of activity should be administered targeting all possible pathological microbes. For the purposes of this chapter, we will focus on BM, encephalitis, ventriculitis and CA as these diseases carry significant mortality and morbidity.

Bacterial Meningitis

BM, defined as an infection of the meningeal layers of the brain, carries a mortality of 30–50%. Fever, headache, and nuchal rigidity form the classic triad of meningitis; however, all three are present in less than 50% of cases. Physical examination findings include the jolt accentuation test (headache worsening with repeated lateral rotation of the neck), Kernig's sign (patient supine, hip flexed, and inability to fully extend knee) and Brudzinski's sign (hip and knee flexion with induced neck flexion). The etiology and risk factors for BM are shown in Box 37.1

Diagnosis requires CSF examination by a lumbar puncture (LP). CSF findings include elevated protein, decreased glucose, and elevated white blood cell count with neutrophil predominance. Gram stain and culture should also be evaluated in all potential BM cases. Head computed tomography should be obtained to evaluate for intracranial hypertension prior to LP in patients at risk of increased intracranial pressure (Box 37.2).

BOX 37.1 Bacterial Meningitis – Etiology and Risk Factors

Microbe	Risk Factors
S. pneumonia	Concomitant respiratory tract/middle ear infection, bacteremia, sinusitis
N. meningiditis	Young adults, splenectomy
H. influenza	Concomitant upper respiratory tract/middle ear infection
L. monocytogenes	Immunocompromised, elderly
S. aureus	Antecent neurosurgical procedure
Gram negatives	Hospitalization

> **BOX 37.2** Consideration for Neuroimaging Prior to Lumbar Puncture
>
> 1. Altered Mental Status
> 2. Focal Neurologic Deficit
> 3. Seizure (within the last week)
> 4. Immunocompromised
> 5. Age > 55
> 6. Papilledema
> 7. Absent Retinal Venous Pulsations

BM requires urgent intravenous antibiotics. Empirical therapy usually includes a third-generation cephalosporin (Ceftriaxone) and Vancomycin. The addition of Vancomycin is used to cover cephalosporin resistance in Streptococcus Pneumoniae, which accounts for approximately 5% to 10% of this species. In immunocompromised patients, antimicrobial coverage for Listeria with Ampicillin should be added. Dexamethasone is indicated for patients with Streptococcus Pneumoniae induced BM who present with a GCS 8–11, as it is associated with decreased mortality, hearing loss, and long-term neurologic sequelae in this patient population. Unfortunately, the use of dexamethasone has not been studied in meningitis caused by other micro-organisms.

Encephalitis

Encephalitis is a primary disorder involving cerebral parenchymal inflammation. Although there is significant overlap with meningitis, altered level of consciousness tends to be more prominent along with signs of personality change, psychiatric symptoms, focal neurological deficits, acute cognitive impairment, speech disturbances, and seizures. CSF examination reveals elevated protein, normal glucose, and increased white blood cell count with a lymphocyte predominance.

Infectious encephalitis most commonly occurs from an invasive viral infection of the cerebral parenchyma, principally enteroviruses, and herpes simplex viruses. Classically, herpes simplex affects the temporal lobe and limbic system (Figure 37.1–3). Enteroviruses can affect variable regions of the cerebrum. Less common causes include Arboviruses which affect the diencephalon, basal ganglia, and limbic system. (Figure 37.1–3) Non-viral causes of encephalitis include Listeria monocytogenes and Mycobacterium tuberculosis, both of which predominantly affect the brainstem.

Management involves administration of antimicrobials targeting underlying pathogens. Antiviral therapy for viral encephalitis is limited to intravenous acyclovir which only has action against herpes simplex virus. Additionally, encephalitis may cause secondary complications such as intracerebral hemorrhage, status epilepticus, and cerebral edema, all of which require aggressive management.

Ventriculitis

Ventriculitis is a primary infection of the ventricular system. Approximately 10–15% of patients with an EVD will develop ventriculitis. Risk factors include concomitant intraventricular hemorrhage, in situ EVD > 5 days, bedside insertion and frequent CSF sampling from the EVD. Culprit gram-positive organisms include *Staphylococcus epidermidis* and

Staphylococcus aureus. The remaining microbiology of ventriculitis is attributable to gram-negative organisms including E. Coli, Klebsiella, Enterobacter, Pseudomonas, and Acinetobacter species.

Clinical signs such as fever, altered mental status, headache, cranial nerve palsies, and meningeal signs should alert the clinician to further detailed evaluation. CSF examination may reveal an increased white blood cell count with a neutrophil predominance. A positive gram stain or culture in the context of clinical findings aid the diagnosis. In select cases, neuroimaging can delineate ependymal enhancement. Empirical antimicrobial therapy includes intravenous high-dose Meropenem and Vancomycin for a duration of 10–14 days. Removal or replacement of the existing EVD and intrathecal antibiotics should be considered.

Infections in Immunocompromised Patients

Cryptococcus

Cryptococcus neoformans and gattii cause a latent pulmonary infection through inhalation of spores. Cryptococcal meningitis may occur in both immunocompromised and immunocompetent hosts. Obstruction of the arachnoid granulations in the superior sagittal sinus can cause communicating hydrocephalus and intracranial hypertension. Therefore, patients may present with headache, altered mental status, cranial nerve palsies, and signs of increased intracranial pressure without meningeal inflammatory signs. Diagnosis requires CSF examination and serum cryptococcal antigen. Classically, the opening pressure is markedly elevated. Routine CSF examination may appear normal in 30% of cases with elevated protein being the only abnormality. Management includes amphotericin with 5-flucytosine for 2 weeks, followed by fluconazole for a total of 10 weeks. Daily LP or a lumbar drain is required for therapeutic CSF diversion.

Toxoplasmosis

Toxoplasmosis gondi encephalitis results from the ingestion of oocytes from felines. A local cerebritis occurs which leads to invasive encephalitis and toxoplasmomas. Classically, HIV patients with CD4 counts less than 100 are affected. Diagnosis requires positive serum IgG levels as well as contrast-enhanced neuroimaging, which reveals ring enhancing intracranial lesions. Stereotactic brain biopsy can also be considered. Treatment with pyrimethamine, folinic acid, and sulfadiazine is the first line therapy with follow up neuroimaging to guide further therapeutic options.

Mycobacterium Tuberculosis

Mycobacterium tuberculosis-associated meningitis is a devastating illness associated with significant mortality. CSF examination reveals a predominance of lymphocytes, low glucose, and markedly elevated protein levels. Acid fast bacilli on CSF gram stain are visible in 50% of cases. CSF polymerase chain reaction for Mycobacterium tuberculosis is the most accurate modality of diagnosis. First line therapy includes isoniazid, pyrazinamide, ethambutol, and rifampin with the addition of intravenous dexamethasone.

Cerebral Abscess

CA is an invasive infection within the cerebral parenchyma by an organism which forms an encapsulated collection of infected liquefied tissue or pus. Risk factors for the formation of a bacterial CA include: male gender, history of immunodeficiency, recent invasive neurosurgical intervention, and a concomitant infection resulting in the spread of microbes into the cerebral parenchyma. CA is thought to result from direct spread of contiguous infection and from hematogenous seeding. Initially, cerebral parenchymal infection ensues with an eventual necrotic center providing the substrate for abscess formation. Thereafter, capsule formation allows for persistent microbial proliferation. Immunocompromised hosts may suffer from similar microbes, but Listeria and fungal species must also be considered.

CA may present with non-specific symptoms. As it evolves, significant neurological signs may develop including depressed level of consciousness, focal neurological deficits, seizures, signs of increased intracranial pressure, and associated meningeal signs. The diagnosis of CA requires neuroimaging with either contrast-enhanced computed tomography or magnetic resonance imaging. Both modalities will typically reveal a ring-enhancing lesion with a 'smooth' capsule in contrast to malignancies, which often appear irregular. Multiple abscesses on imaging indicate a likely hematogenous source.

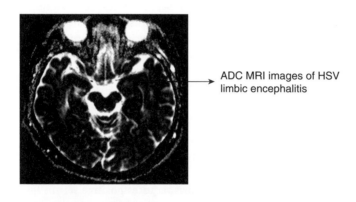

ADC MRI images of HSV limbic encephalitis

Figure 37.1 ADC sequences on magnetic resonance imaging demonstrating acute infarction of the temporal lobe secondary to herpes simplex virus encephalitis.

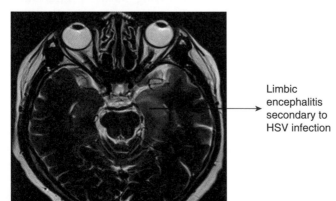

Limbic encephalitis secondary to HSV infection

Figure 37.2 The temporal and uncus are common sites of infection for herpes simplex virus associated encephalitis. Intraparenchymal hemorrhage may also occur concurrently in this location.

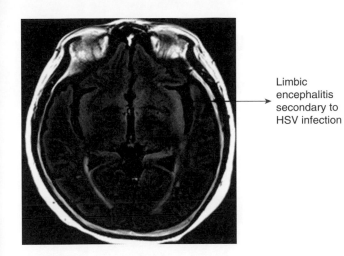

Figure 37.3 Magnetic resonance imaging demonstrating diffuse inflammation in the sylvian fissure, a characteristic location of herpes simplex encephalitis.

Limbic encephalitis secondary to HSV infection

Prompt administration of appropriate empiric antimicrobials should be administered after evaluating the host for the most likely primary source of infection. If cultures are not obtained with a culprit organism, antimicrobials should be continued for 6–8 weeks; repeat neuroimaging should be performed to assess efficacy of treatment. Surgical management involves resection of infected cerebral tissue in cases where the abscess is amendable to drainage.

Further Reading

Beckham, J.D., Tyler, K.L.: Neuro-intensive care of patients with acute CNS infections. *Neurotherapeutics* 2012; 9(1):124–138.

Beer, R., Lackner, P., Pfausler, B., Schmutzhard, E.: Nosocomial Ventriculitis and Meningitis in Neurocritical Care Patients. *J Neurol* 2008; 255(11):1617–1624.

Bhimraj, A.: *Acute Community-Acquired Bacterial Meningitis. CNS Infections.* Cleveland, OH: Springer-Verlag, pp. 17–27.

Schut, E.S., Lucas, M.J., Brouwer, M.C., et al: Cerebral Infarction in Adults with Bacterial Meningitis. *Neurocrit Care* 2012; 16(3):421–427.

Ziai, W.C., Lewin, J.J.: Update in the diagnosis and management of central nervous system infections. *Neurol Clin* 2008; 26(2):427–468.

Chapter

38

Cerebral Venous Sinus Thrombosis

Chris Nixon-Giles and Mypinder Sekhon

Key Points

- Cerebral venous sinus thrombosis is often associated with underlying inherited or acquired thrombophilias.
- Venous sinus thrombosis can cause intracerebral hemorrhage, impaired CSF reabsorption, along with vasogenic and cytotoxic cerebral edema. Ultimately, this pathophysiological cascade can lead to increased intracranial pressure and secondary ischemic cerebral injury.
- Diagnosis requires a careful clinical assessment with supportive neuroimaging. Computed tomography can reveal suggestive findings such as multifocal intracerebral hemorrhage or focal cerebral edema corresponding to the region of anatomical drainage of a major venous sinus.
- Evaluation of the venous vasculature should be sought with a cerebral venogram that may show a filling defect or evidence of intraluminal thrombosis.
- The mainstay of management is therapeutic anticoagulation with unfractionated heparin. In refractory cases, interventional focal thrombolysis may be considered.

Abbreviations

CVST   Cerebral venous sinus thrombosis
CSF   Cerebrospinal fluid
CT   Computed tomography
ICP   Intracranial pressure

Contents

- Anatomy
- Epidemiology
- Pathophysiology
- Thrombophilias and Risk Factors
- Clinical Manifestations
- Diagnosis

- Management
- Further Reading

Anatomy

The cerebral venous sinuses form the major venous drainage from the brain. Each primary venous sinus collects blood from specific anatomical locations within the parenchyma and ultimately delivers it to jugular venous system. The major intracranial venous sinuses are: the transverse, straight, sigmoid, great cerebral vein of Galen, superior and inferior sagittal sinuses (see Figure 2.5 Chapter 2).

Anatomically, the superior sagittal sinus runs in the sagittal plane at the top of the falx cerebrum. Cortical veins drain into it, and it is also the site of the arachnoid granulations that reabsorb cerebral spinal fluid. The inferior sagittal sinus collects blood from perforating cerebral veins that drain the inferior aspect of the frontal and parietal lobes. The transverse sinuses run across the posterior and lateral aspect of the cranium, along the tentorium and drain the cerebellum and inferior aspects of the frontal, temporal, parietal, and occipital lobes. The sigmoid sinuses also drain the venous blood flow from a similar distribution as the transverse sinuses. The deep structures of the brain such as the thalamus, hypothalamus, basal ganglia, and internal capsules return part of their venous blood to the great cerebral vein of Galen, which ultimately empties into the straight sinus. All sinuses drain into the confluence of sinuses, which is located posteriorly. Thereafter, blood enters the jugular bulb and internal jugular vein along its path into the intrathoracic cavity.

Epidemiology

CVST is relatively uncommon with an incidence of approximately five cases per million patients but it can have devastating consequences. The majority of patients (75%) are female, likely due to the increased thrombophilia risk associated with pregnancy, postpartum period, and hormonal therapy. If diagnosed early and appropriately managed, the outcome in 70%–80% of patients can be excellent.

Pathophysiology

The pathophysiology of CVST involves thrombus formation with resultant cerebral edema, intracerebral hemorrhage, increased ICP, and secondary injury.

An underlying hypercoagulable state (inherited or acquired) results in spontaneous thrombus generation. After thrombus formation, venous blood flow becomes limited resulting in increased hydrostatic pressure in the microvasculature. This has three consequences (Figure 38.1): (1) micro vascular flow in the capillary bed becomes compromised, oxygen delivery is impaired, cerebral ischemia ensues with cellular energy failure and eventual cytotoxic edema; (2) cerebral endothelial dysfunction ensues secondary to inadequate oxygen delivery, the integrity of the blood brain barrier is compromised and increased hydrostatic pressure leads to vasogenic edema; and (3) excessive intraluminal hydrostatic pressure leads to damage of the micro vascular and venule walls causing intracerebral hemorrhage. If the thrombus is in the superior sagittal sinus, the CSF flow into the venous vasculature via the arachnoid granulations is impaired, leading to CSF accumulation in an already non-compliant intracranial space.

Ultimately, increased ICP causes inadequate global cerebral perfusion, thereby causing secondary ischemic injury and exacerbating the existing cytotoxic and vasogenic edema.

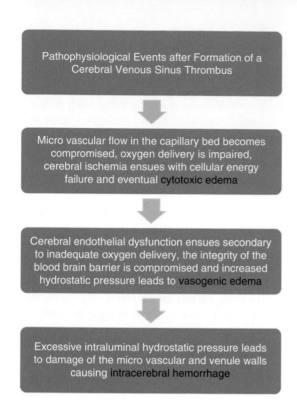

Figure 38.1 Physiological events after formation of a cerebral venous sinus thrombus.

Pathophysiological Events after Formation of a Cerebral Venous Sinus Thrombus

Micro vascular flow in the capillary bed becomes compromised, oxygen delivery is impaired, cerebral ischemia ensues with cellular energy failure and eventual cytotoxic edema

Cerebral endothelial dysfunction ensues secondary to inadequate oxygen delivery, the integrity of the blood brain barrier is compromised and increased hydrostatic pressure leads to vasogenic edema

Excessive intraluminal hydrostatic pressure leads to damage of the micro vascular and venule walls causing intracerebral hemorrhage

Thrombophilias and Risk Factors

An underlying hypercoagulable state is established in approximately 85% of patients with CVST. Inherited (Factor V Leiden, antithrombin III deficiency, protein C or S deficiency, and prothrombin gene mutation) and acquired causes (malignancy, infection, hormonal etiologies, and other systemic diseases) should be sought after the diagnosis of venous sinus thrombosis is established.

Acquired causes of CVST have increased in frequency during the last few decades. Oral contraception medication, hormone replacement therapy, and hormonal therapies for malignancy are major risk factors. Pregnancy and the post-partum period are associated with the highest thrombophilia risk. Other common acquired causes include concurrent infection or preceding cranial trauma.

Clinical Manifestations

The most common manifestation is a severe constant headache that has features of increased ICP such as worsening with coughing, straining and sneezing. The headache is characteristically worse in the morning and in the supine position. Less commonly, intracranial hemorrhage, cerebral venous infarction/ischemia, or focal cerebral edema can result in focal neurological deficits. The deficits usually correspond to the anatomical location of the compromised venous drainage. Finally, seizures and coma can ensue in extreme cases.

Presentation with the above-mentioned symptoms in the setting of a concurrent thrombus elsewhere in the body should prompt immediate consideration of CVST.

Diagnosis

A high clinical suspicion is required to promptly diagnose CVST. CT venography has a slightly higher sensitivity and specificity than magnetic resonance imaging and should be pursued as the imaging modality of choice unless contraindicated. Suggestive findings on non-contrast CT include focal cerebral edema in the distribution of venous drainage of a single or multiple sinuses, multiple petechial hemorrhages, multiple intracerebral hemorrhages located in a lobar distribution, and the dense clot sign at the confluence of sinuses. (Figures 38.2 and 38.3)

Management

The management of cerebral sinus venous thrombosis has four aspects: (1) general measures and supportive care, (2) anticoagulation, (3) interventional thrombolysis, and (4) management of increased ICP.

In the setting of altered consciousness, patients may hypoventilate which can cause a dangerous exacerbation of intracranial hypertension and an absence of protective airway reflexes may lead to aspiration, pneumonia, and systemic sepsis. General management interventions include airway protection and mechanical ventilation in the setting of impaired level of consciousness. Once a definitive diagnosis is made, an attempt to establish a reversible predisposing condition should be sought.

Systemic anticoagulation is the cornerstone of the management of CVST. Anticoagulation to limit propagation of existing thrombus propagation prevents additional intracranial

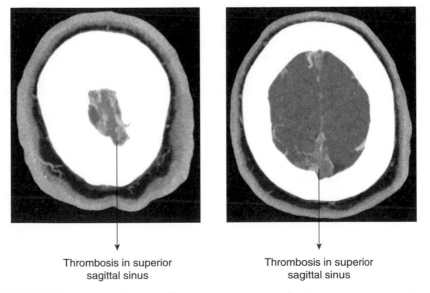

Thrombosis in superior
sagittal sinus

Thrombosis in superior
sagittal sinus

Figure 38.2 Axial plane computed tomography venogram images revealing the presence an acute thrombosis within the superior sagittal venous sinus.

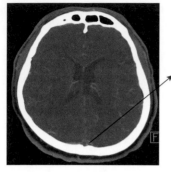

Presence of acute thrombasis on CT venogram in the superior sagittal sinus with extension into the confluence of sinuses

Figure 38.3 Computed venography demonstrating clot extension into the confluence of sinuses from the superior sagittal sinus.

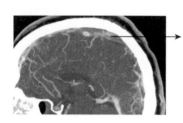

Thrombosis in superior sagittal sinus

Figure 38.4 A sagittal computed tomography venogram image demonstrating extensive clot in the superior sagittal venous sinus.

complications such as hemorrhage, cerebral edema, and herniation. Intravenous unfractionated heparin is the agent of choice as it can be reversed quickly if there is new or worsening intracerebral hemorrhage associated with venous infarcts. In refractory or extensive cases, interventional local administration of thrombolysis can re-canalize the venous sinuses and re-establish venous flow. Current evidence is limited to case series (Figure 38.4).

The management of intracranial hypertension is important and perhaps under-appreciated in CVST. Invasive ICP monitoring is often not possible due to contra-indications from systemic anticoagulation or ongoing local thrombolysis. Non-invasive means of ICP estimation could have an important role in establishing benefit from ICP reducing therapies such as intravenous sedation, temperature control, osmotherapy (hypertonic saline and mannitol), and normocapnic ventilation. All patients should be managed at 30-degree head-up tilt and measures should be undertaken to ensure that endotracheal tube ties or neck position are not restricting jugular venous flow.

Further Reading

Fam, D., Saposnik, G.: Critical care management of cerebral venous thrombosis. *Curr Opin Crit Care*. 2016; **22**(2):113–119.

Filippidis, A1., Kapsalaki, E., Patramani, G., Fountas, K.N.: Cerebral venous sinus thrombosis: Review of the demographics, pathophysiology, current diagnosis, and treatment. *Neurosurg Focus* November 2009; **27**(5):E3.

Saposnik, G., Barinagarrementeria, F., Brown, R.D., Jr, et al: Diagnosis and management of cerebral venous thrombosis: A statement for healthcare professionals from the American Heart Association/American Stroke Association. *Stroke* 2011; **42**:1158.

Stam, J.: Thrombosis of the cerebral veins and sinuses. *N Engl J Med* 2005; **352**:1791–1798.

Chapter 39

Autonomic Dysfunction

Kali Romano and Mypinder Sekhon

Key Points

- PSH is a common clinical entity in neurocritically ill patients and is associated with a wide range of underlying central nervous system disorders, most commonly traumatic brain injury.
- Episodic surges in circulating catecholamines can result in deleterious effects on end organ function.
- Mimicking conditions such as sepsis, opiate, or benzodiazepine withdrawal, neuroleptic malignant syndrome, serotonin syndrome, and malignant hyperthermia should be excluded prior to diagnosing PSH.
- Management is focused on a multi-modal pharmacological approach targeted at the suppression of sympathetic activity and treatment of end organ effects of catecholamine excess.

Abbreviations

CNS   Central nervous system
EIR   Excitatory-inhibitory ratio
GABA   Gamma-aminobutyric acid
NMDA   N-methyl-D-aspartate
PSH   Paroxysmal sympathetic hyperactivity
TBI   Traumatic brain injury

Introduction

Autonomic dysfunction is commonly encountered in neurocritical care. It manifests as a syndrome of uncontrolled surges of sympathetic activity resulting in hyperthermia, diaphoresis (sweating), tachycardia, hypertension, tachypnea, and dystonic posturing. Uncontrolled symptoms can result in end organ dysfunction including secondary brain injury. This constellation of symptoms has previously been termed dysautonomia, reflex autonomic dysfunction, and sympathetic hyper-activity. This lack of standardized nomenclature has precluded development of management guidelines but recent consensus, however, has favored a change to the term "paroxysmal sympathetic hyperactivity" (PSH). While the etiology, risk factors, and pathophysiology of the disease are under researched, the clinical importance is clear.

Etiology and Risk Factors

PSH is a clinical phenomenon occurring in a variety of neurocritical care diseases. TBI is the most representative but it occurs with other causes of acute brain injury. PSH typically occurs 5–7 days post injury, often recognized when weaning from benzodiazepine to opiate sedation making withdrawal a challenging confounder. With respect to frequency, a prospective cohort trial of patients with TBI by Fernandez-Ortega et al. showed that the average number of episodes was 5.6, with a mean duration of 30.8 minutes.

Multiple risk factors for the development of PSH have been identified. Common entities such as TBI represent the highest index of cases. Though a more prevalent condition, TBI in itself may not carry as high a risk for the development of PSH as other diseases such as encephalitis. It is estimated that 70–80% patients with encephalitis demonstrate a syndrome similar to PSH. Specifically, in the case of NMDA receptor encephalitis, a hallmark of the disease is an aggressive PSH-like syndrome that is difficult to control. Demographic risk factors include male gender and young age, both of which are the demographic most often involved in TBI. It is also proposed that because autonomic reflexes are more pronounced in the physiology of younger patients, it may therefore explain the more common occurrence of the condition. Imaging studies have suggested patients with underlying pathologies of diffuse axonal injury, epidural and subdural hemorrhage have a higher predilection for development of PSH. Damage to deep brain structures such as the basal ganglia, thalami, corpus callosum, or brainstem is also associated with a higher incidence of PSH.

Pathophysiology

PSH is a complicated clinical entity, with several pathophysiological hypotheses. The two most prominent include the disconnection theory and the EIR model which will be discussed further.

The disconnection theory, which proposes a functional disconnect in the regulation of autonomic nervous system manifesting as dysregulated activation of the sympathetic nervous system. The underlying cause or pathology for the functional disconnection results from structural or inflammatory damage to CNS structures involved in the regulation of the autonomic nervous system. While the diencephalon is commonly implicated in the loss of higher order inhibitory activity, a definitive anatomic location has yet to be identified. Regardless, the result is excessive adrenergic outflow causing systemic manifestations of PSH.

The EIR model has recently been implicated in the pathophysiology of PSH. Normally, autonomic efferent activity at the level of the spinal cord is modulated both centrally (by interplay of sympathetic and parasympathetic activity) and by spinal cord afferents (stimuli from the environment). Spinal cord afferents have an inherent allodynic tendency whereby peripheral stimuli, noxious or non-noxious, are regulated by central inhibitory signals arising from the diencephalon.

After brain injury, these mechanisms are injured resulting in impaired regulation. Clinically, this results in unopposed sympathetic efferent output from spinal cord afferent stimuli, noxious or non-noxious, forming a positive feedback loop. This phenomenon explains the triggering of PSH episodes in the critical care setting in response to nursing interventions (suctioning, turning) as well as physiological stimuli (bladder distention, pain). The EIR model is not exclusive to PSH, and has been applied to other paradoxical dysautonomias such as the development of allodynia in chronic pain and autonomic dysreflexia in spinal cord injury.

It is important to recognize that regardless of the pathophysiologic mechanism, the end result is increased adrenergic activity resulting in end organ dysfunction. In relation to the brain, this has implications for the development of secondary injury, while for other organs, increased catecholamines and autonomic dysregulation of inflammatory cascades result in a myriad of complications in critically ill patients.

Diagnosis

Diagnosis of PSH is challenging given the non-specific symptomatology that has significant overlap with other sequelae of acute brain injury and critical illness. PSH is therefore a diagnosis of exclusion. Key elements to the diagnosis include:

1. Simultaneous onset of signs of catecholamine excess (tachycardia, tachypnea, dystonic posturing, sweating, pupillary dilatation, hypertension, and fever)
2. Brain injury
3. Daily episodes
4. The paroxysmal nature of symptom onset
5. Recent CNS injury/disease
6. Over two weeks from the initial
7. Absence of parasympathetic features during paroxysms.

Recently, a consensus pinion provided a proposed diagnostic criterion for PSH in neuro-critically ill patients (Tables 39.1 and 39.2).

Management

Treatment of PSH is directed at controlling symptoms as the direct cause has yet to be determined. First, management should be aimed at decreasing the frequency and intensity of episodes. This is achieved by initiating regularly dosed medications aimed at modulating the sympathetic response. A multi-modal approach is most helpful using drugs targeted to adrenergic and GABA receptors (Table 39.3). Second, breakthrough episodes should be

Table 39.1 Clinical Features of Sympathetic Excess

	0	1	2	3	Score
Heart rate	<100	100–119	120–139	>140	
Respiratory rate	<18	18–23	24–29	>30	
Systolic blood pressure	<140	140–159	160–179	>180	
Temperature	<37	37–37.9	38–38.9	>39.0	
Dystonic posturing	Nil	Mild	Moderate	Severe	
Sweating	Nil	Mild	Moderate	Severe	
				Total:	_____

Table 39.2 Features of Disease Episodes/Time Course

Feature	Score (0 or 1)
Simultaneous onset of symptoms	
Paroxysmal episodes	
Sympathetic overactivity to noxious stimuli	
>3 consecutive days with symptoms	
>2 weeks post brain injury	
Symptoms persist despite treatment for alternative diagnoses	
Medication administered to decrease sympathetic features	
>1 episode per day	
Absence of parasympathetic features during episodes	
Absence of alternative diagnosis	
Antecent brain injury	
	Total: _____

The diagnosis of paroxysmal sympathetic hyperactivity is unlikely if the score is less than 8, possible between 8 and 16 and probable if greater than 17.

Table 39.3 The Pharmacologic Approach to the Management of PSH

Pharmacologic Management of PSH		
	Agent	Mechanism of Action
Sympatholytics		
	Propranolol	• Decrease circulating catecholamine effect • Attenuate resting metabolic rate • Agent of choice, non-selective and lipid soluble crossing blood brain barrier
	Clonidine	• Acts at the alpha$_2$ receptor • Enhance sympathetic inhibition in brainstem by decreasing central sympathetic efferent signals • Reduces plasma catecholamine levels in TBI
	Dexmedetomidine	• Acts at the alpha$_2$ receptor • Decreases sympathetic efferent activity
GABA		
	Gabapentin	• GABA analogue • Effective for neuropathy, spasticity, tremor
	Baclofen	• GABA agonist • Decreases number and severity of spasms
	Benzodiazepines	• GABA receptor agonists • Beneficial cardiovascular effect, potent effect on decreasing agitation

Table 39.3 (cont.)

Pharmacologic Management of PSH	
Agent	Mechanism of Action
Opioid	
Morphine	• Benefit in PSH is stimulation of medullary vagal nuclei resulting in parasympathetic stimulation • Analgesia, sedation additional effect

adequately treated by medications with short-acting properties targeted at the predominant symptoms. While short acting benzodiazepines and opioids are most effective, anti-pyretic and direct sympatholytics should also be considered.

Further Reading

Baguely, I.J.: Paroxysmal sympathetic hyperactivity after acquired brain injury: consensus of conceptual definition, nomenclature and diagnostic criteria. *J Neurotrauma* 2014; **31**:1515–1520.

Choi, A.H., Jeon, S.B., Samuel, S., Allison, T., Lee, K.: Paroxysmal sympathetic hyperactivity after acute brain injury. *Curr Neurol Neurosci Rep* 2013; **13**:370–376.

Fernandez-Ortega, J.F., Prieto-Palomino, M.A., Garcia-Caballero, M., et al: Paroxysmal sympathetic hyperactivity after traumatic brain injury: Clinical and prognostic implications. *J Neurotrauma* 2012; **29**:1364–1370.

Lv, L.Q., Hou, L.J., Yu, M.K., et al: Risk factors related to dysautonomia after severe traumatic brain injury. *J Trauma Acute Care Surg* 2011; **71** (3):538–542.

Lump, D., Moyer, M.: Paroxysmal sympathetic hyperactivity after severe brain injury. *Curr Neurol Neurosc Rep* 2014; **14**:494.

Perkes, I., Baguley, I.J., Nott, M.T., Menon, D.K.: A review of paroxysmal sympathetic hyperactivity after acquired brain injury. *Ann Neurol* 2010; **60**:126–135.

Perkes, I.E., Menon, D.K., Nott, M.T., Baguley, I. J.: Paroxysmal sympathetic hyperactivity after acquired brain injury: A review of diagnostic criteria. *Brain Injury* 2011; **25**(10):925–932.

Chapter

Fluid Management

Andrew Wormsbecker and Donald Griesdale

Key Points

- Fluid should be administered with the goal of increasing end-organ perfusion through an increase in cardiac output.
- Response to fluid administration should be monitored with dynamic variables (e.g., systolic pressure variation) and goal-directed resuscitation.
- Many commercially available cardiac output and stroke volume monitors are available but rely on several assumptions, including: normal sinus rhythm and controlled ventilated with tidal volumes of at least 7–8 ml/kg.
- Static markers show poor discrimination to identify patients who are fluid responsive.
- Crystalloids are the preferred initial resuscitation fluid.
- Hypo-osmolar fluids and synthetic colloids should be avoided whenever possible.
- Albumin should be avoided in patients with traumatic brain injury. Its use in acute brain injury requires further study, but may be of benefit in subarachnoid hemorrhage.
- Hyperosmolar therapy is used to treat elevated intracranial pressure. Hypertonic saline may be preferred to mannitol however, the optimal dose and method of administration requires further study.
- Due to familiarity and availability, mannitol remains frequently used for acute herniation syndromes.

Abbreviations

HES   Hydroxyl-ethyl starch
HTS   Hypertonic saline
ICP   Intracranial pressure
IVC   Inferior vena cava
RCT   Randomized controlled trial
SAH   Subarachnoid hemorrhage
TBI   Traumatic brain injury
TCD   Trans cranial doppler

Contents

Introduction

The goal of intravenous fluid administration is to improve end-organ perfusion through an increase in cardiac output. Fluid administration should be targeted to patients who are volume responsive and titrated to improved end-organ perfusion. It is important to avoid volume depletion due to the detrimental effects on cerebral blood flow and oxygenation. However, excessive fluid administration itself results in disruption of the endothelial glycocalyx leading to increased interstitial edema and end-organ dysfunction (e.g., pulmonary edema and abdominal compartment syndrome). Individual goal-directed therapy has supplanted previous fixed-volume maintenance rates of intraoperative crystalloid administration.

Monitoring Volume Responsiveness and Cardiac Output

Static variables, such as central venous pressure, pulmonary capillary wedge pressure, heart rate, and blood pressure, are poor markers of fluid responsiveness. Urine output may also be misleading in the setting of hyperosmolar therapy and sodium disorders seen in patients with neurological illness. Dynamic variables to assess fluid responsiveness (e.g., pulse pressure variation, systolic pressure variation, and stroke volume variation) offer improved discrimination to identify patients who are volume responsive. These variables have gained favor in the perioperative setting. Commonly used commercial devices employ esophageal Doppler of aortic blood flow or pulse contour analysis using an arterial line waveform. Most studies suggest that a variability greater than 10–15% predicts an increase in stroke volume with fluid administration. The accuracy of these devices is predicated on several assumptions: normal sinus rhythm, controlled ventilation with tidal volumes of at least 7–8 ml/kg, and the absence of elevated abdominal pressure or right heart dysfunction.

Change in inferior vena cava (IVC) diameter on ultrasound can also be used to assess fluid responsiveness. While few studies look at the neurocritical care population, in patients with subarachnoid hemorrhage (SAH) with controlled mechanical ventilation at 8 ml/kg tidal volume, IVC distensibility >16% was shown to be predictive of fluid responsiveness. Appropriate fluid administration to volume responsive patients, while limiting unnecessary positive fluid balance, continues to be an evolving area of research.

Choice of Intravenous Fluid

Intravenous fluids can broadly be categorized into crystalloids, colloids (albumin or synthetic), or transfusion of red blood cells. Crystalloids remain the mainstay of fluid administration.

Normal (0.9%) saline is slightly hypertonic to plasma with an osmolality of 308 mmol/L, and is a good initial choice in patients at risk for cerebral edema. Concerns identified with normal saline include: (1) hyperchloremic metabolic acidosis, (2) acute kidney injury, (3) immune dysfunction, and (4) volume overload from sodium accumulation. Balanced crystalloid solutions (e.g., Lactated Ringer's or Plasmalyte®) have gained popularity due to more physiologic ion concentration. Despite this benefit, data is lacking on meaningful clinical outcomes. A multicenter randomized controlled trial (RCT) of fluid resuscitation in 2238 patients compared normal saline versus Plasmalyte 148 and did not find any difference in mortality or renal injury. In the absence of hypoglycemia, glucose-containing solutions should be avoided due to exacerbating effects of hyperglycemia on brain injury.

Albumin is the main protein in human blood accounting for the majority of plasma oncotic pressure. Albumin solutions are available as isotonic (4–5% albumin) or hypertonic (20–25%) solutions and are typically suspended in normal saline. In 2004, the international Saline versus Albumin Fluid Evaluation (SAFE) Study randomized 6997 critically ill patients in a blinded fashion to either Albumin 4% or normal saline for intravenous fluid replacement for 28 days. Despite no overall difference between groups, there appeared to be an increased risk of 28-day mortality in trauma patients (RR 1.36, 95%CI: 0.99–1.86) which was primarily driven by those admitted with a traumatic brain injury (TBI). In a post-hoc analysis of 460 patients (SAFE TBI Study), those who received albumin had a mortality of 33% compared to 20% in the saline group (RR 1.63, 95%CI: 1.17–2.26, P=0.003). Albumin administration was associated with increased intracranial pressure (ICP), which may explain the excess mortality in these patients.

The use of albumin in other neurocritical care patients remains unclear. Albumin 25% in acute ischemic stroke has not demonstrated any improvement in neurological outcomes but led to an increased risk of pulmonary edema. In contrast, patients with aneurysmal SAH may benefit from albumin administration. A recent pilot study demonstrated albumin dose-dependent reductions in vasospasm on trans cranial doppler (TCD), delayed cerebral ischemia and infarction in aneurysmal SAH.

Synthetic colloids are made of starches, dextrans, or gelatins. Initial enthusiasm and widespread adoption has been tempered by concerns of immune dysfunction, coagulopathy, and increased renal failure, particularly with high molecular weight starches. Randomized trials have demonstrated increased risk of mortality (Scandinavian Starch for Severe Sepsis/Septic Shock [6S] Trial), renal failure and renal replacement therapy (Crystalloid versus Hydroxyethyl Starch Trial [CHEST]) in critically ill patients receiving hydroxyl-ethyl starch (HES), particularly among those patients admitted with sepsis. Given this evidence, synthetic colloids should be avoided in critically ill patients.

The optimal transfusion threshold in patients with brain injury remains unknown. The Transfusion in Critical Care (TRICC) trial established a transfusion threshold of 70 g/L in non-bleeding critically ill patients. A randomized trial published in 2014 (Epo Severe TBI Trial) demonstrated no difference in 6-month functional outcomes comparing restrictive (hemoglobin >70 g/L) and liberal (hemoglobin >100 g/L) transfusion thresholds in patients with TBI. However, hemoglobin concentrations in the restrictive group remained above 96 g/L throughout the study period. Observational studies are conflicting. Several studies demonstrate increased mortality with anemia (hemoglobin <90 g/L) in TBI. In contrast, others suggest that the increase in mortality is conferred by red blood cell transfusion itself, rather than anemia. Ongoing research will hopefully offer guidance to this critically important question.

Hyperosmolar Therapy

Elevated ICP is consistently associated with worse outcomes in patients with TBI. As such, control of ICP remains a cornerstone in the management of these patients. In the setting of elevated ICP and impending cerebral herniation, hyperosmolar therapy with mannitol or hypertonic saline (HTS) can be lifesaving. Administration of hyperosmolar fluids leads to egress of water from the cerebral interstitium resulting in decreased ICP. The magnitude of effect depends on the integrity of the blood-brain barrier, the permeability of the hyperosmolar solution, and the concentration gradient established. Hyperosmolar therapy also leads to improved cerebral blood flow, oxygenation, and autoregulation.

Mannitol

Mannitol is effective at decreasing ICP. In addition to reducing cerebral edema by drawing excess water from the brain interstitium into the cerebral vasculature, it improves red blood cell rheology leading to reduced viscosity, vasoconstriction and decreased cerebral blood volume. Notable adverse effects include hypovolemia and hypotension, acute kidney injury, and hypokalemic hypochloremic metabolic alkalosis. Furthermore, mannitol can leak across a disrupted blood-brain barrier, which may exacerbate cerebral edema. Mannitol is given at a dose of 0.25–0.5 g/kg to reduce ICP and at a dose of 1 g/kg as a rescue agent for herniation syndromes. The osmolality should be kept less than 320 mosm/L, though little evidence supports this.

Hypertonic Saline

HTS is typically available at concentrations of 3%, 5%, 7.5%, and 23.4%. Studies suggest that HTS may be more effective at lowering ICP compared to equimolar doses of mannitol. There are additional putative benefits with HTS administration including improved cerebral perfusion pressure, cerebral blood flow, cerebral oxygenation, and favorable immunologic/anti-inflammation effects. In contrast to mannitol, HTS does not cause an osmotic diuresis, thus avoiding the risk of hypovolemia. Compared to mannitol or placebo, HTS is associated with better ICP reduction and lower rate of treatment failure. However, the effect of HTS on neurological outcome remains unclear. Adverse effects of HTS include hypernatremia with volume overload and hyperchloremic metabolic acidosis. It is important to taper HTS therapy and avoid rapid lowering of serum sodium, which can exacerbate cerebral edema and lead to rebound elevation of ICP. HTS can be administered as intermittent bolus dosing, or as a continuous infusion targeting a serum sodium of between of 145–155 mmol/L. We generally administer 1–2 ml/kg of 5% HTS every 4–6 hours. However, the optimal dose and concentration of HTS is unknown.

Further Reading

Finfer, S., Bellomo, R., Boyce, N., et al: A comparison of albumin and saline for fluid resuscitation in the intensive care unit. *N Engl J Med* 2004; **350**(22):2247–2256.

Martin, R.H., Yeatts, S.D., Hill, M.D., et al: Analysis of the Combined Data From Parts 1 and 2. *Stroke*. 2016; **47**(9):2355–2359.

Lazaridis, C., Neyens, R., Bodle, J., DeSantis, S. M.: High-osmolarity saline in neurocritical care:

Systematic review and meta-analysis. *Crit Care Med* 2013; **41**(5):1353–1360.

LeRoux, P.: Haemoglobin management in acute brain injury. *Curr Opin Crit Care* 2013; **19**(2):83–91.

Marik, P.E.: Fluid responsiveness and the six guiding principles of fluid resuscitation. *Crit Care Med* 2015; November 2015 ePub ahead of print.

Mortazavi, M.M., Romeo, A.K., Deep, A., et al: Hypertonic saline for treating raised intracranial pressure: Literature review with meta-analysis. *J Neurosurg* 2012; **116**(1):210–221.

Myburgh, J.A., Mythen, M.G.: Resuscitation fluids. *N Engl J Med* 2013; **369**(13):1243–1251.

Perner, A., Haase, N., Guttormsen, A.B., et al: 6S Trial Group; Scandinavian Critical Care Trials Group Hydroxyethyl starch 130/0.42 versus Ringer's acetate in severe sepsis. *N Engl J Med* 2012; **367**(2):124–134.

Robertson, C.S., Hannay, H.J., Yamal, J.-M., et al: Effect of erythropoietin and transfusion threshold on neurological recovery after traumatic brain injury: A randomized clinical trial. *JAMA* 2014; **312**(1):36–47.

Sekhon, M.S., McLean, N., Henderson, W.R., Chittock, D.R., Griesdale, D.E.G.: Association of hemoglobin concentration and mortality in critically ill patients with severe traumatic brain injury. *Crit Care* 2012; **16**(4):R128.

Suarez, J.I., Martin, R.H., Calvillo, E., Bershad, E.M., Venkatasubba Rao, C.P.: Effect of human albumin on TCD vasospasm, DCI, and cerebral infarction in subarachnoid hemorrhage: The ALISAH study. *Acta Neurochir Suppl* 2015; **120**:287–290.

Thiele, R.H., Bartels, K., Gan, T.-J.: Inter-device differences in monitoring for goal-directed fluid therapy. *Can J Anaesth* 2015; **62**(2):169–181.

Electrolyte Disorders

Simeone Pierre, Nicolas Bruder, and Lionel Velly

Key Points

- CSW and the syndrome of inappropriate antidiuretic hormone secretion are the most common sodium disorders in neurosurgical patients.
- The diagnosis of the syndrome of inappropriate antidiuretic hormone secretion requires hypotonic hyponatremia, high urine osmolality, clinical euvolemia, and the absence of adrenal, thyroid, pituitary, and renal insufficiency.
- CSW is a primary natriuresis characterized by a high renal loss of sodium and a contracted fluid-volume state.
- Postoperative central diabetes insipidis is characterized by a urine output greater than 4 ml/kg/h (or >3 L/day), low urine, high serum osmolality, and hypernatremia (>145 mmol/L), in the absence of other causes of polyuria, and may be diagnosed by measuring serum copeptin levels.
- Management of low serum levels of potassium, magnesium, and phosphate involves treating the underlying cause and administering appropriate replacement therapy.

Abbreviations

ADH	Antidiuretic hormone – arginine vasopressin
CDI	Central diabetes insipidus
CSW	Cerebral salt wasting
DDAVP	1-deamino-8-D-arginine vasopressin
ECG	Electrocardiographic
SIADH	Syndrome of inappropriate antidiuretic hormone secretion
NaCl	Sodium chloride
PH	Postoperative hypernatremia

Contents

- Hypernatremia
  - Postoperative Hypernatremia
  - Central Diabetes Insipidus
  - Hypernatremia Treatment
- Potassium Disorders
- Other Electrolytes Disorders
- Further Reading

Introduction

Major surgery, large perioperative fluid shifts, and brain injury can result in dysfunction of the regulatory pathways that govern water and electrolyte balance. The aim of this chapter is to give a practical guide to screen, investigate, and manage these common electrolyte disorders.

Sodium Disorders

Sodium imbalance is the most common electrolyte disorder in critically ill and surgical patients. As sodium is the major cation in blood, it is an important determinant of extracellular fluid volume. Abnormal fluctuations in this electrolyte can cause brain swelling or shrinkage which can lead to non-specific neurological symptoms and signs that could be difficult to differentiate from other neurosurgical conditions.

Hyponatremia

Hyponatremia is commonly defined as a plasma sodium which is equal or less than 135 mmol/L. Hyponatremia develops acutely within the 2–4 days following surgery and causes non-specific neurological signs such as nausea, vomiting, headache, seizures, and could lead to coma in the most severe cases. The first step in the diagnosis is to rule out hyponatremia with normal or high plasma osmolality (Figure 41.1). The etiologies of hyponatremia with low plasma osmolality may have multiple causes. The SIADH and CSW are two frequent causes of hyponatremia in neurosurgical patients.

Syndrome of Inappropriate Antidiuretic Hormone Secretion

This syndrome has a complex pathophysiology presenting with hypotonic hyponatremia and is due to excessive release of ADH and disordered regulation of osmoreceptors. SIADH is the most frequent cause of euvolemic hyponatremia and several non-osmotic stimuli (e.g., nausea, vomiting, pain, hypoxia, narcotics, and hypovolemia), often experienced in the perioperative period after neurosurgery, increase the risk of SIADH. Other neurological conditions associated with SIADH include CNS infection, intracranial hemorrhage, trauma, brain neoplasm, cerebral vasculitis, and thrombosis. The diagnosis of SIADH requires hyponatremia, hypo-osmolarity, and inappropriately high urine osmolarity in the absence of thyroid and adrenal insufficiency. The diagnosis of SIADH is sometimes difficult to differentiate from CSW (Figure 41.1).

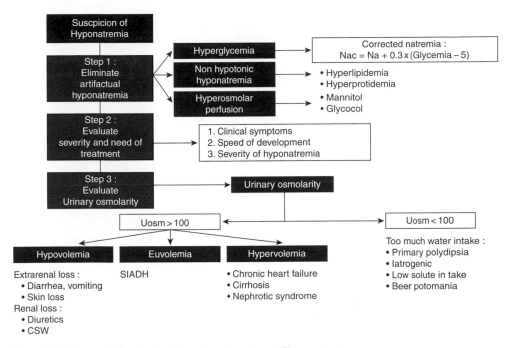

Figure 41.1 Steps to follow for the diagnosis and treatment of hyponatremia.

Cerebral Salt Wasting

CSW is more frequent than SIADH in some neurosurgical conditions such as subarachnoid hemorrhage. The pathophysiology is still unclear but is likely to involve brain secretion of circulating natriuretic factors or decreased sympathetic input to the kidney. The distinction between SIADH and CSW is based mainly on volume and sodium balance (Table 41.1).

Hyponatremia Treatment

The treatment of hyponatremia is determined according to the clinical symptoms, the speed of development, the severity of hyponatremia, and the targets defined in treatment guidelines. In general, guidelines advice excluding hyperglycemic and false hyponatremias by measuring serum glucose concentration, lipids, and proteins.

Hyponatremia resulting from increased water intake, SIADH, and hypervolemia require free water restriction of up to 1–1.5 L/day, whereas CSW requires sodium replacement. Regardless of whether hyponatremia is acute or chronic, a total increase in plasma sodium of 0.5 mmol/L increase per hour or 10–12 mmol/L per day is regarded as a safe limit in an attempt to avoid central pontine myelinolysis and excessive shifts in brain water content. Frequent monitoring of serum sodium is required (2–4 hourly) in the initial period, and if a rise in sodium is not observed with fluid restriction, the addition of fludrocortisone and hydrocortisone is recommended for their mineralocorticoid effects. In patients with chronic refractory SIADH, demeclocycline (150–300 mg twice daily) can be used which interferes with ADH at the renal collecting ducts.

Table 41.1 Clinical Features of CSW and SIADH

Clinical Features of CSW and SIADH	SIADH	CSW
Serum osmolality	Decreased	Decreased
Urine osmolality	Inappropriately high	Inappropriately high
Extracellular fluid volume	Normal or increased	Decreased
Hematocrit	Normal	Increased
Plasma albumin concentration	Normal	Increased
Plasma BUN/creatinine	Decreased	Increased
Plasma K	Normal	Normal or increased
Plasma uric acid	Decreased	Normal or decreased
Fluid balance	Positive	Negative
Treatment	Fluid restriction	Normal saline

Determination of extracellular fluid volume is the main method to differentiate CSW from SIADH. BUN, blood urea nitrogen; CSW, cerebral salt wasting; SIADH, syndrome of inappropriate antidiuretic hormone secretion

In severe hyponatremia (serum sodium <120 mmol/L or severe neurological symptoms) from whatever cause, sodium replacement with hypertonic saline (3% NaCl) may be required. This can be given as a 100–150 ml (2 ml/kg) intravenous bolus (or equivalent 3–4.5 g of NaCl) over 30–60 minutes repeated if necessary, with frequent measurement of the serum sodium. Alternative treatments of hyper- and euvolemic chronic hyponatremia with urea and vasopressin receptor antagonists (vaptans) remain controversial and have not been validated in acute hyponatremia. Vaptans carry the risks of overcorrection of natremia and hepatotoxicity.

Hypernatremia

Hypernatremia can cause neurological signs that could be confused with other neurosurgical conditions such as consciousness impairment, cerebellar syndrome, hypertonia, seizures, and coma. Other non-specific signs may be present such as lethargy, weakness, thirst, fever, and dyspnea. Hypernatremia is defined by a serum sodium concentration >145 mmol/L and is always associated with plasma hypertonicity that leads to cell shrinkage and dehydration. Two common etiologies should to be sought in the postoperative period, namely, postoperative hypernatremia (PH) and central diabetes insipidus (CDI).

Postoperative Hypernatremia

Hypernatremia is frequent after neurosurgery due to infection and fever, inadequate fluid management, and diuretics. It usually appears within five days following surgery especially in elderly patients who frequently develop impairment of thirst sensation and urine concentration capacity.

Central Diabetes Insipidus

CDI is commonly characterized by polyuria (>3 L/day or 4 ml/kg/h) with abnormally dilute urine (<350 mmol/kg), a rise in serum osmolarity (>310 mmol/kg), and serum sodium (>145 mmol/L). A urine specific gravity of 1.005 and rising serum sodium suggests CDI.

CDI is a failure of ADH homeostasis related to dysfunction of the hypothalamopituitary axis. After neurosurgery or traumatic brain injury, the reported incidence of postsurgical CDI varies from 1% to 65%, and factors affecting the likelihood of CDI include surgical approach, surgery of the pituitary region and injury of the hypothalamus. In the intensive care, it is not uncommonly seen after SAH, brain death, and TBI. CDI typically appears early within the first 24 hours postoperatively and recovers within 5 to 7 days. However, it may continue indefinitely particularly in patients after pituitary surgery.

Copeptin is part of the 164 amino acid precursor protein preprovasopressin together with vasopressin and neurophysin II. During precursor processing, copeptin is released together with vasopressin. Copeptin concentrations respond as rapidly as vasopressin to changes in osmolality, hypovolemia, or stress, and there is a close correlation of vasopressin and copeptin concentrations. For these reasons, copeptin is a surrogate marker for vasopressin in the differential diagnosis of the polyuria-polydipsia syndromes. In patients undergoing pituitary procedures, low copeptin levels (<2.5 pmol/L) despite surgical stress reflect postoperative CDI, whereas high levels (>30 pmol/L) virtually exclude it (negative predictive value, 95%; sensitivity, 94%). Copeptin therefore may become a novel tool for early goal-directed management of postoperative CDI (Figure 41.2).

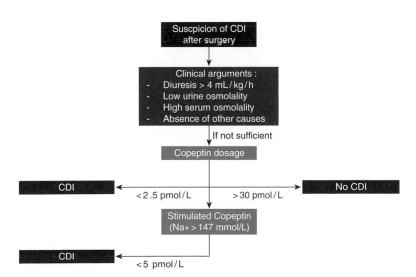

Figure 41.2 Algorythm to use copetin dosage for central diabetes insipidus (CDI) diagnosis. After pituitary surgery, an early dosage (<12 h) <2.5 pmol/l and >30 pmol/L has respectively a positive predictive value of 81% and a negative predictive value of 98% for the diagnosis of CDI. An osmotic stimulated copeptin increase <5 pmol/L has more than 90% sensitivity and specificity for the diagnosis of CDI (not validated in surgical patients) (adapted from ref 5).

Hypernatremia Treatment

Management consists of free water replacement and parenteral or intranasal vasopressin. In cases of acute and severe hypernatremia, free water replacement should match output and aim to reduce serum sodium by 1–2 mmol/h. Sodium should be corrected more slowly (0.5 mmol/h) if hypernatremia is more chronic or the patient is asymptomatic. Desmopressin (1-deamino-8-D-arginine vasopressin – DDAVP) a two amino acid substitute of ADH reduces urine output (aiming to achieve <2 ml/kg/h) and is given intravenously at a dose of 0.5–1 mcg which has a duration of action of 8–12 hours.

Potassium Disorders

Specific causes of potassium disorder after neurosurgery include endocrine disorders after pituitary tumor surgery (e.g., Cushing's disease), corticosteroids, and intentional hypothermia. There are no specific guidelines for the management of hypokalemia, but prevention and monitoring are mandatory in the perioperative period.

Mild hypokaliemia (3 mmol/L ≤ K^+ < 3.5 mmol/L) is often well tolerated and does not need a specific treatment except to avoid a further decrease. The signs of severe hypokalemia (<3 mmol/L) include muscle weakness, paralysis, and cardiac dysrhythmias. Electrocardiographic (ECG) changes include ST depression, T-wave flattening, and U waves. Severe hypokaliemia may be associated with prolonged mechanical ventilation due to muscle weakness, torsades de pointes, and ventricular fibrillation. In addition to treating the underlying cause, oral or intravenous potassium replacement is required. Potassium infusions (usually 20–40 mmol/h) must be given through a central vein. It is important to note that a 1 mmol/L reduction in potassium equates to a total body potassium store deficit of 200–400 mEq and that adequate serum magnesium levels are required for reabsorption by the kidneys. The risk of overtreatment of hypokalemia is rebound hyperkalemia, particularly in cases of potassium shift from the extracellular to the intracellular space due to hypothermia, alkalosis, barbiturate coma, and catecholamine infusions. When the cause of the potassium shift is reversed (e.g., by rewarming), release of potassium from the cells and ongoing potassium infusions may lead to severe hyperkaliemia and cardiac arrest.

The signs of hyperkalemia become apparent when serum potassium levels are greater than 6 mmol/L. Hyperkalemia can result in ECG conduction abnormalities, with peaked T waves, prolonged PR and QRS intervals, bradycardia, and finally, asystole. Treatment includes: (1) intravenous calcium gluconate or chloride to stabilize cardiac myocytes and avoid severe cardiac conduction problems; (2) insulin and glucose, bicarbonate and salbutamol to induce transcellular shifts; and (3) enteral resins, furosemide, or dialysis to increase excretion.

Other Electrolytes Disorders

Other electrolyte disorders are less frequent in neurosurgical procedures. Hypomagnesemia and hypophosphatemia are two electrolytes disorders that can have serious consequences if severe. Hypomagnesemia may occur in patients admitted to intensive care and has been associated with increased mortality. Clinical manifestations include muscle weakness, dysrhythmias, and seizures. Treatment of hypomagnesemia includes correction of the underlying cause and magnesium replacement orally or intravenously (1–2 g of magnesium sulfate over a 5-minute period in case of threatening dysrhythmias). Clinical manifestations of hypophosphatemia generally occur at serum values of less than 0.3 mmol/L and could lead to decreased myocardial contractility and respiratory muscle failure. Treatment is directed at the underlying cause, and replacement of phosphate can be accomplished orally or intravenously in the form of sodium or potassium phosphate.

Further Reading

Adler, S.M., Verbalis, J.G.: Disorders of body water homeostasis in critical illness. *Endocrinol Metab Clin North Am* 2006; **35**:873–894, xi.

Audibert, G., Steinmann, G., de Talancé, N., et al: Endocrine response after severe subarachnoid hemorrhage related to sodium and blood volume regulation. *Anesth Analg* 2009; **108**:1922–1928.

Fenske, W., Störk, S., Blechschmidt, A., et al: Copeptin in the differential diagnosis of hyponatremia. *J Clin Endocrinol Metab* 2009; **94**:123–129.

Palmer, B.F.: Hyponatremia in patients with central nervous system disease: SIADH versus CSW. *Trends Endocrinol Metab* 2003; **14**:182–187.

Fenske, W., Störk, S., Blechschmidt, A., et al: Clinical practice guideline on diagnosis and treatment of hyponatraemia.*Eur J Endocrinol* 2014; **170**:G1–G47.

Winzeler, B., Zweifel, C., Nigro, N., et al: Postoperative copeptin concentration predicts diabetes insipidus after pituitary surgery. *J Clin Endocrinol Metab* 2015; **100**: 2275–2282.

Status Epilepticus

Grant Sanders and John H. Turnbull

Key Points

- SE is a medical emergency that is defined as seizure activity lasting for more than 30 minutes, or two or more seizures occurring within 30 minutes without return to baseline neurologic status in the interim.
- SE has a mortality rate as high as 20%, with prolonged seizure activity resulting in worse outcomes.
- Benzodiazepines are the first-line treatment and can be safely given in the pre-hospital setting.
- Phenytoin and fosphenytoin are common second-line therapies, although emerging data supports the safe use of alternative antiepileptic drugs.
- Anesthetic infusions of propofol, midazolam, or pentobarbital should be considered early for refractory SE.
- Adjuvant therapies that are being studied include ketamine, magnesium, lidocaine, electroconvulsive therapy, ketogenic diet, and vagal nerve stimulation.

Abbreviations

AED	Antiepileptic drugs
GABA	Gamma-aminobutyric acid
GCSE	Generalized convulsive status epilepticus
NMDA	N-methyl-D-aspartate
RSE	Refractory status epilepticus
SE	Status epilepticus

Learning Objectives

1. Define status epilepticus for clinical purposes.
2. Describe the diagnostic approach for a patient with SE.
3. Formulate a treatment approach to a patient with SE.

Contents

- Introduction
- Clinical Presentation
- Epidemiology

Introduction

SE is a commonly encountered, life-threatening medical emergency described as prolonged continuous or multiple intermittent seizure activity. With a high rate of morbidity and mortality, early recognition and treatment of SE is essential to prevent neurologic deterioration and permanent harm.

Broadly, an epileptic seizure is defined as transient and involuntary disturbances of consciousness, movement, behavior, or emotion that are attributable to excessive synchronous electrical brain activity. The clinical presentation of a seizure is broad, ranging from generalized, tonic-clonic convulsions to temporary lapses of awareness (absence seizure). Non-epileptic seizures often mimic the manifestations of epileptic seizures, but are not associated with abnormal electrical brain activity and do not result in SE.

A 1993 task force of the International League Against Epilepsy defined SE as a seizure lasting more than 30 minutes, or two or more consecutive seizures occurring within a 30-minute period without return to baseline neurological function. However, this definition fails to address the urgent need to identify and treat patients with SE prior to such criteria being met, as prolonged seizure duration correlates with resistance to treatment and increased mortality. Therefore, experts are moving toward a more clinically practical definition of SE that allows for more rapid evaluation and treatment implementation. From an operational perspective, the diagnosis of SE occurs when seizure activity persists for more than 5 minutes, or if two or more seizures have occurred within 5 minutes without return to neurological baseline.

Clinical Presentation

Clinical presentation of SE varies among patients, but is generally classified into two broad categories – convulsive and non-convulsive. GCSE – the more obvious of the two presentations – occurs when seizure activity is present in both cerebral hemispheres. Patients present with generalized tonic-clonic movements, mental status impairment and may have focal neurological deficits in the post-ictal period. The definition of non-convulsive SE is less well defined but is broadly considered to be seizure activity on EEG without associated GCSE. Findings may include mental status changes, subtle motor abnormalities, such as rhythmic muscle movements or eye deviation. Finally, RSE occurs in patients whose seizures fail to respond to standard treatment regimens, such as a benzodiazepine and one AED.

Epidemiology

SE is a relatively common medical emergency, with an annual incidence of approximately 10–40 per 100,000 population. Nearly half of all patients who present with a first episode of SE do not have a previous diagnosis of epilepsy. However, patients with a history of SE as compared to those with simple, self-limited seizures are at greater risk of subsequent seizures. RSE occurs in 23%–43% of patients with SE and is often associated with severe underlying etiologies such as stroke, central nervous system infections, and rapidly progressive brain tumors.

Mortality from SE in the adult population is approximately 20%, with the underlying etiology being the most important contributing factor. RSE has a mortality rate that is three times higher than non-refractory SE. Acute, as opposed to chronic, precipitants of SE tend to have the highest mortality. These etiologies include acute stroke, hypoxemia/anoxia, trauma, drug overdose, metabolic disturbances, central nervous infection, and rapidly progressive brain tumors.

Complications of Status Epilepticus

Poor control of GCSE leads to neuronal injury. Abnormal vital signs such as hypertension, tachycardia, hyperthermia, hypoventilation, and hypoxia along with laboratory findings of lactic acidosis may accompany SE. Animal studies link these disturbances during GCSE to cell death from apoptosis, necrosis, and mitochondrial dysfunction. In one animal study, evidence of neuronal injury occurred even when convulsions were terminated with paralysis, specifically implicating excitatory cerebral activity in neurological morbidity. Although there is expert consensus to aggressively treat GCSE to prevent neurological deterioration, evidence to support equally aggressive treatment of non-convulsive SE is less robust.

Diagnostic Workup

EEG monitoring is the gold standard for the diagnosis of SE. Continuous EEG monitoring may be particularly helpful in patients with non-convulsive SE and those with GCSE whose tonic-clonic movements cease despite ongoing EEG evidence of epileptiform activity. CT imaging should be obtained for all patients except children who present with febrile SE. Laboratory studies to consider include blood glucose, complete metabolic panel, toxicology screen, urinalysis, blood and urine cultures, and lumbar puncture. Neurology consultation is necessary to guide workup and treatment.

Treatment

Given derangements to the cardiopulmonary system, initial management of SE focuses on airway management, establishing intravenous access, maintaining hemodynamic stability, and administering pharmacologic therapy to stop seizure activity (Figure 42.1). As new AEDs have entered the market, treatment algorithms for SE continue to evolve with institutional variations. Although care of the SE patient is often protocolized, care should always be case-specific.

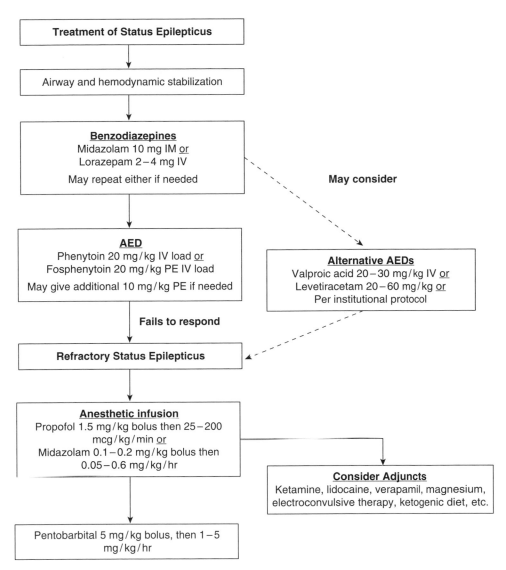

Figure 42.1 Example of a treatment algorithm for status epilepticus.
IM, intramuscular; IV, intravenous; AED, antiepileptic drug; PE, phenytoin equivalents.

Pre-Hospital Treatment

Benzodiazepines are the most effective first-line AEDs for SE and have been extensively studied and utilized. Several studies demonstrate the safe use of pre-hospital benzodiazepines by both home caregivers and first responders. For example, rectal diazepam, used for the in-home treatment of pediatric patients with SE, has a long and established safety record, while buccal and intranasal formulations of midazolam are safe alternatives. Importantly, pre-hospital administration of benzodiazepines is not associated with increased rates of respiratory failure. In fact, when compared to placebo, intravenous treatment with benzodiazepines by first responders decreases the rate of endotracheal intubation, likely due to earlier cessation of seizure activity.

Although intravenous administration of benzodiazepines is preferred, the Rapid Anticonvulsant Medications Prior to Arrival Trial (RAMPART), a randomized double-blind controlled trial published in 2012, demonstrates that pre-hospital intramuscular administration of midazolam is as effective as intravenous lorazepam in stopping SE. Establishing intravenous access in an actively seizing patient can be challenging and time-consuming, and the RAMPART trial supports the use of intramuscular midazolam as a valid first-line treatment of SE.

Initial Hospital Treatment

Patients who present in a hospital setting with GCSE must first be stabilized from a cardiopulmonary standpoint, including adequate airway and hemodynamic support. Many patients with GCSE maintain adequate oxygenation and ventilation with supplemental oxygen and simple interventions, such as a jaw thrust. Suction should be readily available and placement of the patient in a lateral decubitus position may help to prevent aspiration. Endotracheal intubation may be required in the setting of escalating benzodiazepine doses or when airway protection, oxygenation, or ventilation is not adequate.

When IV access is present, lorazepam is the intravenous medication of choice. Lorazepam terminates seizures as effectively as phenobarbital or diazepam plus phenytoin, but with a more favorable pharmacokinetic profile. Typical adult dosing of lorazepam for seizure termination is 2–4 mg intravenously (0.1 mg/kg for pediatric patients), with an expected onset of action in 2–4 minutes and a duration of action of 12–14 hours. Although it has not been robustly studied, many protocols support a repeat dose of lorazepam if the first dose is ineffective. If intravenous or intraosseous access is difficult to obtain, the RAMPART study suggests 10 mg of intramuscular midazolam as the appropriate alternative.

Benzodiazepines exert their effect by enhancing activity of the gamma-aminobutyric acid A (GABA-A) receptor, thereby inhibiting excitatory neurons and helping to abate seizure activity. Side effects may include decreased levels of consciousness, altered mental status, respiratory depression, and hypotension.

Second-Line Treatment

In patients who fail to respond to benzodiazepines, intravenous phenytoin, or fosphenytoin is classically the next drug of choice. A second agent may also be added in patients who initially responded to a benzodiazepine to prevent subsequent seizures when an easily correctable seizure trigger is not evident. By impeding recovery of voltage-gated sodium channels, phenytoin, and fosphenytoin reduce the number of action potentials in epileptic foci. Some institutional protocols preferentially utilize other AEDs, such as, levetiracetam, lacosamide, and valproic acid. These medications have been evaluated in several small SE studies, but currently no robust trials support one second-line agent over another.

The loading dose of phenytoin is 20 mg/kg with an additional 10 mg/kg if needed. Fosphenytoin is a water-soluble prodrug of phenytoin and has 100% bioavailability. Fosphenytoin is often dosed in "phenytoin equivalents", simplifying dosing. Phenytoin has several serious side effects including hypotension, QT prolongation, arrhythmias, and soft-tissue necrosis with extravasation. Although more expensive, fosphenytoin is often preferred over phenytoin as it has a better safety profile. Fosphenytoin is less caustic if extravasation occurs and can be infused more quickly – 150 mg/min as opposed to 50 mg/min for phenytoin.

Third-Line Treatment

In the setting of RSE, many experts encourage rapid progression to anesthetic infusions of either propofol or midazolam. Recognizing that longer seizure duration is associated with increased morbidity, these agents are being turned to earlier than in years past. If not already in place, the patient needs a secure airway for implementation of these treatments.

Propofol, like benzodiazepines, modulates the activity of GABA-A receptors, although its full receptor profile is not entirely understood. It has a short half-life and onset, allowing relatively rapid titration and elimination. Initial dosing is 1.5–3 mg/kg with subsequent infusion of 25–200 mcg/kg/min, titrated to EEG activity. The main side effect of propofol is hypotension, from both vasodilation and direct cardiac depression. Propofol is also associated with hypertriglyceridemia and propofol infusion syndrome (PRIS), a rare syndrome associated with cardiovascular collapse, lactic acidosis, rhabdomyolysis, and renal failure. Prolonged infusions are associated with tachyphylaxis and an increased context-sensitive half-life of up to 48 hr. These characteristics make titration and weaning challenging. When used for RSE, midazolam is given as a loading dose of 0.1–0.2 mg/kg, followed by an infusion of 0.05–0.6 mg/kg/h.

If seizure activity is seen on EEG after the initiation and titration of either propofol or midazolam, then barbiturates such as pentobarbital are often started. Pentobarbital is a short acting barbiturate that has a large volume of distribution and high lipid solubility, leading to prolonged clinical activity after an infusion is stopped. Typical loading dose is 5 mg/kg given slowly, followed by an infusion of 1–5 mg/kg/h. The main side effect of pentobarbital is hypotension, which often requires support with vasopressors.

Additional Treatment Options

For the rare patient where the progression from benzodiazepine, to AED, to anesthetic infusion does not halt electrocorticographic seizure activity, there are several other treatment modalities that have been utilized. The data behind these interventions in the treatment of SE are sparse, but case reports of success have led to increased interest. Isoflurane is a commonly used inhalation anesthetic that has been used to treat RSE with mixed results. The requirement for a gas scavenging system and end-tidal anesthetic monitoring makes the logistics of utilizing volatile anesthetics challenging in the intensive care unit.

Ketamine is a non-competitive NMDA receptor antagonist, with resultant blockade of excitatory neurotransmitter activity through these receptors. Data from a recent systematic review are encouraging and its favorable hemodynamic profile makes it an appealing adjunct to other intravenous anesthetic agents. However, ketamine is known to be neurotoxic with prolonged use and may raise intracranial pressure and cerebral metabolic demand, limiting its widespread use.

Verapamil is a calcium channel blocker that does not have antiepileptic activity, but may modulate activity of other AEDs. Lidocaine, a selective sodium channel blocker, has been trialled in RSE with some success reported in the pediatric literature. Controversy surrounds the use of neuromuscular blockade, which may facilitate ventilation and oxygenation and potentially reduce elevated intracranial pressure.

Non-pharmacologic treatments are also implemented in extreme cases. These treatments include targeting a ketogenic diet, electroconvulsive therapy, vagal nerve stimulation, surgical resection of an epileptic focus, mild hypothermia, and transcranial magnetic stimulation. Further studies are needed before these therapies can be routinely recommended in the treatment of SE.

Further Reading

Al-Mufti, F., Claassen, J.: Neurocritical care: Status epilepticus review. *Crit Care Clin* 2014; 30:751–764.

Betjemann, J.P., Lowenstein, D.H.: Status epilepticus in adults. *Lancet Neurol* 2015; 14:615–624.

Brophy, G.M1., Bell, R., Claassen, J., et al: Guidelines for the evaluation and management of status epilepticus. *Neurocrit Care* 2012; 17:3–23.

Rossetti, A.O., Lowenstein, D.H.: Management of refractory status epilepticus in adults: Still more questions than answers. *Lancet Neurol* 2011; **10**:922–930.

Silbergleit, R., Durkalski, V., Lowenstein, D., et al: Intramuscular versus intravenous therapy for prehospital status epilepticus. *N Engl J Med* 2012; **366**:591–600.

Zeiler, F., Teitelbaum, J., Gillman, L.M.: NMDA antagonists for refractory seizures. *Neurocrit Care* 2014; **20**:502–513.

Chapter	Guillain-Barré Syndrome and Myasthenia Gravis
43	Ashish Agrawal and Kristine E. W. Breyer

Key Points

- GBS is an acute progressive polyradiculoneuropathy resulting in generalized weakness that can last months and even years.
- MG is a chronic autoimmune neurologic disorder characterized by worsening muscle weakness with repeated use.
- Both GBS and MG patients may be treated in the intensive care unit for respiratory failure and both diseases are amenable to plasmapheresis and intravenous immunoglobulin therapy for critical symptoms.

Learning Objectives

1. Learn the common causes or triggers for GBS and MG
2. Understand the pathophysiology of GBS and MG
3. Learn the most common treatment modalities for GBS and for MG, as well as their impact on the respective diseases
4. Understand the symptoms indicating the need for admission of Guillain-Barré and MG patients to the intensive care unit

Abbreviations

AChR	Acetylcholine Nicotinic Receptor
AIDP	Acute inflammatory demyelinating polyneuropathy
AMAN	Acute motor axonal neuropathy
AMSAN	Acute motor and sensory axonal neuropathy
DTRs	Deep tendon reflexes
GBS	Guillain-Barré Syndrome
IVIG	Intravenous Immunoglobulin
LRP4	Lipoprotein-related Protein 4
MC	Myasthenic Crisis
MFS	Miller Fisher Syndrome
MG	Myasthenia Gravis
MUSK	Muscle-specific Tyrosine Kinase
NIPPV	Non-invasive Positive Pressure Ventilation
NMBDs	Neuromuscular Blocking Drugs

NMJ	Neuromuscular Junction
NSAIDs	Non-steroidal Anti-inflammatory Drugs
PLEX	Plasma exchange

Contents

Guillain-Barré Syndrome

GBS is an umbrella term to describe a heterogeneous group of syndromes all characterized by acute immune-mediated polyradiculoneuropathy. The overall incidence is 1–2 per 100,000 adults and increases with age. Males are affected slightly more often than females and subtype incidence varies by geographical location.

Clinical Subtypes

GBS is subdivided into demyelinating GBS, axonal GBS and MFS based upon pathophysiology and clinical symptoms. AIDP is the most common variant in the United States and

Europe. AIDP is characterized by demyelination starting at the nerve roots resulting in symmetric ascending muscle weakness with decreased or absent DTRs. AIDP affects motor nerves more than sensory but both are involved. Axonal subtypes are characterized by demyelination at the axonal level with preservation of peripheral nerve myelination. AMAN only involves ventral motor axons whereas the more severe AMSAN affects both dorsal sensory and ventral motor axons. Differentiation between AIDP, AMAN, and AMSAN can only be performed with nerve conduction studies.

MFS is a separate GBS subtype characterized by a triad of acute onset ataxia, areflexia, and ophthalmoplegia. Demyelination in MFS occurs at the peripheral nerve level. A variant of MFS called Bickerstaff's brainstem encephalitis also includes hyper-somnolence. Treatments of GBS do not differ by subtype but disease progression and prognosis do.

Causes

All types of GBS are immune mediated. Antecedent infection is diagnosed in over half of all cases and the resultant immune response cross-reacts with peripheral neural components due to cross-reactive epitopes (molecular mimicry). Campylobacter jejuni is the most common organism but cytomegalovirus, Epstein-Barr virus, *Mycoplasma pneumonia*, *Haemophilus influenza*, human immunodeficiency virus and influenza A virus have all been implicated. New data also suggest a relationship between GBS and Zika virus.

Clinical Features

GBS is characterized by acute onset and progression. Within 2 weeks over 70% of patients will have reached a nadir in their symptoms and by definition all patients reach their clinical nadir and plateau phase by 4 weeks. The plateau can last weeks to months until clinical recovery slowly begins.

Neurological

Patterns of weakness vary with subtype; however, the most common neurologic symptoms include symmetric ascending weakness and areflexia. Over two-thirds of patients will be unable to ambulate independently. Many patients also present with distal parasthesia. Pain, especially severe radicular back pain or neuropathic pain is also common.

Respiratory

Ten to thirty percent of patients require mechanical ventilation. Predictors of respiratory failure include rapidity of decline, quadriplegia, neck, and bulbar weakness, vital capacity <20 ml/kg or reduction of greater than 30%, and maximal inspiratory pressure greater than negative 30 cm H_2O.

Autonomic

Dysautonomia is common (70%) and is due to demyelination of peripheral autonomic nerves. Tachycardia, orthostatic hypotension, hypertension, urinary retention, ileus, severe bradycardia, conduction blocks, and other arrhythmias have all been described. Arrhythmias are a cause of sudden death in these patients.

Diagnosis

Diagnosis of GBS is clinical. Progression occurs within 4 weeks of onset. Other core features include symmetric weakness and absent or decreased reflexes. CSF analysis classically reveals elevated CSF protein level (>400 mg/L) in the presence of normal CSF cell counts (cytoalbuminologic dissociation), although this is not present in all patients. Other supportive features include dysautonomia, pain, and sensory involvement (Table 43.1). Nerve conduction studies (reduced conduction velocities and evidence of demyelination) can aid in diagnosis but alternative diagnoses must be excluded (Table 43.2).

Management

Supportive Care

Approximately one third of GBS patients will require intensive care. Early tracheostomy is reasonable for those requiring mechanical ventilation. Succinylcholine should be avoided due to the risk of hyperkalemia. Management of dysautonomia includes avoidance of triggers (e.g., suctioning and postural changes), and short acting medications (e.g., labetalol, esmolol, or nitroprusside) should be used to treat hypertensive episodes. Anti-thromboembolic prophylaxis, nutrition, and physical therapy are all of critical importance in the management of these patients. Gabapentin or carbamazepine is recommended for pain management.

Table 43.1 Diagnostic Criteria of GBS

Core Features:	Supportive features:	Features *Inconsistent* with Guillian-Barre Syndrome
Symmetric progressive weakness in legs and/or arms	Mild sensory signs	Marked asymmetry
Areflexia or hyporeflexia	Autonomic involvement	Bladder or bowel dysfunction at onset
	Cranial nerve involvement	Sharp spinal cord level
	Pain	Severe sensory symptoms with limited weakness
	Nerve conduction study consistent with demyelination or axonal degeneration	Severe respiratory symptoms without limb involvement
	Elevated CSF protein and normal WBCs (albuminologic dissociation)	
Progression < 4 weeks		Progression beyond 4 weeks (consider subacute or chronic inflammatory demyelinating polyneuropathy)

Table 43.2 Differential Diagnosis of GBS

Mimics of Guillian-Barre Syndrome	Examples:
Flaccid paralysis	Polio, West Nile, Herpes, Cytomegalovirus, Epstein Barr Virus (EBV), Rabies, HIV
Transverse myelitis	Mycoplasma pneumonia, EBV, CMV
Spinal cord injury	Trauma, spinal stenosis, anterior spinal artery occlusion, epidural abscess
Central nervous system injury	Stroke (basilar)
Acute peripheral neuropathies	Infections, toxins (heavy metal poisoning), shellfish poisoning, Lyme disease, Porphyria
Neuromuscular junction disorder	Myasthenia Gravis, Lambert-Eaton, Botulism
Critical illness myopathy	
Muscle disorders	Myositis, periodic paralysis, electrolyte abnormalities

Immune therapy

Both high dose intravenous immune globulin (IVIG, 400 mg/kg for 5 days) and PLEX (four to five exchanges of 1.5x plasma volume) are effective in speeding recovery and reducing disability in patients with GBS. There is no benefit for PLEX over IVIG, though IVIG is more commonly available at smaller hospitals. Patients with IgA deficiency are at risk for anaphylaxis with PLEX and IVIG. There is no role for corticosteroids in treating GBS.

Prognosis

Mortality from GBS ranges from 4% to 20%, and risk factors include elderly patients, severity of disease at nadir, mechanical ventilation, and rapid onset of symptoms. Recovery takes months with only 80% of patients able to walk independently at 6 months and some patients never regaining full strength.

Myasthenia Gravis

MG is a chronic autoimmune neurological disease at the post-synaptic neuromuscular end plate with a waxing and waning clinical course. MG is the most common disorder of neuromuscular transmission with a prevalence of 70–165 per million. Incidence is bimodal generally affecting females aged 20–30 years old and males over 50 years old.

Pathophysiology

MG is classically characterized as seropositive and seronegative. Over 80% of patients are seropositive, meaning they have IgG antibodies to the AChR. These IgG antibodies are thought to accelerate cross-linking of AChR, increasing degradation of Ach or to prevent binding by ACh. Seronegative MG patients do not have IgG AChR antibodies; however, many of these patients do have autoantibodies to other portions of the neuromuscular end plate (MUSK and LRP4). Differences in pathophysiology may account for variations in presentation between different subtypes; for example, the MUSK MG patients have less ocular symptoms, are less likely to have thymomas and are less responsive to antic-holinesterase therapy and immunosuppressive medications. A drug-induced form of MG can be triggered most commonly by penicillamine, and it responds to cessation of that drug.

Clinical Features

Clinical subtypes of MG are ocular (15%) and generalized (85%). Ocular MG patients display oculomotor paresis, ptosis, and diplopia without generalized weakness. Patients with generalized MG also present with ocular symptoms, however, they will progress to have fluctuating skeletal muscle weakness in the rest of the body including muscles of the neck, head, face muscles, intercostal, diaphragmatic, and those muscles related to bulbar function. Both ocular and generalized forms are characterized by worsening muscle fatigue with repeated use, or fatigability. MG is chronic and involves symptomatic relapses with intervening periods of normal strength.

Diagnosis

The diagnosis of MG is based on clinical history and physical examination. Serologic testing for AChR, MUSK, and LRP4 are important in confirming a diagnosis of MG, though a10% of patients remain seronegative. Electromyographic testing is especially important in cases of seronegative MG. Repeated stimulation of a motor nerve may diagnose progressive fade in compound muscle action potentials, suggesting fatigability. Imaging including a CT scan of the chest may reveal thymic hyperplasia (60%) or a thymoma (15%) which may be associated with MG.

Edrophonium (Tensilon) is a short-acting acetylcholinesterase inhibitor that can be used to detect clinical improvement in suspected MG. Edrophonium is also used to distinguish between weakness resulting from MC and cholinergic crisis. MC improves with edrophonium due to increased availability of Ach while cholinergic crisis worsens or remains the same. Edrophonium administration can cause life threatening side effects such as bradycardia and atropine should be immediately available.

Management

Acetylcholinesterase Inhibitors

Acetylcholinesterase inhibitors, such as pyridostigmine or neostigmine, limit breakdown of acetylcholine at the NMJ.

Immunosuppressive Therapy

MG patients with persistent symptoms, despite acetylcholinesterase inhibitors, may benefit from immunosuppressive therapy. Initial options include prednisone (0.75–1 mg/kg/day), prednisolone, and azathioprine (2–3 mg/kg/day). Second-line immunosuppressive drugs include mycophenolate mofetil, rituximab, cyclosporine, methotrexate, and tacrolimus. Caution should be used when initiating prednisone as there are reports of prednisone triggering an MC in some patients.

BOX 43.1 Medications to Use with Caution in Patients with Myasthenia Gravis

Antibiotics: *Aminoglycosides, Clindamycin, Fluoroquinolones, Ketolides, Vancomycin*
Cardiovascular Medications: *Beta-blockers, Procainamide, Quinidine*
Botulinum toxin
Chloroquine/Hydroxychloroquine
Magnesium
Penicillamine
Quinine

Thymectomy

Thymectomy is recommended for early-onset MG or patients with a thymoma on imaging. Patients with MUSK or LRP4 antibodies or ocular-only symptoms are less likely to benefit from thymectomy.

Plasma Exchange and High-Dose Immunoglobulin Therapy

Both IVIG (400 mg/kg for 3–5 days) and PLEX (4–5 exchanges of 1.5x plasma volume over 10 days) are equally effective. Benefit can be seen in 2–5 days and can last 2–3 months.

Triggering Medications

Certain drugs trigger or unmask symptoms and should be avoided (Box 43.1).

Myasthenic Crisis

Approximately 10–20% of MG patients will experience a MC. This is a clinical diagnosis defined by the requirement of mechanical ventilator support for either respiratory or bulbar muscle weakness. MC can be triggered by infections, emotional stress, and surgery. Respiratory failure may be due to obstruction or due to respiratory muscle fatigue. Signs of bulbar muscle weakness include inability to manage secretions, decreased cough, dysphagia, facial paresis, and staccato speech. Hypercapnia is an ominous finding and hypoxemia appears very late. Patients with forced vital capacity less than 20 ml/kg or maximal inspiratory pressure greater than negative 30 cmH$_2$0 are likely to benefit from intubation.

NIPPV is emerging as a modality to assist with respiratory failure early in a MC to avoid intubation. NIPPV can off-load the fatigued muscles so they can regain strength. Bi-level NIPPV is the preferred mode and must be applied at early signs of respiratory failure. Hypercapnia is highly predictive of NIPPV failure. Bi-level NIPPV is also helpful post-extubation in patients recovering from a MC.

Anesthetic Considerations

MG patients undergoing elective surgery should be medically optimized. Continuation of pyridostigmine on the morning of surgery is debated; discontinuation reduces the risk of prolonged neuromuscular blockade after chemical paralysis but puts the patient at risk for pre-operative weakness. Risk factors for post-operative ventilation include forced vital capacity less than 2.9 L, chronic lung disease, greater than 6-year history of MG, or daily

Table 43.3 Causes of Neurological Weakness

	Guillian-Barre (GBS)	Myasthenia Gravis (MG)	Lambert Eaton Syndrome (LES)	Critical Illness Myopathy (CIM)
Presenting Symptom	Symmetric weakness (can vary with subtypes)	Ocular-bulbar weakness	Proximal muscle weakness, legs	Symmetric limb weakness, can involve phrenic nerve (spares cranial nerves)
Progressive Symptoms	Often involves respiratory muscles; areflexia, sensory loss, autonomic dysfunction	proximal to distal muscles; cranial to caudal; (rare autonomic dysfunction); 15–20% develop crisis (respiratory failure)	Spreads proximal to distal muscles; caudal to cranial; autonomic dysfunction; areflexia	Decreased/loss reflexes, sensory loss
Etiology	Acute inflammatory polyneuropathy	Autoimmune: antibodies to AchR, (Post-synaptic at NMJ)	Autoimmune: antibodies to voltage gated calcium channels (Pre-synaptic at NMJ)	(Unknown mechanism) Acquired during critical illness, hyperglycemia, NMB, corticosteroids, aminoglycosides
Diagnostic Test	CSF studies, EMG	Serum antibody	EMG: repetitive nerve stimulation (RNS); 85–90% all cases are Ab+	EMG
Histology	Most common: demyelination peripheral nerves, perifascicular lymphocytic small cuffing (varies)	(Non-diagnostic, varies with Ab subtype) Type I &II muscle filament patchy atrophy	Type II fiber atrophy	Necrosis /loss thick filaments, preservation of thin filaments, Z-discs and nerves
Unique Features	CSF: cytoalbuminologic dissociation	Post-exercise fatigability	Areflexia, Post-exercise facilitation, posttetanic potentiation	Elevated creatinine phosphate kinase (CPK)

Additional Workup	Arrhythmia monitoring	CT Chest for thymoma, arrhythmia monitoring	50% cases due to paraneoplastic syndrome, perform chest CT to evaluate for small cell lung cancer	
Therapy	IVIG, PLEX	Meds: cholinesterase inibitors, immunosuppresives, IVIG, PLEX; thymectomy	Tumor rx; Meds: 3, 4-DAP, cholinesterase inhibitors, immunosuppresives, IVIG, PLEX	Treat underlying causes, physical and occupational therapy

NMJ: neuromusclular junction, CT: computed tomography scan. Ab+/-: antibody positive/negative, 3, 4-DAP: 3, 4- diaminopyridine, IVIG: intravenous immunoglobulin, PLEX: plasma exchange, NMB: neuromuscular blocking agent pyridostigmine dose greater than 750 mg. Whenever possible, patients should be investigated for other autoimmune conditions including thyroid disorders as they coexist with MG in 15% of cases.

Routine use of NMBDs should be avoided. A thoracic epidural can be helpful for thoracic or abdominal cases to facilitate muscle relaxation. Remifentanil can be considered as an infusion to reduce intraoperative respiratory effort. When required, short acting non-depolarizing NMBDs are preferred, as the MG patient is very sensitive to their effects. The dose of non-depolarizing NMBDs should be reduced by at least half. Succinylcholine should be used with caution. MG patients are often very resistant to succinylcholine with reports of such high requirements that a Phase II block is produced.

There are several case reports in the literature on the use of Sugammadex to reverse deep neuromuscular blockade with rocuronium or vecuronium in patients with MG without complications. Standard reversal with neostigmine should be avoided if the patient is on pre-operative acetylcholinesterase inhibitors as that enzyme may be maximally inhibited. High doses may also trigger a cholinergic crisis that may also present with weakness.

The patient should be evaluated for extubation at the end of surgery as per normal but emphasis should be placed on avoiding residual neuromuscular blockade. A maximal inspiratory pressure greater than negative 30 cm H_2O predicts failure with extubation. Pain should be treated effectively as it can trigger an MC. Regional techniques such as epidurals or nerve blocks and multimodal analgesic therapy including acetaminophen (Paracetamol) and NSAIDs should be used to reduce the need for opioid analgesics.

Prognosis
With optimum surgical and medical management, the prognosis for patients with myasthenia gravis is excellent.

Further Reading
Blichfeldt-Lauridsen, L., Hansen, B.D.: Anesthesia and myasthenia gravis. *Acta Anaesthesiol Scand* 2012; **56**(1):17–22.

Gilhus, N.E., Verschuuren, J.J.: Myasthenia gravis: Subgroup classification and therapeutic strategies. *Lancet Neurol* 2015; **14**(10):1023–1036.

Godoy, D.A., Mello, L.J., Masotti, L., Di Napoli, M.: The myasthenic patient in crisis: An update of the management in neurointensive care unit. *Arq Neuropsiquiatr* 2013; **71**(9A):627–639.

Hoffmann, S., Kohler, S., Ziegler, A., Meisel, A.: Glucocorticoids in myasthenia gravis – if, when, how, and how much?. *Acta Neurol Scand* 2014; **130**(4):211–221.

Rabinstein, A.A.: Acute neuromuscular respiratory Failure. *Continuum (Minneap Minn)* 2015; **21**(5 Neurocritical Care):1324–1345.

Rabinstein, A.A.: Noninvasive ventilation for neuromuscular respiratory failure: When to use and when to avoid. *Curr Opin Crit Care* 2016; **22**(2):94–99.

Wakerley, B.R., Yuki, N.: Mimics and chameleons in Guillain-Barré and Miller Fisher syndromes. *Pract Neurol* 2015; **15**(2):90–99.

Willison, H.J., Jacobs, B.C., van Doorn, P. A.: "Guillain-Barré syndrome." *Lancet* 2016.

Yuki, N., Hartung, H.P.: "Guillain-Barré syndrome." *N Engl J Med* 2012; **366**(24):2294–2304.

Chapter

44

Brain Death

Joyce Chang and David Shimabukuro

Key Points

- Although there are US federal and European legal standards for the diagnosis of brain death, there are also state, regional, institutional, cultural, and religious standards to consider.
- The determination of brain death by clinical criteria is widely accepted as standard of care, but the need for ancillary tests varies from country to country.
- For ancillary tests, 4-vessel cerebral catheter angiography is the gold standard in the assessment of intracranial blood flow.

Abbreviations

AAN   American Academy of Neurology
CNS   Central nervous system

Contents

- History and Legal Considerations
- Diagnosis
    - Preconditions
    - Clinical Examination
- Ancillary Tests
- Further Reading

History and Legal Considerations

For a long time, death was simply defined as a permanent cessation of circulatory and respiratory function. However, with the advances in cardiopulmonary resuscitation and the introduction of organ transplantation, the concept of death as complete and irreversible loss of brain function became an important consideration. The process started in 1968 when a committee at Harvard Medical School sought to define death as an irreversible coma. In 1981, the President's Commission for the Study of Ethical Problems in Medicine and Biomedical and Behavioural Research issued a report that subsequently formed the basis for the Uniform Determination of Death Act in the USA where brain death was legally recognized as an acceptable indication of death. Since then, given the controversies in the determination of brain death, the neurological standard has been re-examined multiple times with the most recent consensus guidelines by the AAN published in 2010.

The Uniform Determination of Death Act states an individual who has sustained either (1) irreversible cessation of circulatory and respiratory function or (2) irreversible cessation of all functions of the entire brain, including the brain stem, is dead. A determination of brain death must be made with accepted medical standards. Practice varies around the world and even from state to state in the United States as to what constitutes accepted medical standards in the determination of brain death. It is therefore advisable to determine the guidelines or requirements that are specific to the area or institution.

Diagnosis

Preconditions

Prior to the clinical evaluation to determine brain death, multiple prerequisites must be met. These include the establishment of:

(1) Coma with a known irreversible cause
(2) Absence of CNS-depressant drugs and/or neuromuscular blocking agents
(3) Exclusion of other medical conditions that may mimic coma
(4) Absence of electrolyte, acid-base, or endocrine abnormalities
(5) Core temperature >36 degrees Celsius
(6) Normalized hemodynamics with systolic blood pressure > 100 mmHg

A patient in a coma is defined as unresponsive, without evidence of seizures, absence of limb movement (except for spinal reflexes) and ventilator dependent. The most common causes of coma include severe traumatic brain injury, subarachnoid or intracerebral hemorrhage, extensive ischemic strokes, cerebral edema secondary to fulminant hepatic failure, and hypoxic ischemic brain injury. The cause of the coma can typically be ascertained from history, examination, laboratory tests, and neuroimaging.

Common drugs that can cause CNS-depression include anesthetic agents, benzodiazepines, barbiturates, opiates, and tricyclic antidepressants. In general, the time allowed for drug clearance should be four to seven times the half-lives of the agents concerned but patients with renal or hepatic dysfunction may require longer.

Many conditions may mimic coma including Guillain-Barre syndrome, locked-in syndrome and severe hypothyroidism. Abnormalities in electrolytes, acid-base status, endocrine hormones as well as hypothermia can also lead to CNS-depression.

Clinical Examination

After the clinical prerequisites have been made, clinical examination and, in some countries, ancillary tests are performed to confirm brain death. Key components of the clinical examination are summarized in Table 44.1. No evidence of motor responses, withdrawal/extensor or flexor posturing are all consistent with brain stem death but movements related to spinal reflexes are allowed.

The apnea test is performed to confirm the loss of spontaneous respiratory effort. Brainstem respiratory control depends on centrally located chemoreceptors that sense changes in $PaCO_2$ and pH of the cerebral spinal fluid. Current research identifies $PaCO_2$ levels > 60 mmHg (6.5 kPa) as producing maximum stimulation of the brainstem and

Table 44.1 Brainstem Reflex Examination

Cranial Nerve	Examination	Technique	Brain Death Finding
1) CN II	2) Pupillary light reflex	Shine sustained bright light into each pupil	3) Fixed, dilated pupils with no response to light
4) CN III, IV, VI, VIII	5) Oculocephalic reflex 6) Oculovestibular reflex	7) Rapidly turn head from midline to one and then the other side. Observe for lateral movement of eyes, contralateral to the direction of head turn 8) Elevate head to 30 degrees. Irrigate each tympanic membrane with 50 ml ice water. Observe tonic eye deviation toward the side of ice water irrigation. Wait 5–10 minutes between each tympanic membrane evaluation. (Ensure no rupture of tympanic membrane prior to test)	9) No movement of eyes with head turn 10) No eye movement to injection of ice water
11) CN V, VII	12) Corneal reflex	13) Stimulate cornea with swab or gauze, look for reflexive eye blink	14) No corneal response on either side
15) CN IX, X	16) Cough reflex 17) Gag reflex	18) Stimulate larynx with suction device, insert suction catheter through endotracheal tube 19) Stimulate posterior pharynx with suction device	20) No cough response to laryngeal or bronchial stimulation 21) No gag response to pharyngeal stimulation bilaterally

therefore is the threshold used for the apnea test by current AAN guidelines. There are no guidelines for the threshold in patients with chronic elevated baseline $PaCO_2$.

Prior to initiating the apnea test, the patient is pre-oxygenated with 100% inspired oxygen for at least 10 minutes until PaO_2 > 200 mm Hg. (~26kPa). This will minimize potential complications of hypoxia during the test. The patient should be normothermic (core temperature >36.5 degrees Celsius), have adequate cerebral perfusion pressure, and $PaCO_2$ should be in the normal range (35–45 mmHg/5–5.5 kPa). The patient is disconnected from the ventilator to avoid detection of false-respiratory efforts. Oxygen can be delivered either via t-piece or a suction catheter placed at the level of the carina. Vasopressors can be used to maintain adequate perfusion pressures (mean arterial pressure 60–80 mmHg). Respirations defined as abdominal or chest excursions should be observed for. If observed, the apnea test should be terminated. If no respiratory efforts are visualized, apnea can be continued for 5–10 minutes with repeat arterial blood gases performed at the end of the test. A $PaCO_2$ > 60 mmHg (8 kPa) or an increase of > 20 mmHg (~3 kPa) with no respiratory efforts confirms brain death. If significant cardiac dysrhythmia, hypoxia, or refractory hypotension occurs the apnea test should be terminated.

Ancillary Tests

Brain death is a clinical diagnosis. There are times when confirmatory ancillary tests are needed because a clinical determination cannot be made or is required by a certain area or institution practice. These ancillary tests are performed to evaluate cerebral blood flow. The absence of cerebral blood flow means the brain is not viable. Current ancillary tests are divided into the assessment of cerebral blood flow or the assessment of cerebral function. They include cerebral angiography, transcranial doppler ultrasonography (TCD), nuclear medicine scintigraphy, single-photon computed tomography (SPECT), cerebral magnetic resonance angiography, cerebral computed tomographic angiography, electroencephalography, and somatosensory evoked potentials.

Cerebral angiography is considered the gold standard but is an invasive procedure performed by injection of contrast into the aortic arch. Contrast reaching both anterior and posterior circulations with absence of intracranial filling starting at the level of entry of the carotid and vertebral arteries (4 vessels) into the skull is consistent with brain death.

Transcranial doppler is quick and non-invasive but is operator dependent. Signals consistent with brain death include reverberating flow, isolated systolic spikes with no or reversal of diastolic flow, or small peaks in early systole. Absence of TCD signals cannot be interpreted because some patients do not have temporal windows to perform the examination.

There is currently insufficient data to dictate the observation waiting period and the utility of serial neurologic examinations. Practice varies widely, but most centers require a minimum of two examinations consistent with brain death separated by a certain time interval. The AAN original practice parameters for determination of brain death was published in 1995 and updated guidelines were published in 2010. There are no published case reports in the academic literature detailing the recovery of brain function in a patient who has fulfilled the clinical criteria of brain death per AAN practice guidelines.

Further Reading

Kramer, A.H.: Ancillary testing in brain death. *Semin Neurol* 2015; **35**:125–138.

Rincon, F.: Neurologic criteria for death in adults. In Parrillo, J., Dellinger, R. (Eds.). *Critical Care Medicine: Principles of Diagnosis and Management in the Adult*. Philadelphia, PA, USA: Elsevier-Saunders; 2014: 1098–1105.

Roberts, P., Todd, S. *Comprehensive Critical Care: Adult*. Mount Prospect, IL: Society of Critical Care Medicine; 2012.

Smith, M.: Brain death: The United Kingdom perspective. *Semin Neurol* 2015; **35**(2):145–151.

Spinello, I.M.: Brain death determination. *J Intensive Care Med* 2015; **30**(6):326–337.

Uniform Determination of Death Act, 12 uniform laws annotated 489 (West 1993 and West suppl 1997).

Wijdicks, E.F.: Brain death guidelines explained. *Semin Neurol* 2015; **35**:105–115.

Wijdicks, E.F., Varelas, P.N., Gronseth, G.S., et al: Evidence based guideline update: determining brain death in adults: Report of the Quality Standards Subcommittee of the American Academy of Neurology. *Neurology* 2010; **74**:1911–1918.

Chapter

45

Intracranial Pressure Monitoring

Marek Czosnyka and Karol Budohoski

Key Points

- ICP has four components, associated with: (1) arterial blood inflow, (2) venous blood outflow, (3) cerebrospinal fluid circulation, and (4) volumetric changes in brain tissue or lesion.
- Continuous measurement of ICP is an important parameter in the management of traumatic brain injury.
- Common methods of monitoring ICP are either by intraparenchymal pressure sensors or an intraventricular catheter.
- The pressure-reactivity index reflects the autoregulatory reserve of cerebral blood vessels and gives useful information regarding adequate and optimal cerebral perfusion pressures.
- ICP pulse waveforms provide dynamic information about cerebrospinal compensatory reserve.
- Noninvasive measurcment of ICP and cerebral perfusion pressure, though of limited accuracy, is possible.

Abbreviations

ABP   Arterial blood pressure
CBF   Cerebral blood flow
CPP   Cerebral perfusion pressure
CSF   Cerebrospinal fluid
EVD   External ventricular drain
ICP   Intracranial pressure
MAP   Mean arterial pressure
MCA   Middle cerebral artery
PRx   Pressure reactivity index
SAH   Subarachnoid hemorrhage
TCD   Transcranial doppler

Contents

Introduction

ICP is an essential parameter in most brain-monitoring systems and requires the use of an invasive sensor. Measurement of ICP also allows estimation of CPP:

$$\text{Mean CPP} = \text{MAP} - \text{Mean ICP}.$$

ICP is a complex signal derived from volumetric changes of cerebral blood, CSF, brain parenchyma, and in pathological conditions, volume of space occupying lesions. ICP has dynamic (changing in time) and static components (which may still change in time but at a much slower rate). Both fast and slow changes in ICP can be associated with a change of volume of arterial blood, venous blood, CSF circulation, as well as volumetric changes of brain tissue (edema formation) or other space-occupying lesions (e.g., hematomas, tumors, and abscesses). ICP also provides information regarding autoregulation of CBF, pressure reactivity of cerebral vessels, and compliance of the cerebrospinal system.

It is important to distinguish between different components of ICP, as clinical strategies to treat intracranial hypertension depend on which component is elevated. For example, arterial blood volume may elevate ICP to very high levels in a matter of seconds and these elevations are known as plateau waves, secondary to intrinsic arterial dilatation. Rapid, short-term hyperventilation causing cerebral vasoconstriction usually reduces ICP in such cases. The CSF-circulatory component may elevate ICP in acute hydrocephalus. In such cases, an EVD is helpful. Venous outflow obstruction may also elevate ICP, and neutral head positioning or investigation of possible venous thrombosis may be useful strategies. Finally, if ICP is elevated due to brain edema or space-occupying lesions, osmotherapy, or surgical intervention (including decompressive craniectomy) may be beneficial.

Methods of Measurement

Microtransducers

Modern ventricular, subdural, or intraparenchymal microtransducers have a low risk of infection, and have demonstrated excellent metrologic properties during bench tests. Intraparenchymal systems are inserted through a burr hole via an airtight support bolt or tunneled subcutaneously. With the intraparenchymal microtransducers, the measured pressure may be local and not necessarily representative of ventricular CSF pressure. Microtransducers cannot generally be recalibrated after insertion, and zero drift may occur with long-term monitoring.

Intraventricular Drains

An external pressure transducer connected to a catheter ending in the ventricular system that allows direct pressure measurement is still the "gold standard" for ICP measurement. Additional advantages include the capability of periodic external calibration and CSF drainage. However, insertion of a ventricular catheter may be difficult or impossible in patients with advanced brain swelling, and the risk of infection is increased significantly after 3 days of monitoring. Care should be taken that the EVD is not open to drainage when measurements are recorded, and the EVD should be closed for at least 15 minutes prior to measurement.

Other Sensors

The least invasive systems use epidural probes, Contemporary epidural sensors are much more reliable than older versions but there is uncertainty about their accuracy. Manometric lumbar CSF pressure measurement is not considered a reliable method in neurointensive care.

Non-invasive Intracranial Pressure Measurement

It would be very helpful to measure ICP or CPP without invasive transducers. To this end, TCD examination of ophthalmic artery, tympanic membrane displacement, and ultrasound "time-of-flight" techniques have been suggested. There is reasonable correlation between the pulsatility index of MCA velocity and CPP after head injury, but absolute measurements of CPP cannot be accurately extrapolated. However, recently, a method for non-invasive assessment of CPP has been reported: mean ABP multiplied by the ratio of diastolic to mean flow velocity. This estimator can predict actual CPP – in the adult range (60–100 mmHg) – with an error of less than 10 mmHg for more than 80% of measurements. Non-invasive approaches do yet not yield useful ICP data.

Events and Trends Seen in Intracranial Monitoring

Specific patterns of the ICP waveform can be identified when mean ICP is monitored continuously. Patients with a low and stable ICP (<20 mmHg) characteristically have no ICP vasogenic waves, with the exception of a phasic response of ICP to variations in ABP. The most common picture after head injury consists of vasogenic waves of limited amplitude when ICP is high and stable (>20 mmHg). Vasogenic waves, plateau waves, or waves related to changes in arterial pressure and hyperemic events are common in post injury recordings (see Figure 45.1).

Cerebrovascular Pressure Reactivity

The correlation between spontaneous waves in ABP and ICP is dependent on the ability of cerebral vessels to autoregulate. With intact autoregulation, a rise in ABP produces

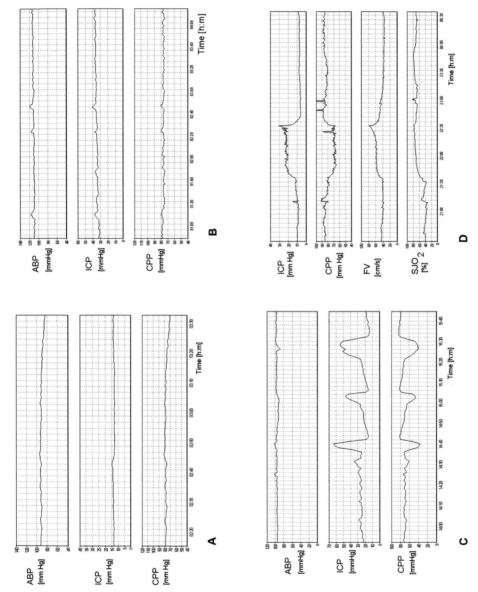

Figure 45.1 Examples of monitored ICP, arterial blood pressure (ABP) and cerebral perfusion pressure (CPP) after TBI: (A) low and stable ICP, (B) elevated and relatively stable ICP, (C) elevations of ICP with plateau waves, and (D) "hyperemic wave" elevation of ICP secondary to a rise in cerebral blood flow, here depicted as an increase in doppler blood flow velocity (FV) and jugular bulb oximetry (SJO2).

vasoconstriction, a decrease in cerebral blood volume and a fall in ICP. With disturbed autoregulation, changes in ABP are transmitted to the intracranial compartment and result in a passive pressure effect. The correlation coefficient between slow changes in mean ABP and ICP (termed the "pressure reactivity index" [PRx]) is negative when cerebral vessels are pressure reactive and retain the ability to autoregulate (Figure 45.2A). A positive correlation coefficient (+PRx) indicates disturbed cerebrovascular pressure reactivity and a passive system (Figure 45.2B).

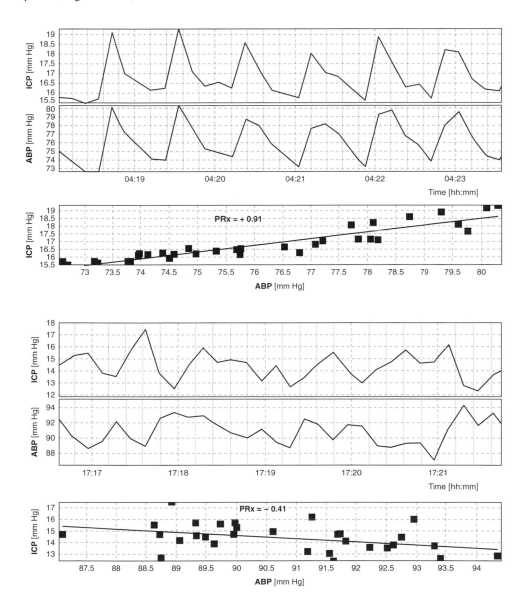

Figure 45.2A and B Principles of calculating pressure reactivity index (PRx). Shown is the correlation coefficient between 30 consecutive 10-second averages of ICP and ABP. **A:** Negative PRx (–0.41), indicating excellent reactivity and autoregulation. **B:** Positive PRx (+0.91) indicating disturbed pressure reactivity and poor autoregulation.

Optimal Cerebral Perfusion Pressure

In adults with head trauma, PRx plotted against CPP gives a "U-shape" curve that indicates, for the majority of patients, a value of CPP for which pressure reactivity is optimal (Figure. 45.3). This optimal pressure can be estimated by plotting and analyzing the PRx-CPP curve in sequential 4-hour periods; the greater the distance between the current and the "optimal" CPP, the more likely that the outcome will be poor (Figure 45.4). This potentially useful methodology attempts to refine our current approach to CPP- oriented therapy by helping to avoid periods when CPP is too low (i.e., ischemia) or too high (i.e., hyperamia and secondary increase in ICP).

Pulse Waveform Analysis of Intracranial Pressure

To adequately identify potentially harmful intracranial hypertension in individual patients, an analysis of the amplitude of ICP waveforms can be performed. The pulse waveform of ICP provides information about the transmission of arterial pulse pressure through the arterial walls to the CSF space. As CPP decreases, the wall tension in reactive brain vessels decreases. This in turn increases transmission of the arterial pulse to ICP. Therefore, when cerebral vessels are normally reactive, a decrease in CPP should provoke an increase in ABP-to-ICP pulse transmission. If this relationship is disturbed, the cerebral vessels are no longer pressure reactive.

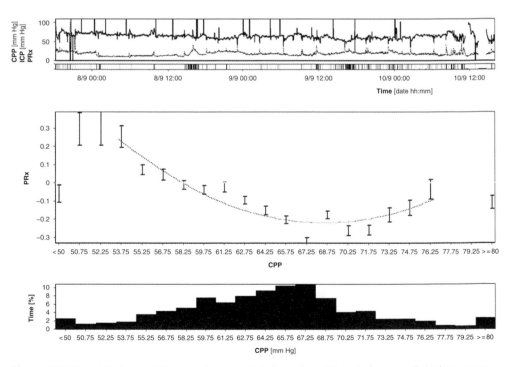

Figure 45.3 PRx, plotted against CPP over a longer period of time (here: 2.5 days), shows usually U-shape curve- medium panel. Minimum point of this curve indicates "optimal CPP" in this period. If this minimum overlaps maximum of CPP histogram (lower panel), it indicates that on average management of CPP in a given period was correct.

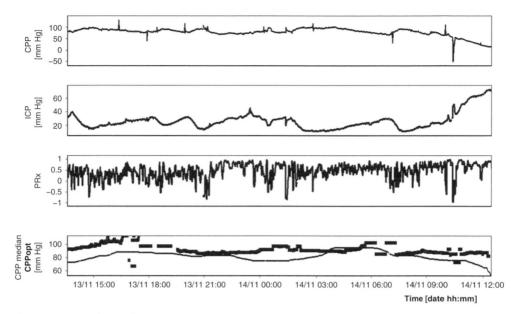

Figure 45.4 Calculation of optimal CPP may be shortened to a 4 hours moving window. Current value may be displayed on bedside computer screen and compared with current (median) CPP value. Displayed is a monitoring trace of a patient who developed high ICP and subsequently died. Periods when median CPP is far below optimal CPP can be observed, particularly at the end phase of monitoring.

A moving linear correlation coefficient between mean ICP and ICP pulse amplitude values (termed the RAP index: R, symbol of correlation; A, amplitude; P, pressure) calculated over a 3–5-minute time window is used for continuous detection of the amplitude-pressure relationship. The advantage is that the coefficient has a normalized value from −1 to +1 and thus allows comparison between patients. In a pooled analysis of patients with head injury, the value of RAP was close to +1. This is expected in head-injured patients with moderately raised ICP (>15 mmHg) and CPP (>50 mmHg) and indicates decreased compensatory reserve with preserved cerebrovascular reactivity. A decrease in RAP to 0 or negative values, found with very high ICP and very low CPP, indicates loss of cerebrovascular reactivity with a risk of brain ischemia and is also predictive of a poor outcome (Figure 45.5).

Is Intracranial Pressure Monitoring Useful?

ICP monitoring should be regarded as "more than a number". End-hour instant values of ICP from the bedside monitor are not an efficient method to manage intracranial hypertension. It has never been shown conclusively that monitoring ICP and using treatment protocols based on these monitored values improves outcome. As ICP monitoring is regarded as "standard of care" in most neuroscience units caring for acute brain injury patients, it would be unethical to conduct a prospective randomized control trial of management of patients with or without monitoring. However, there is evidence that there is an almost two-fold lower mortality in neurosurgical centers where ICP is usually monitored versus general intensive care units where it is not monitored.

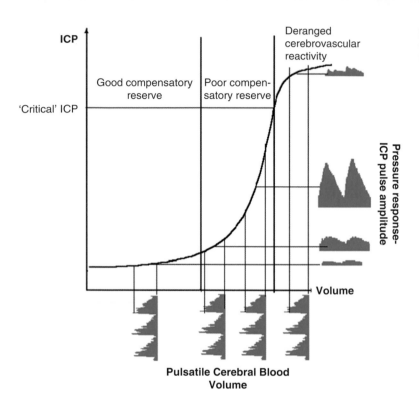

Figure 45.5 Pulse waveform analysis of intracranial pressure.

The ICP waveform contains valuable information about the nature of cerebrospinal pathophysiology. Autoregulation of CBF and compliance of the CSF system are both expressed in ICP. Methods of waveform analysis are useful both to derive this information and to guide the management of patients.

The value of ICP in acute states such as head injury, poor-grade SAH, and intracerebral hematoma depends on a close link between monitoring and therapy. Interventions to manage acute brain injury cannot be conducted correctly without inspection of the trend of ICP and, preferably, by information derived from its waveform.

Further Reading

Aries, M.J., Czosnyka, M., Budohoski, K.P., et al: Continuous determination of optimal cerebral perfusion pressure in traumatic brain injury. *Crit Care Med* 2012 August; **40**(8):2456–2463.

Castellani, G., Zweifel, C., Kim, D.J., et al: Plateau waves in head injured patients requiring neurocritical care. *Neurocrit Care* 2009; **11**:143–150.

Czosnyka, M., Guazzo, E., Whitehouse, M., et al: Significance of intracranial pressure waveform analysis after head injury. *Acta Neurochir (Wien)* 1996; **138**(5):531–541.

Czosnyka, M., Smielewski, P., Kirkpatrick, P., et al: Continuous assessment of the cerebral vasomotor reactivity in head injury. *Neurosurgery* 1997 July; **41**(1):11–17.

Dias, C., Maia, I., Cerejo, A., et al: Pressures, flow, and brain oxygenation during plateau waves of intracranial pressure. *Neurocrit Care* 2014 August; **21**(1):124–132.

Donnelly, J., Czosnyka, M., Harland, S., et al: Cerebral haemodynamics during experimental intracranial hypertension. *J Cereb Blood Flow Metab* 2016 March 18.

Koskinen, L.O., Grayson, D., Olivecrona, M.: The complications and the position of the Codman MicroSensor™ ICP device: An analysis of 549 patients and 650 sensors. *Acta Neurochir (Wien)* 2013 November; **155**(11):2141–2148.

Lazaridis, C., DeSantis, S.M., Smielewski, P., et al: Patient-specific thresholds of intracranial pressure in severe traumatic brain injury. *J Neurosurg* 2014 April; **120**(4):893–900.

Lu, C.W., Czosnyka, M., Shieh, J.S., Smielewska, A., Pickard, J.D., Smielewski, P.: Complexity of intracranial pressure correlates with outcome after traumatic brain injury. *Brain* 2012 August; **135**(Pt 8):2399–2408.

Robba, C., Bacigaluppi, S., Cardim, D., et al: Non-invasive assessment of intracranial pressure. *Acta* 2015 October 30. Review.

Vik, A., Nag, T., Fredriksli, O.A., et al: Relationship of "dose" of intracranial hypertension to outcome in severe traumatic brain injury. *J Neurosurg* 2008 October; **109**(4):678–684.

Zweifel, C., Castellani, G., Czosnyka, M., et al: Noninvasive monitoring of cerebrovascular reactivity with near infrared spectroscopy in head-injured patients. *J Neurotrauma* 2010 November; **27**(11):1951–1958.

Chapter 46

Jugular Venous Oximetry

Arun Gupta

Key Points

- $SjvO_2$ is a global measure of the balance of cerebral blood flow and metabolism.
- The insertion technique and complications for the placement of a $SjvO_2$ monitor are similar to those of an internal jugular central venous catheter.
- Measurement can be either intermittent or continuous.
- $SjvO_2$ is particularly useful in monitoring interventions such as hyperventilation therapy.
- Lack of sensitivity to regional changes in cerebral metabolism is a major limitation.

Abbreviations

$AVDO_2$	Arterio-jugular venous difference of the oxygen content
$CMRO_2$	Cerebral metabolic requirement for oxygen
CBF	Cerebral blood flow
ICP	Intracranial pressure
IJV	Internal jugular vein
$SjvO_2$	Jugular venous oxygen saturation

Contents

- Introduction
- Anatomy
- Insertion Technique
- Choice of Internal Jugular Vein
- Intermittent Monitoring
- Continuous Monitoring
- Rationale of Measuring
    - Management of Patients in Neurocritical Care
    - Monitoring Adequacy of Cerebral Blood Flow
    - Guiding Therapy
    - Intraoperative Monitoring
- Complications and Limitations
- Further Reading

Introduction

Jugular venous oximetry is a bedside method for measuring the saturation of cerebral venous blood. The procedure involves insertion of a jugular venous bulb catheter, percutaneous sampling allowing analysis of cerebral venous blood, and continuous measurement of cerebral venous oxygen saturation with the use of fiberoptic catheters. This technique can give an estimation of global cerebral oxygenation and metabolism which can be employed as part of routine multimodal monitoring in neurocritical care.

Anatomy

Deoxygenated blood from the brain is collected by the major cranial venous sinuses. The majority of this blood then drains into the left or right sigmoid sinuses. These follow a curved path in the posterior fossa passing caudally and forwards to form the IJV in the posterior jugular foramen on each side.

The venous outflow from left and right hemispheres is mixed with approximately 30% of the IJV blood arising from the contralateral side. In most cases, one side (usually the right) is dominant although subcortical areas tend to drain preferentially to the left. A percentage of the blood is extracranial in origin from anatomically variable emissary veins and the cavernous sinus.

At its origin in the posterior part of the jugular foramen, the IJV is dilated and known as the (superior) jugular bulb. Several veins carrying extracerebral blood, of which the facial vein is the most significant, empty into the IJV a few centimeters below. From its origin, the vein runs down the neck within the carotid sheath, lateral to the vagus nerve and carotid artery, where it can be conveniently cannulated. Caudally it dilates again forming the inferior jugular bulb before joining the subclavian vein to become the brachiocephalic vein behind the medial clavicle at the thoracic inlet.

The vein is related anterolaterally to the superficial cervical fascia, platysma, deep cervical fascia, and sternomastoid muscle. The transverse processes of the cervical vertebrae, cervical plexus, phrenic nerve, and (on the left) thoracic duct lie posterior to the vein. A bicuspid valve is typically found just above the inferior bulb, the central venous system cephalad being valveless.

Insertion Technique

Using a Seldinger technique, a catheter is inserted and advanced cephalad into the internal jugular vein beyond the inlet of the common facial vein to lie in the jugular bulb at the base of the skull (Figure 46.1). The site is selected, prepared, and infiltrated with local anesthetic using a strict aseptic technique, as for conventional central venous cannulation. Ultrasound visualization, which has been demonstrated to reduce complications in central venous access, may be particularly helpful in avoiding the need for significant head-down tilt which may otherwise have deleterious effects on ICP. Correct placement is confirmed when the catheter tip is level with the mastoid air cells on the lateral neck radiograph (level with the bodies of C1/C2).

Choice of Internal Jugular Vein

As described above, there is often a dominant side of venous drainage, and this can be determined by sequential manual compression of the IJV on each side. The side with the

---

BOX 46.1 Factors Affecting Jugular Venous Oxygen Saturation

Decrease in $SjvO_2$

Decrease in Oxygen Delivery	Increase in Oxygen Consumption
Increase in intracranial pressure, decrease in cerebral perfusion pressure	Increased metabolism
Excessive hypocapnia	Hyperthermia
Vasospasm	Pain
Hypotension	Light plane of anesthesia
Hypoxia	Seizures
Cardio-respiratory insufficiency	
Anemia	
Hemorrhage	
Hemoglobin abnormalities	
Sepsis	

Increase in $SjvO_2$

Increase in Oxygen Delivery	Decrease in Oxygen Consumption
Decrease in intracranial pressure, increase in cerebral perfusion pressure	Coma
Hypercapnia	Hypothermia
Drug-induced vasodilation	Sedative drugs
Arterial hypertension	Cerebral infarction
Arteriovenous malformation	Brain death
Increase in PaO_2	

---

largest rise in ICP is the dominant side and should be cannulated. If the dominant side is not easily detected, the side of the brain with the most pathology is used. In many centers, it is still common practice to cannulate the right side which is often the dominant internal jugular vein.

Intermittent Monitoring

Jugular venous oxygenation can be measured intermittently by serial blood sampling or continuously by fiberoptic oximetry. Intermittent sampling has the advantage of low cost and additionally allows $AVDO_2$, and the arteriovenous glucose and lactate difference to be measured by oximetry, co-oximetry, and blood biochemical analysis. Since venous flow velocities are low, it is essential to draw the sample slowly (<2 ml/min) to avoid contamination with extracranial blood.

Continuous Monitoring

Continuous monitoring of $SjvO_2$ can be performed with spectrophotometric catheters that employ either two or three wavelengths of light. Those with two wavelengths, need to be calibrated against a sample of the patient's own blood whereas catheters using three wavelengths have in-built calibration, thus allowing continuous monitoring. Both types of catheter are double lumen. One lumen contains transmit and receive optical fibers which measure $SjvO_2$ optically. The other lumen is available for blood sampling and may be continuously flushed with saline at 2–4 ml/h to maintain patency. The spectrophotometric determination of $SjvO_2$ relies on the different absorption properties of oxygenated and deoxygenated hemoglobin in the red and near infrared range.

Rationale of Measuring

Measurement of $SjvO_2$ can determine adequacy of the balance between global CBF and cerebral metabolic demands. Under physiological conditions, $CMRO_2$ and CBF are coupled such that the ratio of these two parameters remains constant. The difference between the cerebral arterial and mixed venous (i.e., internal jugular) oxygen content (C [a–v] O_2) represents the oxygen extraction. $CMRO_2$ can be calculated using the equation:

$$CMRO_2 = CBF \times C(a-v)O_2.$$

Assuming hemoglobin concentration is the same in arterial and venous blood and the amount of dissolved oxygen is minimal, arterio-venous oxygen content difference can be substituted for arterio-venous oxygen saturation difference i.e.

$$CMRO_2 = CBF \times \left(SaO_2 - SjvO_2\right)$$

Thus, a low $SjvO_2$ (i.e., a high oxygen extraction ratio) may indicate low CBF in relation to $CMRO_2$, as $SjvO_2$ is proportional to CBF/$CMRO_2$. While the normal $SjvO_2$ is 60%–70%, changes in trends of measured $SjvO_2$ can reveal useful information about adequacy of CBF. An increase in $AVDO_2$ greater than 9 ml/dl has been shown to provide a useful marker of inadequate CBF or an increased oxygen extraction by the brain. A variety of physiological and pathological conditions can alter the relationship between brain oxygen demand (as indicated by $CMRO_2$) and supply (i.e., CBF) thereby affecting $SjvO_2$ (Box 46.1).

In addition to measuring venous oxygen saturation, jugular bulb catheters allow estimation of substances such as lactate and glucose by intermittent sampling, thereby giving further information of the metabolic wellbeing of the brain.

Management of Patients in Neurocritical Care

$SjvO_2$ has many potentially useful applications in the management of patients in neurocritical care.

Monitoring Adequacy of Cerebral Blood Flow

$SjvO_2$ monitoring allows detection of episodes of desaturation associated with raised ICP and hyperventilation therapy. Episodes of jugular venous desaturation ($SjvO_2 < 50\%$) have been reported in patients with severe head injury generally caused by intracranial hypertension and systemic causes such as hypoxia, hypotension, and pyrexia. These indicate hypoperfusion states. Conversely, values of $SjvO_2$ greater than 85% suggest a state of hyperemia (e.g., secondary to hypercapnia), or failing oxygen utilization due to either a state of cellular dysoxia or shunting of arterial blood. Both hypo and hyperperfusion states can be associated with a poor outcome.

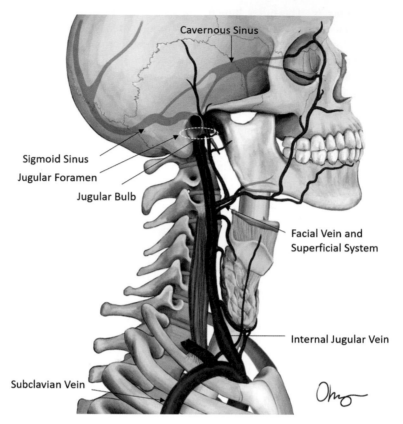

Figure 46.1 Placement of the jugular bulb catheter in the internal jugular vein. Note the tip of the sensor should be above the common facial vein.

Hyperventilation therapy for reduction of ICP in patients with acute intracranial hypertension can be associated with significant reduction in CBF as an acute fall in $PaCO_2$ can cause profound vasoconstriction. Assuming a constant brain metabolism, this will lead to reduction in global brain oxygenation. $SjvO_2$ monitoring is therefore useful in optimizing the use of hyperventilation. $SjvO_2$ should be kept above 55% if hyperventilation is indicated. There are also benefits in measuring $SjvO_2$ to assess cerebral hypoperfusion during the perioperative management of patients with subarachnoid hemorrhage.

Guiding Therapy

The use of $SjvO_2$ monitoring to guide hyperventilation therapy is common place. Barbiturate-induced cerebral metabolic suppression in patients with severe brain injury can be guided by $SjvO_2$ monitoring. Global cerebral oxygenation can be evaluated using $SjvO_2$ before and after intravenous administration of pentobarbital for the management of refractory intracranial hypertension in comatose patients with traumatic brain swelling.

Outcomes are significantly better in patients whose SjvO$_2$ remains above 45% compared to those in whom it drops to below this value.

Intraoperative Monitoring

Cerebral oxygenation has been studied by jugular bulb cannulation during aneurysm clipping surgery. It was demonstrated that many patients exhibit a critical threshold for MAP below which SjvO$_2$ falls. This was a more common finding in patients in which aneurysm rupture had occurred acutely suggesting a state of altered autoregulation.

Complications and Limitations

There are a few potential complications associated with insertion of the SjvO$_2$ catheter (carotid artery puncture, thrombosis, and raised ICP) but these are rare. Inaccuracies in SjvO$_2$ can occur for several reasons. For example, there may be no blood draining from an infarcted area of the brain, resulting in a normal SjvO$_2$ value. Serial sampling gives a "snapshot" of the state of cerebral oxygenation and metabolism at the time of sampling. Samples may be contaminated by factors such as extracranial venous blood, catheter placement which is too low or against the petrosal veins, or if blood sampling is too rapid. These can be avoided if blood is sampled at a site within 2 cm of the jugular bulb and at a rate of <2 ml/min. Continuous SjvO$_2$ monitoring, however, also has some limitations. The continuous fiberoptic catheters may give inaccurate readings if impacted against the vessel wall, if a thrombosis develops on the catheter tip, or if the sensor is curled within the vessel. Up to half of measured desaturations below 50% might be false positives.

The main limitation of this form of monitoring is that it represents a global measure of cerebral oxygenation while a regional change may not be detected unless it is of sufficient magnitude to affect overall brain saturation. Evidence from Positron Emission Tomography studies have shown significant volumes of brain below an ischemic CBF threshold even when SjvO$_2$ is above 55%. Clinicians will need to be mindful of the global nature of SjvO$_2$ monitoring and may need to employ other monitors that can detect focal or regional changes in oxygenation to help manage the clinical situation.

Further Reading

Coles, J.P., Minhas, P.S., Fryer, T.D., et al: Effect of hyperventilation on cerebral blood flow in traumatic head injury: Clinical relevance and monitoring correlates. *Crit Care Med* 2002;**30**:1950–1959.

Croughwell, N.D., White, W.D., Smith, L.R., et al: Jugular bulb saturation and mixed venous saturation during cardiopulmonary bypass. *J Card Surg* 1995;**10**:503–508.

Dearden, N.M., Midgley, S.: Technical considerations in continuous jugular venous oxygen saturation measurement. *Acta Neurochir* 1993; **59**(Suppl):91–97.

Feldman, Z., Robertson, C.S.: Monitoring of cerebral hemodynamics with jugular bulb catheters. *Crit Care Clin* 1997; **13**:51–77.

Gupta, A.K., Bullock, M.R.: Monitoring the injured brain in the intensive care unit: Present and future. *Hosp Med* 1998; **59**:704–713.

Obrist, W.D., Langfitt, T.W., Jaggi, J.L., Cruz, J., Gennarelli, T.A.: Cerebral blood flow and metabolism in comatose patients with acute head injury: Relationship to intracranial hypertension. *J Neurosurg* 1984;**61**:245–253.

Robertson, C.S., Narayan, R.K., Gokaslan, Z., et al: Cerebral arteriovenous oxygen difference as an estimate of cerebral blood flow in comatose patients. *J Neurosurg* 1989;**70**:222–230.

Robertson, C.S., Gopinath, S.P., Goodman, J.C., et al: SjvO$_2$ monitoring in head injured patients. *J Neurotrauma* 1995;**1**:891–896.

Sheinberg, M., Kanter, M.J., Robertson, C.S, et al: Continuous monitoring of jugular venous oxygen saturation in head injured patients. *J Neurosurg* 1992; **76**(2):212–217.

Chapter 47

Cerebral Oxygenation

Lingzhong Meng and Shaun E. Gruenbaum

Key Points

- Both cerebral tissue oxygenation saturation ($SctO_2$) and brain tissue oxygen tension ($PbtO_2$) monitor cerebral oxygenation, i.e., the balance between cerebral tissue oxygen consumption and supply. The technologies used in both these monitoring modalities are different. $SctO_2$ monitoring is non-invasive whereas $PbtO_2$ is intraparenchymal and invasive.
- Cerebral oxygenation is a physiological parameter that is characterized by versatility (functionally active), vulnerability (easily deranged), and virulence (adversely consequential if jeopardized).
- $PbtO_2$ and $SctO_2$-guided interventions are available and useful in treating cerebral hypoxia, but necessitates an appropriate differential diagnosis.
- The contribution of cerebral oxygen monitoring technology to improving outcomes in neuroanesthesia and intensive care requires further prospective evaluation.

Abbreviations

CBF   Cerebral blood flow
CPP   Cerebral perfusion pressure
$CMRO_2$ Cerebral metabolic rate of oxygen
FiO_2 Inspired oxygen fraction
NIRS   Near-infrared spectroscopy
$PbtO_2$ Brain tissue oxygen tension
$SctO_2$ Cerebral tissue oxygen saturation

Contents

   – Altering Cerebral Blood Flow
- Cerebral Perfusion Pressure Augmentation
- Manipulation of Arterial Carbon Dioxide Tension
- Increasing Arterial Blood Oxygen Content
- Clinical Considerations
- Patient Outcome and Cerebral Oxygenation Monitoring
- Further Reading

Learning Objectives

1. Define cerebral oxygenation and explain the technologies used for cerebral oxygenation monitoring.
2. Describe the physiological characteristics that are examined by cerebral oxygenation monitoring.
3. Discuss the clinical care guided by cerebral oxygenation monitoring.
4. Discuss the patient outcomes associated with cerebral oxygenation monitoring – guided care.

Introduction

Cerebral oxygenation is the balance between the rates of cerebral tissue oxygen consumption and supply. Inadequate cerebral oxygen supply relative to the $CMRO_2$ results in cerebral hypoxia. $SctO_2$ and $PbtO_2$ monitoring are two modalities that are currently used to monitor cerebral oxygenation in clinical care.

Cerebral Oxygenation Monitoring

Cerebral Tissue Oxygen Saturation

$SctO_2$ can be measured using cerebral oximetry based on NIRS. $SctO_2$ monitoring utilizes two adhesive probes that are typically placed on the left and right upper forehead, which is non-invasive, continuous, and portable.

There are some similarities between the working mechanisms used by cerebral oximetry and pulse oximetry. Near-infrared light with a wavelength between 700 and 1000 nm can penetrate into tissue over a distance of a few centimeters. A typical cerebral oximeter has an emitter that sends light into the tissue and a detector that receives it coming from the tissue by chance (Figure 47.1A). The majority of the light is lost in the tissue due to either absorption or scattering in multiple directions. The emitted light that returns to the detector travels from the emitter to the detector with a "banana-shaped" trajectory. Nonetheless, based on the difference of the light intensities between the emitter and detector, a determination of the quantity of light absorbed into the brain can be calculated.

The technology of continuous wave NIRS does not differentiate light absorption and scattering well, while technologies based on frequency domain or time domain do. All technologies use at least two different wavelengths of light to determine the tissue concentration of oxyhemoglobin and deoxyhemoglobin, respectively, based on the differential absorbers. $SctO_2$ is calculated as the percentage of oxyhemoglobin relative to the total hemoglobin, or the sum of oxyhemoglobin and deoxyhemoglobin.

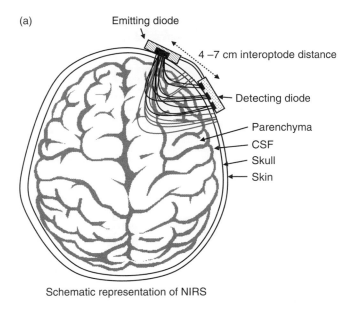

(a) Emitting diode

4 –7 cm interoptode distance

Detecting diode

Parenchyma

CSF

Skull

Skin

Schematic representation of NIRS

(b) 795 mV polarization

e⁻

0.8 mm

Figure 47.1 The working mechanism of SctO₂ monitoring (A) and PbtO₂ monitoring (B).

47.1(A) In SctO₂ monitoring, the photons that penetrate into tissue fly through a zigzag pathway due to scattering (deflected but non-absorbed). The photon disappears if it is absorbed by an absorber such as oxyhemoglobin, deoxyhemoglobin, or other absorbers. Some of the photons are able to escape the absorption, exiting out of the head, and are lost in the environment. Some of the photons are lost in the extracranial tissue. Only a small portion of the emitted photons are collected by the detector of the oximetry probe.

47.1(B) In PbtO2 monitoring, the dissolved oxygen molecules diffuse through the semi-permeable membrane that encases the Clark cell. The oxygen reduction on the surface of the gold polarographic cathode generates a current flow with the magnitude of the flow determined by the oxygen partial pressure or conventration.

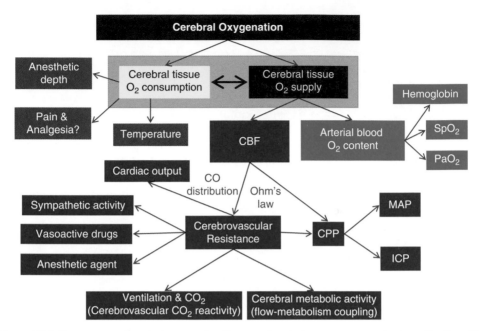

Figure 47.2 Determinants of cerebral oxygenation. The rate of cerebral oxygen consumption is readily affected by anesthesia, hypothermia, and disease processes such as traumatic brain injury (TBI). Cerebral oxygen supply is jointly determined by CBF and arterial blood oxygen content. CBF is robustly regulated by multiple yet integrated factors including cerebral metabolic activity, cerebral perfusion pressure, cardiac output, and carbon dioxide, to name a few. Arterial blood oxygen content is primarily determined by hemoglobin concentration and oxygen saturation, which can be readily deranged by anemia or hypoxemia. Lastly, it is well known that the brain requires a continuous supply of oxygen, and cerebral hypoxia is associated with poor outcomes depending on the severity and duration of the derangement.
CBF, cerebral blood flow; CPP, cerebral perfusion pressure; CO_2, carbon dioxide; SpO_2, pulse oximetry oxygen saturation; PaO_2, arterial blood oxygen partial pressure.

One of the major differences between cerebral oximetry and pulse oximetry is that cerebral oximetry measures the hemoglobin oxygen saturation of mixed arterial, capillary and venous blood in the brain tissue illuminated by the light; while pulse oximetry targets arterial blood only. The value of $SctO_2$ is closer to the hemoglobin oxygen saturation of venous blood than arterial blood because the majority of cerebral blood volume is contributed by capillary and venous blood.

NIRS-based cerebral oximetry has limitations one of which is the "contamination" by the extra-cranial tissue, especially the blood in the scalp, which unavoidably sits over the light pathway. In order to minimize the contamination, modern technology typically adds a detector that is much closer to the emitter in addition to the detector that is farther. The closer detector targets the superficial tissue (i.e., the scalp) while the farther one samples the deeper tissue (i.e., the brain). An algorithm can be developed to minimize the measurement imprecision caused by the extracranial tissue. Another limitation is that cerebral oximetry has poor spatial differentiation even though it has great temporal resolution. When it is applied on the forehead, it monitors a region of the frontal lobe that is jointly perfused by the anterior and middle cerebral arteries (i.e., the watershed zone). Therefore, it can be difficult to tell which artery is the source of a flow-related decrease in $SctO_2$.

Brain Tissue Oxygen Tension

In contrast to $SctO_2$ monitoring, which measures hemoglobin oxygen saturation in cerebral blood, $PbtO_2$ monitoring measures oxygen partial pressure in brain tissue. The flux of oxygen through the extracellular compartment arises from a concentration gradient which is maintained by a balance between supply at the capillaries and consumption within the cells. The oxygen sensor is normally inserted into the frontal white matter via a burr hole or under direct vision during surgery. The monitor employs a closed polarographic (Clark-type) cell containing a gold polarographic cathode and a silver polarographic anode, encased by a semi-permeable membrane (Figure 47.1B). The diffusion of the dissolved oxygen into the Clark cell via the semi-permeable membrane leads to oxygen reduction on the platinum surface and a current flow in proportion to the dissolved oxygen tension. Temperature compensation is achieved in the most recent generation of devices by means of an integral sensor which also allows the instrument to display brain temperature. The device does not require calibration but results may be unreliable for the first two hours after insertion as a result of microtrauma in the region immediately adjacent to the surface of the sensor. $PbtO_2$ monitoring is invasive and carries the potential risk of causing cerebral hemorrhage and infection.

Monitored Cerebral Oxygenation Parameters

The wellbeing of the brain is dependent on adequate cerebral oxygenation which reflects the balance between cerebral oxygen consumption and supply. In the perioperative and intensive care settings, a valuable monitor should target a physiological variable that is versatile (robust and dynamic), vulnerable (easily deranged), and virulent (adversely consequential if deranged); the so-called "VVV" attributes. Cerebral oxygenation is one such variable that encompasses these three attributes and can be monitored by both $SctO_2$ and $PbtO_2$ in a specific brain region. Thus care guided by these monitors may lead to improved outcomes.

Clinical Interventions Guided by Cerebral Oxygenation Monitoring

A monitor benefits a patient only when effective interventions guided by the monitoring are available to restore the deranged physiology. Currently, $SctO_2$ monitoring is normally used in high-risk surgical patients or during cardiac or other major surgery; while $PbtO_2$ monitoring is normally used in patients with traumatic brain injury.

A normal $SctO_2$ ranges from 60% to 80% in a healthy and neurologically intact human. However, there are large variations between individuals and even for the same individual, there are variations between different monitoring locations. It is thus prudent to make a clinical decision based on the trend of change in $SctO_2$ monitored at the same location. There is currently no consensus on the threshold for intervention for a compromised cerebral oxygenation. Some practitioners use a 20% decrease from the baseline value while more liberal and conservative thresholds are also used.

In contrast, the intervention based on $PbtO_2$ monitoring relies on the absolute (not relative) value. $PbtO_2$ values in normal brain tissue value ranges from 20 to 35 mmHg. Although prospective data of threshold values is limited, it is accepted by most practitioners that a $PbtO_2$ of 15–20 mmHg can be used as the threshold for intervention.

Decreasing Cerebral Metabolic Rate of Oxygen

The practice of decreasing $CMRO_2$ via hypothermia or increasing anesthetic depth is logical. However, its effectiveness relies on the functional integrity of the mechanism of cerebral metabolism-flow coupling. If the mechanism is intact, a decrement of consumption will lead to a corresponding decrement of supply. The ratio between cerebral oxygen consumption and supply is subsequently maintained, which is perceived as an ineffective treatment of cerebral hypoxia. The coupling mechanism is maintained during propofol anesthesia, volatile anesthesia, and hypothermic cardiopulmonary bypass. Therefore, the $CMRO_2$-suppressing strategy is normally ineffective in treating compromised cerebral oxygenation monitored using $SctO_2$ because $SctO_2$ is the monitoring modality used in neurologically intact patients during major surgery. In contrast, in patients with severe head injury, interventions based on $CMRO_2$-suppressing strategies have a higher probability of being effective in treating cerebral hypoxia based on $PbtO_2$ monitoring. This is likely due to the fact that the cerebral metabolism-flow coupling mechanism is frequently impaired in patients with traumatic brain injury.

Altering Cerebral Blood Flow

Cerebral Perfusion Pressure Augmentation

When cerebral autoregulation, is intact, CBF is maintained within a CPP range (normally quoted as 50–150 mmHg). In a patient with impaired cerebral autoregulation, an increase in CPP will lead to an increase in CBF and a corresponding increase of cerebral oxygenation, even if the CPP is within the autoregulatory range. If $PbtO_2$ is below 20 mmHg or $SctO_2$ is trending downwards, a possible intervention to improve these parameters is to increase CPP either by fluid resuscitation or vasoconstrictor therapy.

Manipulation of Arterial Carbon Dioxide Tension

Carbon dioxide is a powerful modulator of cerebral vasomotor tone. Impaired cerebral tissue oxygenation may be improved by increasing arterial CO_2 thereby increasing CBF. However, it should be noted that the increase in cerebral blood volume consequent to a rise in arterial CO_2 may increase ICP in a swollen non-compliant brain. In patients where hyperventilation therapy (hypocapnia) is used in the management of intracranial hypertension, cerebral oxygenation monitoring can detect reductions in tissue oxygenation and can therefore be used to optimize ventilation strategy.

Increasing Arterial Blood Oxygen Content

Increasing FiO_2 and red blood cell transfusion can both improve cerebral oxygenation because hemoglobin and its oxygen saturation are the two major determinants of arterial blood oxygen content. The improvement of cerebral oxygenation via FiO_2 increment occurs in patients with normal arterial blood hemoglobin oxygen saturation ($SpO_2 \approx 100\%$). Therefore, it appears that the underlying mechanism may not simply reflect the addition of extra oxygen (dissolved in the blood and not bound to hemoglobin), but rather results from the diffusion of oxygen into cerebral tissue that is enhanced by oxygen partial pressure augmentation.

Clinical Considerations

It should be emphasized that the effective treatment of cerebral hypoxia necessitates an appropriate differential diagnosis. The same treatment may have differing therapeutic effects between $PbtO_2$- and $SctO_2$-guided care due to the different patient populations in which these monitors are typically used. Every intervention has both desirable and undesirable effects. The final decision should be made based on the risk-benefit ratio and ideally outcome-oriented evidence. The goal of monitor-guided care is to maintain the patient's physiological homeostasis and improve clinical outcomes, and not to chase a perceived "better" number on the monitor.

Patient Outcome and Cerebral Oxygenation Monitoring

At present, $SctO_2$ monitoring is primarily used during surgeries that pose a high risk of cerebral ischemia/hypoxia, e.g., cardiac surgery, carotid endarterectomy, major vascular surgery, and surgeries in sitting position. However, the application has also been expanded to other disciplines such as liver transplantation, thoracic surgery, certain neurological procedures, and cardiopulmonary resuscitation. In contrast, $PbtO_2$ monitoring is primarily used in the intensive care and not the perioperative care setting, due to its invasive nature. $PbtO_2$ is normally used in patients with severe intracranial pathologies such as TBI, ischemic stroke, and hemorrhage.

The fundamental question that should be asked about a clinical monitor is whether the monitor-guided care improves the clinical outcomes that matter most to patients. The available evidence pertaining to the effect of $PbtO_2$-guided care on outcomes is primarily based on retrospective studies conducted in patients with TBI. These studies have various methodological limitations, as well as inconsistent conclusions. Therefore, a consistent statement on the outcome effect associated with $PbtO_2$-guided care cannot be made at this time. In contrast, most studies on the impact of $SctO_2$-guided care on outcome are randomized controlled trials, and primarily conducted in patients undergoing cardiac surgery. However, these studies also have various methodological limitations. While the use of NIRS may be useful in neurosurgical anesthesia, its use in neurointensive care is less certain.

Further Reading

Meng, L., Gelb, A.W.: Regulation of cerebral autoregulation by carbon dioxide. *Anesthesiology* 2015; **122**(1):196–205.

Meng, L., Hou, W., Chui, J., Han, R., Gelb, A.W.: Cardiac output and cerebral blood flow: The integrated regulation of brain perfusion in adult humans. *Anesthesiology* 2015; **123**(5):1198–1208.

Chapter

Microdialysis

Mathew Guilfoyle, Ivan Timofeev, and Peter Hutchinson

Key Points

- Microdialysis allows in vivo measurement of biochemical substances in extracellular fluid.
- The system consists of perfusion pump, catheter implanted in the tissue, microvials for dialysate collection, and analyzer.
- Recovery of the substances is a proportion of true extracellular concentration and depends on flow rate and catheter length.
- Glucose, lactate, and pyruvate are bedside markers of energy metabolism.
- Lactate/Pyruvate ratio is a sensitive marker of impaired aerobic metabolism.
- Glutamate and glycerol are additional markers of adverse tissue conditions.
- Trends, rather than individual values, provide useful clinical information.
- Catheter location in relation to injured tissue areas needs to be considered, when interpreting results.
- Microdialysis can be used to investigate secondary brain injury mediators in vivo, e.g., inflammatory cytokines.

Abbreviations

aSAH   Aneurysmal subarachnoid hemorrhage
ATP   Adenosine triphosphate
ECF   Extracellular fluid
LP   Lactate/Pyruvate
RR   Relative recovery
TBI   Traumatic brain injury

Contents

- Introduction
- Principles
- Recovery
- Common Microdialysis Markers
  - Glucose, Lactate, and Pyruvate

Introduction

Microdialysis is a monitoring method that allows measurement of extracellular chemistry in living tissue. For several decades, following its invention in the 1970s, it was used predominantly in laboratory research. Since the 1990s, microdialysis was introduced into clinical practice and is now used by many specialties. Monitoring cerebral tissue chemistry in neurointensive care remains one of its main applications.

Principles

Microdialysis catheters consist of concentric outer and inner polyurethane tubes with a semipermeable membrane at the distal end (Figure 48.1). A microinfusion pump perfuses the catheter with solution isotonic to normal ECF at a typical flow rate of 0.3 µl/min. As the perfusion fluid passes the semipermeable membrane molecules passively diffuse from the ECF driven by their concentration gradients. Membrane pore size defines the maximal molecular weight that can cross the membrane. Catheters commonly used in clinical practice have a membrane permeability which ranges from 20 to 100 kDa and are similarly effective for measuring small molecules and larger macromolecules such as proteins.

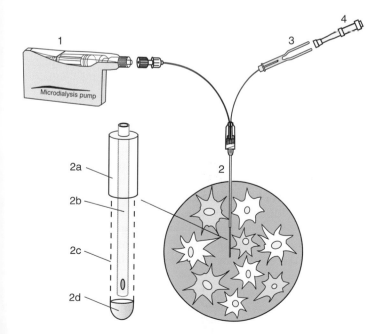

Figure 48.1 Microdialysis principle. (1) Precision pump. (2) Microdialysis catheter implanted in tissue. The catheter consists of outer (2a) and inner (2b) tubes and semipermeable membrane at the distal end (2c). Golden tip (2d) facilitates visualization on CT. (3) Microvial holder, with needle that on insertion of the vial penetrates its lid. (4) Microvial for collection of dialysate.

Perfusion fluid from the catheter (microdialysate) is collected in microvials and analyzed at regular intervals.

Key biochemical markers including glucose, lactate, pyruvate, glutamate, glycerol, and urea can be assayed immediately using bedside analyzers or the microdialysate can be stored for later analysis of other molecules of interest. Adding drugs or other substances to the perfusion fluid so that they diffuse into the extracellular space allows direct delivery into the brain, a technique known as retrodialysis.

Recovery

Constant exchange of perfusion fluid at the membrane helps to maintain a concentration gradient, but at the same time, prevents complete equilibration between ECF and perfusate. RR defines the concentration of the substance in the dialysate after it leaves the membrane area expressed as the percentage of its total ECF concentration. RR increases at lower perfusion flow rates due to the longer time available for diffusion and approaches 100% of ECF concentration as the flow rates tends to zero. Catheters with larger membrane areas provide higher recovery at the same flow rate due to increased area of diffusion. Unfortunately, the reduction in flow rates limits the amount of dialysate available for analysis, and increasing the length of membrane leads to difficulties with catheter implantation. It has been estimated that the standard catheters with membrane length of 10 mm at a flow rate of 0.3 μl/min provide RR of substance at 70% of tissue concentration. Other factors that may influence recovery include, charge of the molecule or the membrane, pH, temperature, pressure, and osmolarity of the ECF.

Common Microdialysis Markers

Clinical application of microdialysis as a monitoring modality is based on early detection of changes in tissue biochemistry which represent impending or ongoing tissue injury due to a variety of causes. In some situations, microdialysis can be the only modality to detect unfavorable tissue conditions at an early stage. The most commonly used bedside microdialysis markers include glucose, lactate, pyruvate, glutamate, and glycerol. Changes in these markers reflect the general pathophysiology of cellular injury and therefore can be applied to many organs. In cerebral tissue, they are predominantly used to detect ischemia, impaired mitochondrial function as well as excitotoxic and structural damage.

Glucose, Lactate, and Pyruvate

Adequate aerobic production of ATP in the brain relies on a constant supply of glucose and oxygen with preserved mitochondrial function (Figure 48.2). Under normal conditions, glucose is metabolized to pyruvate and lactate, and the former is used as substrate for the mitochondrial Krebs cycle. There is a relative balance among glucose, lactate, and pyruvate concentrations in ECF under baseline conditions. A cellular oxygen deficit caused by ischemia, hypoxemia, or impaired mitochondrial function due to injury or toxic effects, may lead to failure of oxidative phosphorylation despite preservation of glycolysis. In this situation, pyruvate is not used to the same extent by the mitochondria, but increasingly converted to lactate, leading to its accumulation. The ratio of lactate to pyruvate (LP ratio) reflects this changing balance and benefits from being independent of the absolute values. LP ratio has been proven to be a sensitive marker of impaired energy metabolism.

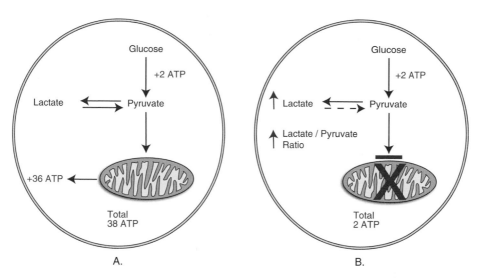

Figure 48.2 Simplified energy metabolism in the cell and microdialysis markers (1) adequate delivery of oxygen and mitochondrial function (2) ischemia or hypoxemia leading to reduced availability of tissue oxygen or impaired mitochondrial function.

A low cerebral extracellular glucose concentration can result from an increase in its consumption or a reduction in cerebral blood flow. Low extracellular glucose levels are associated with a poor outcome after TBI and are indicative of poor perfusion in aneurysmal aSAH. Lactate to glucose ratio can also serve as a marker of ischemia or increased glycolysis.

Glutamate

Cerebral extracellular glutamate levels increase in tissue ischemia and hypoxia and carry prognostic information. Glutamate is believed to play a role in secondary brain injury due to the phenomenon of excitotoxicity. This process may manifest as raised extracellular gluta-mate in the absence of ischemia even though the origin of extracellular glutamate is generally extrasynaptic.

Glycerol

One of the manifestations of cellular distress and injury is the degradation of its membrane which may be an early sign of necrotic or apoptotic cell death. An increase in metabolism of membrane phospholipids leads to a rise in ECF glycerol concentration, making it an important marker of brain injury. Although, the main source of cerebral glycerol is cellular membrane, systemic increases in glycerol, due to peripheral lipolysis or administration of glycerol containing drugs, may also affect cerebral levels.

Catheter Location

A cerebral microdialysis catheter monitors only a few cubic millimeters of brain tissue. Knowledge of the catheter location in relation to the pathological areas is important for the interpretation of the microdialysis data. The tip of a standard microdialysis catheter

Table 48.1 Values of Microdialysis Markers in Normal Brain and in Different Catheter Locations in Relation to Traumatic Contusions

Biochemical Marker	Normal Brain, Awake Patient	Microdialysis Catheter Located in the Minimally Injured Brain Contralateral to the Lesion in TBI.	Microdialysis Catheter Located in the Penumbra of the Lesion in TBI.
Glucose (mmol/l)	1.7±0.9	3.1±0.1	1.2±0.1
Pyruvate (mmol/l)	166±47	160±50	170±80
Lactate (µmol/l)	2.9±0.9	2.9±0.1	6.3±0.1
Lactate/Pyruvate Ratio	23±4	20±0.3	45±1
Glutamate (µmol/l)	16±16	17±1	63±2
Glycerol (µmol/l)	35±11	38±1	175±6

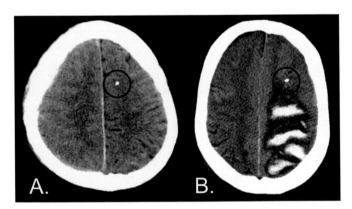

Figure 48.3 Catheter locations on CT. (1) Less injured brain (2) peri-contusional tissue.

contains gold and can be visualized on computed tomography (Figure 48.3). The values obtained with the catheter located in the diffusely injured brain correlate with the whole brain metabolism, whereas a catheter located in the vicinity of contusional or ischemic penumbrae, provides focal information on the state of this vulnerable tissue (Table 48.1). In many cases, concurrent use of two catheters in different locations is recommended for optimal biochemical monitoring. No catheter should be placed into necrotic tissue.

Clinical Applications

TBI and subarachnoid hemorrhage are the two most common conditions where cerebral microdialysis has been used. In TBI, its application along with other methods of multi-modality monitoring, allows early detection of ischemia, hypoxia, and seizures, all of which may lead to secondary injury (Figure 48.4). Microdialysis markers can be used to individualize cerebral perfusion pressure targets, evaluate the adequacy of tissue perfusion and oxygenation and assess physiological responses to therapy (e.g.,

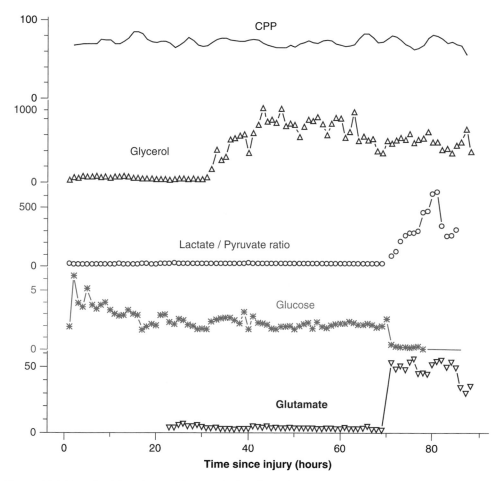

Figure 48.4 Example of clinical microdialysis trends. Significant elevation in extracellular glycerol concentration is seen on the second day after severe TBI, followed by other biochemical markers despite absence of significant changes in cerebral perfusion pressure. The patient did not survive.

hyperventilation, sedation, surgical interventions, etc.). In a large series of TBI patients, increased LP ratio has been shown to be an independent predictor of mortality and neurological outcome. In SAH, microdialysis offers the possibility of detecting ischemic damage before the development of clinical symptoms from delayed cerebral ischemia due to vasospasm.

Microdialysis is also used to monitor stroke (ischemic penumbra or malignant brain edema in areas of major vessel occlusion), intracranial hemorrhages, epilepsy, tumors, infections, and hepatic encephalopathy. Intraoperative use of microdialysis helps evaluate the safety of manipulations and duration of hypoperfusion (e.g., during temporary clipping in aneurysm surgery or anastomosis formation for cerebral bypass procedures).

Research Applications

Microdialysis remains a useful tool in basic and clinical science. Its main research applications include evaluation of pharmacokinetics and tissue bioavailability of pharmacological agents, exploring pathophysiology of tissue injury and developing and validating novel biochemical markers. The advent of high molecular weight cut-off catheters (~100 kDa) has extended the possibilities of investigating protein signaling pathways in vivo, in particular, inflammatory mediators such as cytokines and chemokines, which have important roles in secondary injury following TBI. Microdialysis plays an important role in translational research, helping to test pre-clinical research findings in a clinical setting. In bedside research, microdialysis markers can be used as surrogate endpoints to evaluate the physiological benefits of therapeutic interventions in early phase studies.

Limitations

Microdialysis provides retrospective measurement of biochemical markers which depends on the rate of vial change and therefore cannot be considered as a truly online technique. Many factors can affect recovery and tissue concentration of biochemical substances in vivo and analysis of the trends requires experience. The invasiveness of the procedure, in addition to dependence on trained and motivated personnel, limits its widespread use. Despite this, microdialysis provides a unique ability to monitor tissue biochemistry in vivo and, therefore, is likely to remain an integral part of multimodality monitoring.

Further Reading

Hutchinson, P.J., O'Connell, M.T., Al-Rawi, P. G., et al: Clinical cerebral microdialysis: A methodological study. *J Neurosurg* 2000; **93**(1):37–43.

Vespa, P., Bergsneider, M., Hattori, N., et al: Metabolic crisis without brain ischemia is common after traumatic brain injury: A combined microdialysis and positron emission tomography study. *J Cereb Blood Flow Metab* 2005; **25**(6):763–774.

Hlatky, R., Valadka, A.B., Goodman, J.C., et al: Patterns of energy substrates during ischemia measured in the brain by microdialysis. *J Neurotrauma* 2004; **21**(7):894–906.

Reinstrup, P., Stahl, N., Mellergard, P., et al: Intracerebral microdialysis in clinical practice: Baseline values for chemical markers during wakefulness, anesthesia, and neurosurgery. *Neurosurgery* 2000; **47**(3):701–709; discussion 709–710.

Engstrom, M., Polito, A., Reinstrup, P., et al: Intracerebral microdialysis in severe brain trauma: The importance of catheter location. *J Neurosurg* 2005; **102**(3):460–469.

Hutchinson, P.J., Jalloh, I., Helmy, A., et al: Consensus statement from the 2014 International Microdialysis Forum. *Intensive Care Med* 2015; **41**(9):1517–1528.

Timofeev, I., Carpenter, K.L., Nortje, J., et al: Cerebral extracellular chemistry and outcome following traumatic brain injury: A microdialysis study of 223 patients. *Brain* 2011; **134**:484–494.

Sarrafzadeh, A., Haux, D., Sakowitz, O., et al: Acute focal neurological deficits in aneurysmal subarachnoid hemorrhage: Relation of clinical course, CT findings, and metabolite abnormalities monitored with bedside microdialysis. *Stroke* 2003; **34**(6):1382–1388.

Shannon, R.J., Carpenter, K.L., Guilfoyle, M.R., et al: Cerebral microdialysis in clinical studies of drugs: Pharmacokinetic applications. *J Pharmacokinet Pharmacodyn* 2013; **40**(3):343–358.

Helmy, A., Carpenter, K.L., Menon, D.K., et al: The cytokine response to human traumatic brain injury: Temporal profiles and evidence for cerebral parenchymal production. *J Cereb Blood Flow Metab* 2011; **31**(2):658–670.

Electromyography and Evoked Potentials

Chapter 49

Jeremy A. Lieberman

Key Points

- Electromyography monitors cranial and peripheral nerve integrity.
- Electromyography is not affected by anesthetics, but muscle relaxants should be avoided.
- Evoked potentials use a stimulus to elicit a distant response. Changes in response may indicate injury along any part of the sensory neurological pathways.
- Evoked responses are adversely affected by anesthetics in the following order: Visual > Somatosensory/Motor > Brainstem Auditory.
- Volatile anesthetic agents suppress evoked potentials most and propofol less so; opiates, ketamine, and etomidate are minimally suppressive or neutral.
- Physiologic alterations such as hypotension, anemia, hypoxia, or hypothermia may affect evoked responses and result in inaccurate interpretation.

Abbreviations

BAEP   Brainstem Auditory Evoked Potentials
EMG   Electromyographic
MAC   Minimal Alveolar Concentration
MEP   Motor Evoked Potentials
SSEP   Somatosensory Evoked Potentials
VEP   Visual Evoked Potentials

Contents

Introduction

Electromyography and evoked potentials are monitors of neurological function that are used during many neurosurgical procedures (Table 49.1). These techniques can identify reversible changes in neurological function intraoperatively, thereby allowing intervention and possible prevention of injury. However, no randomized prospective trials have clearly demonstrated that such techniques improve outcome.

Table 49.1 Lesions for which EMG or Evoked Potential Monitoring Might Be Used

Sensory Evoked Potentials		
VEP	BAEP	SSEP
Pituitary or suprasellar lesions	Acoustic neuroma	Spinal deformity
Retro-orbital lesions	Vth nerve compression – Trigeminal neuralgia	Spinal cord tumors or vascular lesions
Lesions near occipital cortex	VIIth nerve compression – facial spasm	Lesions of the posterior fossa
Neurovascular lesions in the posterior circulation	Lesions in the posterior fossa	Lesions near the thalamus
	Lesions of the temporal or parietal cortex	Lesions of the parietal cortex
EMG and Motor Evoked Potentials		
EMG	Motor evoked potentials	
Acoustic neuroma	Spinal deformity	
Posterior fossa lesions	Intramedullary spinal cord tumors	
Cervical or lumbar spine defects	Cerebral tumors or vascular structures near motor cortex	

Electromyography

Electromyography allows continuous assessment of cranial and peripheral motor nerves by placing needle electrodes near specific muscles. If a nerve is touched or stretched during surgery, EMG activity will occur in the muscle that is innervated by that nerve. Mild nerve irritation leads to transient EMG discharges that resolve rapidly. More serious nerve irritation may produce sustained EMG discharges. Electrocautery and saline irrigation are major sources of interference.

Electromyography is used when trying to preserve the facial nerve (cranial nerve VII) during procedures involving the base of the skull, such as resection of acoustic neuromas. EMG activity may also be recorded from other motor cranial nerves, including nerves III, IV, VI, IX, X, XI, and XII.

EMG activity may be recorded from muscles of the upper and lower extremities and used to detect injury to the spinal cord and spinal nerve roots during spine surgery. Electrodes are placed in muscles most at risk from surgically induced neurological injury. In addition, vertebral pedicle screws may be electrically stimulated to determine whether they are wholly within the bony pedicle and vertebral body. If there is a breach into the spinal canal, EMG activity will occur with lower stimulation current.

Anesthetic Considerations

Anesthetic agents do not interfere with EMG responses. Muscle relaxants block the neuromuscular junction and should be avoided during periods of EMG recording.

Evoked Potentials

These techniques apply a stimulus to evoke a response. Sensory evoked potentials may be recorded after various types of sensory input: somatosensory (SSEP), visual (VEP), or auditory (brainstem auditory [BAEP]). Sensory evoked potential amplitudes are small relative to background EEG activity. Therefore, it is necessary to evoke many responses to permit "signal averaging", which filters out this background and yields a more distinct evoked potential waveform. MEPs involve stimulation of the motor cortex to elicit a response in the spinal cord, peripheral nerves, or muscles. All evoked potential responses are described in terms of latency (the time from the stimulus until the response) and amplitude (the size of the response) (Figure 49.1). Neurological injury may prolong latency and decrease amplitude.

Visual Evoked Potentials

VEPs monitor the visual pathway from the eye through the optic nerve to the visual cortex. The eyes are exposed to a series of bright lights while scalp electrodes record the VEPs. VEPs may be useful in assessing visual pathway integrity for surgery near the optic nerve and chiasm (e.g., pituitary resection). They may also help when resecting tumors in the occipital cortex or neurovascular lesions involving the posterior circulation. VEPs are technically difficult to obtain and are exquisitely sensitive to most anesthetic agents, so consistent responses are hard to obtain and interpret under general anesthesia. Thus, they are not commonly used in the operating room.

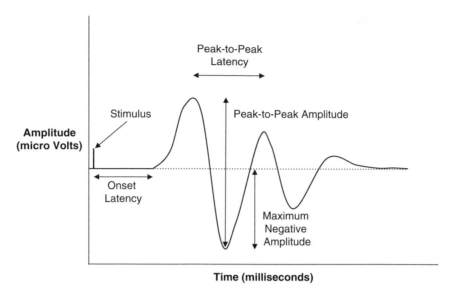

Figure 49.1 Example of an evoked potential response curve depicting latency and amplitude measurements. Note that "onset latency" is the time from the stimulus to the beginning of the response. "Peak-to-peak" or "interpeak" latency is the time between various amplitude peaks. Peak amplitude may be characterized as either the largest voltage deviation in one direction from baseline or as the maximum total voltage spread (maximum positive maximum negative amplitude).

Brainstem Auditory Evoked Potentials

BAEPs record the integrity of the auditory pathway, starting from the ear and including nervous system structures such as hair cells, spiral (cochlear) ganglion, cranial nerve VIII, cochlear nuclei, superior olivary complex, lateral lemniscus, inferior colliculus, and medial geniculate thalamic nuclei.

An auditory stimulus, a series of clicks in the ear, produces responses measured across electrodes placed over the scalp. Multiple signals are averaged (≈2000) to yield a series of six or seven positive waves, each given a Roman numeral designation (Figure 49.2). Each wave was originally believed to arise from a specific structure along the auditory pathway, but studies have shown that many waves originate from multiple structures. Thus, pathologic lesions or surgical trauma may affect several waves.

Interpretation

To elicit interpretable BAEPs, the patient must have adequate hearing function. With middle ear or cochlear deficits, no waves will be generated. Eighth nerve injury affects all waves after wave I. Cerebellar retraction often causes prolongation of interpeak latency between waves I and V. Transient changes are not predictive of hearing loss, but when complete loss of these later waves occurs, permanent auditory tract damage is more likely.

Typical Procedures

BAEPs are most commonly used during microvascular decompression of cranial nerves V or VII. BAEPs may help reduce hearing loss during resection of acoustic neuromas.

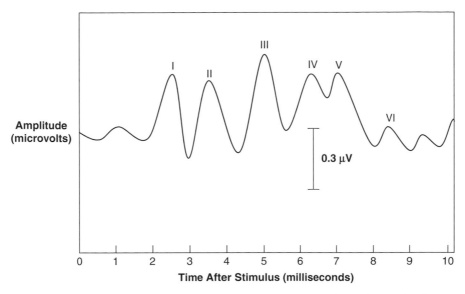

Figure 49.2 Brainstem auditory evoked potential tracing demonstrating multiple waveform peaks after an auditory stimulus. Loss of wave amplitude and prolongation of interpeak latency may suggest injury.

Auditory tract injury is due to brainstem compression, direct trauma to the eighth nerve, or ischemia of the nerve. BAEPs are less useful for posterior fossa tumors. They may miss focal brainstem injury because abnormal BAEPs might occur only with global brainstem damage.

Anesthetic Considerations

BAEPs are resistant to most anesthetics. Volatile inhalational agents are most suppressive, but the effects are minimal and signals are easily obtained with any regimen. Muscle relaxants have no effect on BAEPs.

Somatosensory Evoked Potentials

SSEPs monitor the integrity of sensory pathways, including peripheral nerves, the spinal cord, the brainstem, subcortical structures, and the sensory cortex. Disruption along any part of this pathway may disrupt normal SSEP responses. A repetitive electrical stimulus is applied to a peripheral nerve and responses are measured over the cerebral cortex with scalp electrodes. Subcortical responses may be recorded by placing electrodes near the upper cervical spine. A transcutaneous electrical stimulus is applied to a peripheral nerve, typically the median or ulnar nerve of the upper extremity or the posterior tibial nerve of the lower extremity. The main sensory pathways travel up the spinal cord in the dorsal columns. Some sensory tracts from the lower extremities travel along ventral and lateral pathways as well. The fibers cross at the brainstem and proceed up through the thalamus to the postcentral gyrus of the cortex. Scalp electrodes record the evoked potentials. SSEPs have small amplitude, and averaging of more than 1000 responses is needed to produce a clear signal.

Typical Procedures

SSEPs are commonly used during spine surgery when injury to the spinal cord may be due to ischemia secondary to spinal distraction and disruption of perforating radicular vessels. Direct trauma may occur during pedicle screw placement or other instrumentation or while resecting a pathological lesion that is proximate to the sensory tracts. SSEPs may be used to ensure adequate perfusion to the cortex during intracranial or extracranial vascular surgery (e.g., aneurysm, carotid endarterectomy).

Interpretation of Responses

SSEP responses elicited from posterior tibial nerve stimulation are mediated by cortex supplied by the anterior cerebral artery. In contrast, stimulation of the median nerve evokes responses in the cortex supplied by the middle cerebral artery. Changes in SSEPs may indicate inadequate blood flow. Loss or decrease of SSEP responses may be due to disruption of any component of the sensory pathway. A significant change is typically a 50% fall in amplitude or a 10% increase in latency, or both. Asymmetric changes are also suspicious.

Frequent causes of false-positive changes (i.e., changes but without resulting injury) include anesthetics, hypothermia, acute changes in $PaCO_2$, hypotension, hypovolemia, and anemia. Because SSEPs monitor the integrity of sensory tracts, isolated injury to motor tracts might be missed (i.e., a false-negative response).

Anesthetic Considerations

Cortical SSEPs are sensitive to anesthetic agents, and avoidance of rapid changes in anesthetic depth is warranted, especially at critical stages of the operation. Volatile agents and N_2O are the most suppressive agents (Table 49.2). It is difficult to obtain reliable SSEPs

Table 49.2 Relative Effects of Anesthetic Agents on Somatosensory and Motor Evoked Potentials

Agent	Cortical SSEPs		MEPs
	Latency	Amplitude	Amplitude
Volatile Agents*	↑↑↑	↓↓↓	↓↓↓
Nitrous Oxide	↑	↓↓	↓
Barbiturates*	↑↑	↓↓↓	↓↓
Propofol*	↑↑	↓↓	↓↓
Benzodiazepines	↑	↓	↓↓
Narcotics/opioids	+/-	+/-	+/-
Ketamine	↑	↑	+/-
Etomidate	↑	↑↑	↑
Muscle Relaxants*	0	0	↓↓↓

↑ = mild increase; ↑↑ = moderate increase; ↑↑↑ = significant increase
↓ = mild decrease; ↓↓ = moderate decrease; ↓↓↓ = significant decrease
=/-, minimal or no effect
* The degree of suppression is highly dose-dependent.

when giving more than 0.5 to 1 MAC of these agents. Intravenous anesthetics, such as propofol, are less suppressive. They are commonly used with opioids, which have minimal effects on SSEPs. Ketamine and etomidate do not depress SSEP responses. Muscle relaxants do not interfere with SSEP responses.

Motor Evoked Potentials

MEPs involve stimulation of the motor cortex to activate the motor pathways and elicit a movement response. For spine surgery, MEP, SSEP, and EMG monitoring has reduced the need for intraoperative wake-up tests. MEPs are also used to reduce motor deficits during cranial surgery near the motor cortex.

Magnetic stimulation of the motor cortex is less painful but difficult to use in the operating room. Electrical stimulation using electrodes placed into the scalp is preferred. A brief train of pulses directly depolarizes cortical motor neurons. This creates activity in the descending corticospinal tracts of the spinal cord. These signals summate at the ventral horn, synapse with alpha motor neurons, and the resulting compound motor action potential triggers muscle movement. Responses are usually recorded as muscle movement (myogenic MEPs). These responses are strong, and often cause patient movement.

Interpretation of Responses

A decrease in the amplitude of MEP responses suggests neurologic injury, as do acute increases in the threshold voltage needed to obtain an MEP response. Acute and asymmetric changes are more suggestive of true injury. Changes in the duration or complexity of the morphology of the myogenic response may also suggest motor damage.

Several physiologic factors depress MEP responses, including hypothermia, hypotension, and hypovolemia. MEP responses may be difficult to obtain from patients with pre-existing muscle weakness. In addition, young children require stronger stimuli to elicit MEP responses, probably because of lack of complete myelinization of immature motor pathways.

Anesthetic Considerations

Myogenic MEPs are highly susceptible to suppression by anesthetics (Table 49.2). Volatile inhalational agents are the most suppressive. Nitrous oxide appears to be less depressing than the MAC equivalent of volatile agents. Intravenous agents, such as propofol, are less suppressive but produce dose-dependent MEP amplitude reduction. Ketamine and etomidate are well tolerated, as are narcotics. Gradual decreases in MEP response amplitudes occur over time while under general anesthesia – a process described as "anesthetic fade". Muscle relaxants clearly weaken myogenic responses; they should not be used during critical parts of the operation. However, if required, partial neuromuscular blockade is compatible with MEP monitoring if a constant depth of blockade is carefully maintained.

Further Reading

Lall, R., Lall, R.R., Hauptman, J.S., et al: Intraoperative neurophysiological monitoring in spine surgery: Indications, efficacy, and role of the preoperative checklist. *Neurosurg Focus* 2012; **33**:1–10.

Lieberman, Feiner, J., Lyon, R., et al: Effect of hemorrhage and hypotension on transcranial motor-evoked potentials in swine. *Anesthesiology* 2013; **119**:1109–1119.

Lotto, M., Banoub, M., Schubert, A., et al: Effects of anesthetic agents and physiologic changes on intraoperative motor evoked potentials. *J Neurosurg Anesthesiol* 2004; **16**:32–42.

Lyon, Feiner, J., Lieberman, J.A., et al: Progressive suppression of motor evoked potentials during general anesthesia: The phenomenon of 'Anesthetic Fade'. *J Neurosurg Anesthesiol* 2005; **17**:13–19.

Rabai, F., Sessions, R., Seubert, C.N., et al: Neurophysiological monitoring and spinal cord integrity. *Best Pract Res Clin Anaesthesiol* 2016; **30**:53–68.

Shils, J., Sloan, T.: Intraoperative neuromonitoring. *Int Anesthesiol Clin* 2015; **53**:53–73.

Simon, M.: Neurophysiologic intraoperative monitoring of the vestibulocochlear nerve. *J Clin Neurophysiol* 2011; **28**:566–581.

Electroencephalography and Nervous System Function Monitoring

Oana Maties and Adrian Gelb

Key Points

- Neuron activity produces voltage differences between different places on the brain surface or scalp.
- The scalp EEG is a recording over time of the summation of the extracellular postsynaptic potentials generated mainly by the pyramidal neurons in the cerebral cortex.
- An electrocorticogram is obtained by placing electrodes on the surface of the cerebral cortex intraoperatively for recording.
- Intense, uncontrolled brain electrical activity that alters brain function is called a seizure.
- Intraoperative EcoG recordings help identify the origin of the seizures and their relationship to cortically mapped regions that control speech and motor activity.
- The unprocessed EEG and various forms of processed EEG have been used to monitor the depth of anesthesia.
- Different monitors exist to measure depth of anesthesia but to date there is no clear evidence of superiority of one over the others.

Abbreviations

AEP	Auditory evoked potential
BIS	Bispectral Index
CBF	Cerebral blood flow
CSA	Compressed spectral array
DSA	Density spectral array
EcoG	Electrocorticography
EEG	Electroencephalogram
Hz	Hertz
SEF	Spectral edge frequency

Contents

- Basic Features and Normal Patterns
- Effects of Anesthetic Drugs

- Processed Electroencephalogram – Concept and Devices
- Current Uses in Clinical Practice
  - Neurovascular Surgery
  - Seizure Focus Localization and Surgery
  - Monitoring Depth of Anesthesia
- Further Reading

Basic Features and Normal Patterns

The first human electroencephalogram (EEG) recordings were reported in 1929. The scalp EEG is a recording over time of the summation of the extracellular postsynaptic potentials generated mainly by the pyramidal neurons in the cerebral cortex. However, because of the complex connections between the cortical and subcortical structures, the EEG may reflect the state of all of these structures. The EEG signal is much smaller than the action potential recorded over nerves or muscles.

Surface EEG recordings can be made with scalp electrodes or with subdermal needle electrodes. In order to minimize impedance, electrodes can also be applied to the surface of the brain (EcoG) or they can be placed transcortically to record from selected deeper neuron groups (e.g., during surgery for Parkinson's disease).

An EEG consists in a set of tracings from specific electrodes at designated scalp locations, called a montage. The International 10–20 Electrode Placement Protocol represents a standardized montage of 20 scalp electrodes distributed symmetrically and systematically, based on the distances from the nasion to the inion and between the pretragal bony indentations associated with both temporomandibular joints. They therefore encompass all the cerebral regions (Frontal, Temporal, Parietal, and Occipital). Their locations are designated with letter-number combinations that reflect the distance from the midline and their left-right orientation, that is, left-sided electrodes have odd number while the right sided electrodes have even number subscripts. The numbers increase with the distance from the sagittal sinus. Midline electrodes are designated with a z subscript (Figure 50.1). A channel represents the voltage between any two electrodes. The standard diagnostic EEG uses at least 16 channels of information. Intraoperative recordings have been reported to use between 1 and 32 channels.

The EEG signal is characterized by three parameters: amplitude, frequency, and time. Amplitude (or voltage) represents the size of the recorded signal, typically between 5 microV and 500 microV. Frequency refers to the number of times per second the signal oscillates and is expressed in Hertz (Hz). Time is the duration of the recording. The scalp EEG recordings detect signals in the frequency range of 0.5–30 Hz (Table 50.1).

EEG tracings vary among normal individuals depending on their age and state of arousal, but there are certain elements that define them. For example, the amplitude of the EEG decreases with age but the recordings remain symmetrical in both frequency and amplitude, with patterns consistent with the clinical scenario and without spike waveforms.

Signals in the alpha frequency range seen best in the occipital region are typical for the EEG of a normal subject lying awake with their eyes closed. This is the baseline awake pattern and is described as having occipital dominance. With eye opening, higher frequency, lower amplitude signals in the beta range can be recorded from all cortical regions.

Table 50.1 Characteristics of EEG Wave Bands

EEG waves	Frequency (Hz)	Amplitude (microV)
α (alfa)	8–13	20–60
β (beta)	13–30	2–20
γ (gamma)	30–70	3–5
δ (delta)	0.5–4	20–200
θ (theta)	4–7	20–100

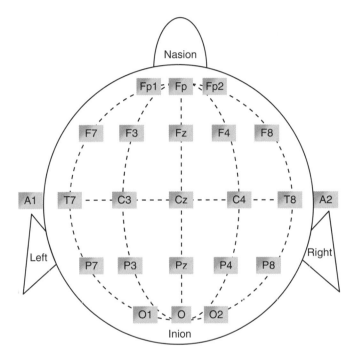

Figure 50.1 Scalp locations for electrode placement in the international 10–20 protocol.

The EEG during sleep has patterns characteristic for the various sleep stages. REM sleep is characterized by high frequency low amplitude rhythms and non-REM sleep by low frequency high amplitude rhythms.

Effects of Anesthetic Drugs

Anesthetic drugs affect the EEG in a drug-specific and dose-dependent way. Small doses of intravenous anesthetics such as propofol, etomidate, or barbiturates produce initially a paradoxical excitation characterized by an increase in the frontal beta activity and a reduction in the occipital alpha activity (frontal dominance). Light general anesthesia is characterized by a decrease of the beta activity and increase of the alpha and delta activity. The next phase sees the same pattern but with anteriorization, that is, alpha and delta activity increases in the anterior leads compared to the posterior leads. Thereafter an isoelectric EEG ensues with bursts of alpha and beta activity called burst suppression. In the deepest state of anesthesia, the EEG is isoelectric. Not all anesthetic drugs can produce burst suppression.

Processed Electroencephalogram – Concept and Devices

General anesthesia produces a transition from the state of wakefulness to a state of unconsciousness and this is reflected in the changes of the EEG recordings. However, adjusting the anesthetic based on the changes in the raw EEG data to obtain the desired level of anesthetic depth is cumbersome and challenging. The development of microcomputers with signal processing algorithms has permitted the analysis of EEG signals in almost real time and thereby development of "depth of anesthesia" monitors.

There are several approaches that may be used. All use digitally recorded EEG over a defined period of seconds called an epoch that is then processed and displayed with a small delay. The approaches may use amplitude, frequency, phase shift, and wave shape in some combination. A common technique is Fourier analysis of the frequencies so that one can "see" the power of different frequency ranges. The spectral edge frequency (SEF) is the frequency below which 90% of activity occurs. As anesthesia deepens, the SEF moves to lower frequencies. This information can also be displayed as a compressed spectral array (CSA) or density spectral array (DSA). The latter is usually color coded so that blue indicates little activity and red much activity. The frequency analysis can be coupled with other analyses such as phase coherence, entropy, and percent burst suppression to produce patented indices giving the clinician a single number that has supposedly integrated all this complex information. The algorithms are empirically calibrated against large anesthesia related EEG databases. These databases are composed of mainly vapor and/or propofol anesthesia. The devices have been shown to be quite useful trend monitors but not as useful when the anesthetic is composed of agents such as dexmedetomidine, ketamine, nitrous oxide, or large dose opioids. The skilled clinician using these devices should be able to make an elementary interpretation of a one to two lead EEG to enhance use of a single index number.

Muscles also generate voltage signals and their tracings constitute the electromyogram. The scalp muscles and extraocular muscles are responsible for some background noise on the EEG, with frequencies generally above 25 Hz. This "noise" can also be useful in assessing the anesthetic depth because muscle activity increases with light anesthesia. The auditory evoked potentials (AEPs) evaluate the response of the auditory pathway to the application of a repetitive stimulus. The evoked potential obtained 40–60 ms after the application of the stimulus represent neural activity within the thalamus and the primary auditory cortex and can be used as a measure of the anesthetic effect.

There are several commercial depth-of-anesthesia monitors currently on the market. They all attempt to convert the frontal EEG signal into a dimensionless index, with values ranging from 0 to 100, with 0 representing no electrical activity and 100 a fully responsive patient. Among the more common are Bispectral index (BIS, Covidien, Mansfield, MA), SedLine (Masimo Inc, Irvine California), Narcotrend (MT MonitorTechnik GmbH, Bad Bramstedt, Germany), and MEntropy (GE Healthcare, Chalfont St Giles, UK) that all use the processed spontaneous EEG. The aepEX device (Medical Device Management, Braintree, UK) uses auditory-evoked potentials (AEP) to calculate the depth of anesthesia (see Figures 50.2–50.4).

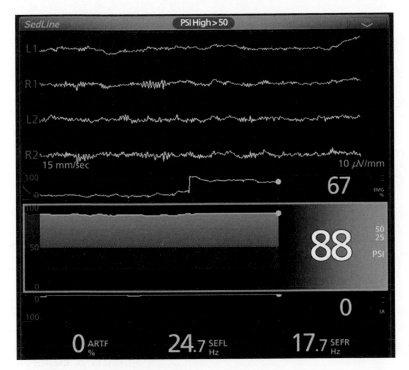

Figure 50.2 High frequency, low amplitude waves prior to induction of general anesthesia. The EMG activity is also recorded and is high.

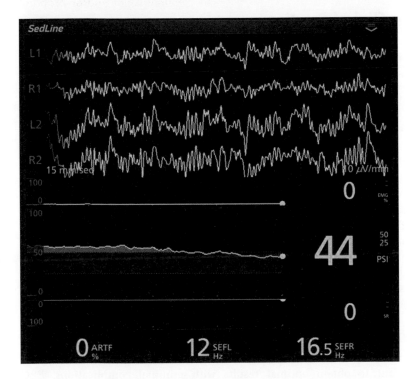

Figure 50.3 General anesthesia characterized by low frequency, high amplitude waves. The EMG activity has dropped to zero.

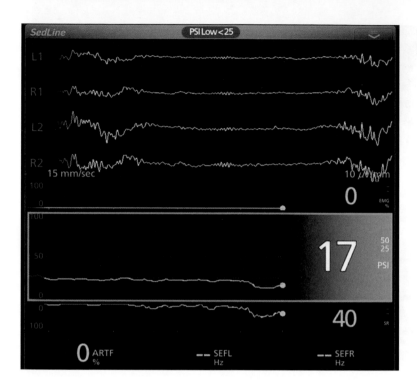

Figure 50.4 Burst suppression pattern. The EMG is quiet.

Current Uses in Clinical Practice

The EEG is used to monitor and help control the brain's electrical activity in the context of an existing or impeding traumatic or ischemic insult, to diagnose, monitor, and treat epilepsy and to monitor depth of anesthesia.

Neurovascular Surgery

Normal CBF is 50 ml/100 g tissue/min. Ischemia typically is considered below 20 ml/100 g/min and cellular survival is threatened at 12 ml/100 g/min. At these CBF levels, there is initially a loss of high frequency waves followed by progressive slowing until an isoelectric EEG occurs approximately concurrent with cell damage.

The use of the EEG to monitor CBF during carotid endarterectomy to direct selective shunting has been discussed for years. EEG monitoring does provide information about the CBF but has not been proven to improve outcome mainly because most perioperative strokes with all types of surgery are thromboembolic rather than hemodynamic and occur more frequently postoperatively. In aneurysm surgery, EEG and evoked potentials may detect intraoperative cerebral ischemia when temporary occlusion of the cerebral circulation is planned. They can be useful as a guide to blood pressure management while the blood flow is interrupted and also to titrate the anesthetic agents to pharmacologic metabolic suppression.

Seizure Focus Localization and Surgery

For patients who are candidates for epilepsy surgery, precise localization of the seizure focus is extremely important to obtain optimal results with minimal complications. EEG recordings, especially in combination with video recordings are crucial to this process. In certain cases, EcoG recordings from subdural electrodes inserted during a craniotomy are also used as they provide signals directly from the surface of the brain that have a high signal-to-noise ratio and a high spatial and temporal resolution.

Monitoring Depth of Anesthesia

The unprocessed EEG and various forms of processed EEG have been used to monitor the depth of anesthesia. Ideally this information could help optimize drug titration to the needs of the individual patient to avoid awareness under anesthesia and the long-term consequences that may be related to inadequate or excessive anesthetic depth. Currently there are at least seven different monitors in use. To date there is no clear evidence of any one superiority over the others.

The Bispectral index monitor (BIS) is by far the most studied monitor on the market. It combines power spectral analysis with analysis of the phase relationships between the frequencies of the EEG signal. The BIS monitor lacks sensitivity to the hypnotic effects of ketamine, nitrous oxide, xenon, and opiates.

There is consistent evidence that the BIS monitor is superior at reducing the intraoperative awareness events in a high-risk population compared to routine clinical care alone, but not superior to alarms based on the end-tidal anesthetic concentration.

A depth of anesthesia monitor may be most useful for patients maintained with total intravenous anesthesia especially if neuromuscular blockers are used. There is a higher incidence of awareness in this group due to the variability of sedative-hypnotic response and the inability to measure effect site anesthetic levels in real time.

The utility of the depth of anesthesia monitors is limited by a variety of factors, including electrical interference, individual variability of the baseline EEG characteristics, clinical conditions including hypothermia, hypoglycemia, cortical atrophy, dementia, advanced age, seizures, and cerebral ischemia as well as by the interactions between different anesthetic agents used. The currently available monitors focus mainly on the hypnotic effect of a general anesthetic, leaving the other aspects (amnesia, analgesia, immobility, and autonomic stability) largely uncharted.

Further Reading

Brown, E.N., Lydic, R., Schiff, N.D.: General anesthesia, sleep, and coma. *N Engl J Med* 2010 December 30; 363(27):2638–2650.

Marchant, N1., Sanders, R., Sleigh, J., et al: How electroencephalography serves the anesthesiologist. *Clin EEG Neurosci* 2014 January; 45(1):22–32. Epub 2014 January 10.

Mashour, G.A., Avidan, M.S.: Variability indices of processed electroencephalography and electromyography. *Anesth Analg* 2012 April; 114(4):713–714.

Mashour, G.A., Avidan, M.S.: Intraoperative awareness: Controversies and non-controversies. *Br J Anaesth* 2015 July; 115(Suppl 1):i20–i26. Epub 2015 March 3. Review.

Purdon, P.L., Pavone, K.J., Akeju, O., et al: The Ageing brain: Age-dependent changes in the electroencephalogram during propofol and sevoflurane general anaesthesia. *Br J Anaesth* 2015 July; 115(Suppl 1):i46–i57.

Purdon, P.L., Sampson, A., Pavone, K.J., Brown, E.N.: Clinical electroencephalography for anesthesiologists: Part I: Background and basic signatures. *Anesthesiology* 2015 October; 123(4):937–960.

Transcranial Doppler Ultrasonography and Cerebral Blood Flow Measurement

Andrea Lavinio and Antoine Halwagi

Key Points

- The detection of cerebral hypoperfusion in anesthetized and sedated patients relies on instrumental assessment.
- TCD can provide non-invasive, continuous measurement of blood flow velocity in major intracranial vessels.
- A sudden drop in flow velocity indicates a reduction of CBF of the same magnitude.
- TCD can diagnose vasospasm but cannot determine the size of ischemic penumbra or adequacy of regional blood flow.
- A CTP can quantify regional blood flow and identify areas of cerebral infarction and reversible hypoperfusion.
- CTP criterion of size of penumbra is more accurate than time from onset of symptoms in identifying patients likely to benefit from thrombolysis and endovascular treatment following ischemic stroke.
- CTP should be performed at target blood pressure to confirm adequacy of CBF in response to blood pressure manipulation.

Abbreviations

aSAH	Aneurysmal subarachnoid hemorrhage
CA	Cerebrovascular autoregulation
CBF	Cerebral blood flow
CBFV	Cerebral blood flow velocities
CBV	Cerebral blood volume
CPP	Cerebral perfusion pressure
CR	Cerebrovascular reactivity
CT	Computed tomography
CTP	Computed tomography perfusion scan
dFV	Diastolic flow velocity
HITS	High-intensity transient signal
ICP	Intracranial pressure

LI   Lindegaard index
LLA   Lower limit of autoregulation
MCA   Middle cerebral artery
mFV   Mean flow velocity
MR   Magnetic resonance
MTT   Mean transit time
PET   Positron emission tomography
PI   Pulsatility index
sFV   Systolic flow velocity
TCD   Transcranial Doppler
TTP   Time to peak
TTD   Time to drain
ULA   Upper Limit of autoregulation

Contents

Introduction

Cerebral hypoperfusion is defined as a mismatch between CBF and cerebral metabolic demand. Insufficient delivery of oxygen and metabolic substrates results in cellular energy failure, neuronal dysfunction and in the absence of prompt intervention, neuronal death. Rapid correction of cerebral hypoperfusion and the prevention of cerebral ischemia are cornerstones of neuroanesthesia and neurocritical care. Given the time-sensitive vulnerability of the central nervous system to ischemic insults, it is essential that cerebral hypoperfusion is promptly identified. Although clinical observation and neurological examination can reliably identify signs of cerebral hypoperfusion in awake self-ventilated patients, the detection of cerebral hypoperfusion in anesthetized and sedated patients relies on instrumental assessment. Two diagnostic modalities, essential to current clinical practice, include TCD ultrasonography and CTP.

Transcranial Doppler Ultrasonography

Basic principles

TCD allows non-invasive, real-time monitoring of blood flow velocities in major intracranial vessels. TCD technology is based on the Doppler effect, i.e., an apparent increase (or decrease) in the frequency of a wave when the source of said wave moves towards (or away from) the observer. Using a hand-held emitting-receiving probe, a pulsed range-gated ultrasonic beam is directed towards the perceived anatomical location of a target vessel. Ultrasound waves are echoed back towards the probe by the skull contents. When the ultrasound beam hits a cerebral vessel, the frequency of the echo originating from flowing blood cells differs from the frequency of the wave emitted by the probe. The frequency of the echoed wave is higher than the frequency of the emitted wave when blood flows towards the emitting-receiving probe, and lower than the frequency of the emitted wave when blood flows away from the probe. When such a frequency-shift is detected, the TCD apparatus calculates the velocity (relative to the probe) of moving red blood cells. CBFV and intensity of the echo signal are represented graphically as a continuous waveform on a computer screen and acoustically (acoustocerebrography), conveying flow velocity by sound pitch and intensity by sound volume.

Technique

Two-dimensional echoencephalography is of limited clinical relevance in adults with intact skulls due to attenuation of ultrasound by bony skull and poor image quality. Although modern diagnostic equipment allows for 2D imaging, TCD examinations are typically performed as a blind technique using a 2-MHz pulsed range-gated ultrasound probe. Insonation of cerebral vessels is performed at specific anatomical locations that allow reliable intracranial penetration and reflection of the ultrasound beam. The use of pulsed-range gated probes allows to discriminate the distance at which the echo signal originates from (i.e., the operator can adjust the "depth" and "sample size" of insonation). Acoustic windows and normal TCD findings are summarized in Table 51.1.

Cerebral vessels can be identified based on anatomical landmarks, probe angulation, insonation depth, direction of flow and responses to dynamic maneuvers such as carotid compression. Continuous monitoring of CBFV can be performed by means of specially designed headbands and probe holders. Most commonly, the MCA is monitored by securing TCD probes at the temporal acoustic window. This can be done unilaterally (this is often the preferred configuration during intraoperative monitoring for carotid endarterectomies) or bilaterally. The most relevant recorded variables are peak sFV, end dFV and time-averaged mean maximum-flow velocity, commonly referred to as mean flow velocity (mFV). Important derived parameters are the Lindegaard index (LI = MCA mFV/ICA mFV) and the pulsatility index (PI = (sFV – dFV)/mFV).

Cerebrovascular Autoregulation

CA is a complex homeodynamic process whereby cerebral vasculature modulates its regional resistances to distribute and maintain cerebral perfusion to meet cerebral metabolic demand over a wide range of CPP. The term "cerebrovascular reactivity" refers to the

Table 51.1 Acoustic Windows and Normal TCD Findings in Adults. MCA: Middle Cerebral Artery. ACA: Anterior Cerebral Artery. PCA: Posterior Cerebral Artery. ICA: Internal Carotid Artery. VA: Vertebral Artery. BA: Basilar Artery. OA: Ophthalmic Artery. (T) towards. (A) away

Window	Technique	Vessel	Depth [mm]	mFV [cm/s]
Temporal	The probe is positioned on the superior edge of the zygomatic process between the cantus and the external auditory meatus and is directed anteriorly for MCA/ACA and posteriorly for PCA	MCA (M1)	45–60	45–75 (T)
		ACA (A1)	60–65	40–60 (A)
		PCA (P1)	60–75	30–50 (T)
Submandibular	The probe is paratracheal and parallel to ipsilateral ICA	ICA	45–60	25–45 (A)
Suboccipital	Probe at the atlanto-occipital space and directed towards the glabella, paramedian approach for VA and median for BA	VA	60–90	30–50 (A)
		BA	80–110	30–50 (A)
Transorbital	The probe is positioned on closed eyelid and directed posteriorly	OA	40–50	15–25 (T)

ability of the cerebrovascular bed to modulate its resistances in response to various stimuli, such as changes in regional metabolic demand, CO_2 and blood pressure. TCD is used in clinical practice and clinical research to assess CA and CR using a multitude of methods yielding highly predictive prognostic information in a variety of clinical settings including stroke, subarachnoid hemorrhage and traumatic brain injury.

The term static autoregulation refers to TCD methodologies based on slow manipulation of CPP and simultaneous measurement of CBFV. Static autoregulation is quantified as a percentage of full autoregulatory capacity in the pressure range studied. In other words, static CA is 100% when CBFV remains constant irrespective of changes in perfusion pressure and static CA is 0% when CBFV changes linearly with changes in perfusion pressures. Extreme manipulations of CPP can also identify the LLA and ULA, CPP levels below and above which CBFV becomes linearly dependent on changes in CPP. Such extreme manipulations of perfusion pressure have limited applications in clinical practice and should be restricted to experimental studies.

The term "dynamic cerebral autoregulation" refers to TCD methods based on rapid reduction in perfusion pressure (tilt test, sudden release of thigh blood pressure cuffs, compression and release of the carotid artery). Dynamic CA methods do not identify the LLA-ULA range but capture the ability of cerebral autoregulation to compensate for rapid fluctuations in perfusion pressure. Dynamic CA methods provide robust prognostic information in a variety of clinical scenarios and are better suited for routine clinical use due to their practicality and safety profile (Figure 51.1).

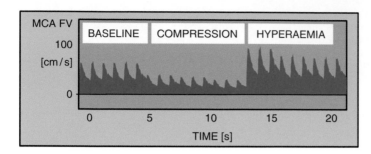

Figure 51.1 The transient hyperemic response (THR) test evaluates the hypersemic response of MCA CBFV following a brief carotid compression. An increase in systolic FV of 10% or more from baseline following compression indicates preserved dynamic autoregulation.

Interpretation and Pitfalls

The most appropriate use of TCD in modern practice is as a screening tool. Normal parameters are arbitrarily set to detect abnormal CBF with high sensitivity. Summarily, symmetrical velocities within normal ranges in all the major arteries of the Circle of Willis indicate normal CBF. Further prognostic reassurance is provided by preserved dynamic autoregulation. Abnormal TCD findings should be integrated, in the appropriate clinical context, by further instrumental assessment of regional CBF using complementary methods such as CTP.

The main limitations of TCD-based techniques arise from the fact that TCD quantifies flow velocities rather than absolute flow. CBFV and CBF are linearly correlated when the cross-sectional area [A] of the insonated vessel is constant [CBF = A · CBFV]. The assumption of a constant vessel diameter generally holds true over time periods measured in seconds to minutes. Thus, a sudden reduction in CBFV reflects a reduction in CBF of the same magnitude. Intraoperative TCD monitoring can therefore accurately reveal a critical reduction in CBF, for example, as the result of arterial clamping in the absence of adequate collateral flow or inadequate CPP.

The assumption of a constant cross sectional area of cerebral arteries does not necessarily hold true over periods of hours or days. The finding of abnormally elevated CBFV can indicate a critical reduction in vessel diameter with compromised CBF. Typical TCD findings associated with cerebral vasospasm are high-velocity, turbulent CBFV in the spastic vessel with reduced CBFV in the extracranial carotid artery feeding the spastic territory. Abnormally elevated CBFV may also indicate cerebral hyperemia, which is also a common occurrence in patients with resolving vasospasm and iatrogenic hypertension exceeding the ULA. The differential diagnosis between vasospasm and hyperemia relies on the simultaneous assessment of CBFV in the MCA and in the terminal extracranial ICA, which is generally not affected by the vasospastic process. In the case of vasospasm and compromised flow, ICA CBFV will be reduced, whereas in the case of hyperemia ICA CBFV will be increased. The ratio between intracranial CBFV and extracranial ICA CBFV (LI) will therefore be elevated in the case of vasospasm (LI > 3) and low-normal in the case of cerebral hyperemia (LI < 3).

A second important consideration is that flow velocities are measured relative to the probe and are underestimated depending on the angle between the probe and the direction of flow. Accurate assessments can only be obtained when the ultrasound beam is precisely aligned with the vessel and blood is flowing directly towards (or away) from the probe. At a 30-degree angle, velocities are underestimated by approximately 15%. When the ultrasound beam hits a vessel perpendicularly to the direction of flow, the estimated velocity will be zero irrespective of the actual flow velocity. TCD cannot overestimate CBFV so the maximum velocity recorded is the most accurate.

Other factors affecting TCD accuracy include vascular tortuousness and thickness of the acoustic widow with insufficient penetration of ultrasound making TCD assessment impossible in approximately one in ten patients. Although recent technical improvements mitigate the problem, prolonged monitoring is technically challenging as minimal inadvertent movements of the probe can result in complete loss of the echo signal.

Interpretation of TCD findings should also take into account age, gender and other physiological variables known to affect normal CBFV. MCA mFV is lowest at birth (25 cm/s), peaks at the age of 6 (100 cm/s) and decreases to about 40 cm/s during the seventh decade of life.

Indications

Intraoperative Monitoring

TCD can be used to monitor the adequacy of cerebral perfusion in surgical procedures known to compromise carotid blood flow such as carotid endarterectomy and aortic arch surgery. In carotid endarterectomy, TCD can be useful in identifying critical hypoperfusion following arterial clamping, guiding blood pressure augmentation to maximize collateral flow or indicating arterial shunting. A drop in MCA mFV below 50% of baseline (or below 25 cm/s) during clamping is associated with severe ischemia and high risk of postoperative stroke. Use of TCD monitoring during carotid endarterectomy can also detect shunt malposition or occlusion, intraoperative emboli (generating characteristic high-intensity transient signal – HITS), postoperative carotid occlusion and hyperemia.

Aneurysmal Subarachnoid Hemorrhage

Delayed cerebral ischemia is a clinical syndrome of focal neurological and/or cognitive deficits occurring unpredictably in a third of patients 3–21 days following aSAH as a result of cerebral vasospasm. Daily TCD monitoring can allow early identification of vasospasm. The finding of mFV >100 cm/s with LI >3 should trigger consideration of treatment or confirmatory tests such as CTP or digital subtraction angiography, depending on local protocols.

Traumatic Brain Injury

TCD can estimate ICP in patients at risk of intracranial hypertension. Elevation in ICP gradually impairs CBF by compressing cerebral arteries with a typical TCD pattern (Figure 51.2). Continuous TCD monitoring also allows the identification of LLA and CA assessment, guiding treatment and providing useful prognostic information.

Identification of right-to-left shunt. Following intravenous injection of an agitated saline solution, the appearance of microembolic signals on TCD monitoring suggests presence of a right-to-left shunt. This technique is useful in identifying patients at risk of paradoxical embolism from positioning during surgery (e.g., neurosurgical procedures in sitting position and paradoxical air embolism) or surgical manipulation (e.g., intramedullary nailing and paradoxical fat embolism).

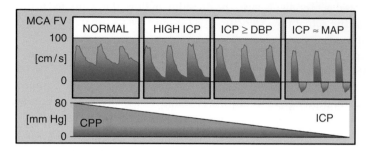

Figure 51.2 Typical TCD findings with increasing intracranial pressure (ICP) and progressively compromised cerebral perfusion pressure (CPP). **NORMAL:** continuous diastolic flow with pulsatility index (PI) < 1.2. **HIGH ICP:** as ICP increases, diastolic CBFV becomes progressively compromised. PI positively correlates with ICP (1 mmHg increase in ICP is reflected by a 2.4% increase in PI). **ICP ≥ DBP:** as ICP exceeds diastolic blood pressure (DBP) diastolic flow drops to zero. **ICP ≈ MAP:** as ICP approaches mean arterial pressure and CPP approaches zero cerebral circulatory arrest can be demonstrated by a pattern of diastolic reversal of flow.

Brain Death

Although the confirmation of death following irreversible cessation of brainstem function is a clinical diagnosis, cerebral circulatory arrest can be confirmed with high specificity by demonstrating diastolic flow reversal with an oscillating systolic forward flow and diastolic reversed flow.

Computed Tomography Perfusion

TCD bedside monitoring is complemented by imaging modalities (CT, MR, PET) that can assess the adequacy of regional CBF and differentiate between areas of reversible cerebral hypoperfusion and infarcted brain. CTP is the preferred modality in the acute clinical setting due to its accessibility and rapidity of image acquisition.

Basic Principles

Following rapid administration of intravenous iodinated contrast, the cranium and its contents are repeatedly scanned at regular intervals over a period of approximately 10 seconds. As contrast travels through the intracranial vasculature and cerebral parenchyma, CT attenuation transiently increases as a function of regional blood flow. Attenuation time curves are generated in an arterial region of interest, in a venous region of interest and in each pixel. Post-processing software generates color-coded perfusion maps depicting MTT, TTP, TTD, CBF and CBV.

Interpretation

CTP can be interpreted qualitatively by visual inspection of perfusion maps or quantitatively using commercially available software. Normal CTP findings include symmetrical time parameters within expect time ranges for grey and white matter. Delayed time parameters (TTP, MTT, and TTD) can identify areas with compromised flow with high sensitivity. Areas of salvageable brain parenchyma (penumbra) are identified by areas of reduced CBF with preserved or increased CBV. Infarcted brain (core) is identified by areas of matching critical reduction in CBF and CBV. Following ischemic stroke, the optimal approach to define the infarct and the penumbra is a combined approach using relative MTT and absolute CBV, with optimal thresholds of rMTT > 145% and CBV < 2.0 ml/100 g, respectively.

Limitations

The main limitations of the technique relate to radiation exposure and to the risks associated with the administration of iodinated contrast, limiting the number of scans that can be safely performed within individual patient and therefore limiting the usefulness of this modality for the assessment of response to treatment or dynamic changes in CBF. Further technical limitations include poor detail in the posterior fossa due to bone attenuation, movement artefacts in non-cooperative patients and vulnerability to post-processing errors.

Indications

Acute Stroke

A growing body of clinical evidence reveals that imaging, not time, determines patients likely to benefit from thrombolysis and endovascular treatment following ischemic stroke. Patients with a large penumbra (i.e., mismatch between CBF and CBV) may benefit from clot retrieval up to 18 hours following onset of symptoms. Conversely, patients with large established infarcts and small penumbra may suffer the side effects of thrombolysis and clot retrieval without any significant benefit despite early intervention.

Aneurysmal Subarachnoid Hemorrhage

CTP can identify areas of regional hypoperfusion. In order to assess response to treatment and adequacy of CBF, CTP should be performed at target blood pressure. Images can also be reconstructed to generate CT angiograms, identifying areas of critical vasospasm and indicating endovascular treatment.

Further Reading

Alexandrov, A.V., Sloan, M.A., Tegeler, C.H., et al: Practice standards for transcranial Doppler (TCD) ultrasound. Part II. Clinical indications and expected outcomes. *J Neuroimag* 2012; **22**(3):215–224.

Allmendinger, A.M., Tang, E.R., Lui, Y.W., et al: Imaging of stroke: Part 1, Perfusion CT–overview of imaging technique, interpretation pearls, and common pitfalls. *Am J Roentgenol* 2012; **198**(1):52–62.

Budohoski, K.P., Guilfoyle, M., Helmy, A., et al: The pathophysiology and treatment of delayed cerebral ischaemia following subarachnoid haemorrhage. *J Neurol Neurosurg Psychiatry* 2014; **85**(12):1343–1353.

Cremers, C.H.P., van der Schaaf, I.C., Wensink, E., et al: CT perfusion and delayed cerebral ischemia in aneurysmal subarachnoid hemorrhage: A systematic review and meta-analysis. *J Cereb Blood Flow Metab* 2014; **34**(2):200–207.

Kumar, G., Shahripour, R.B., Harrigan, M.R.: Vasospasm on transcranial Doppler is predictive of delayed cerebral ischemia in aneurysmal subarachnoid hemorrhage: A systematic review and meta-analysis. *J Neurosurg* 2016; **124**(5):1257–1264.

Chapter

52

Neuroanesthesia in Pregnancy

Mark D. Rollins and Mark A. Rosen

Key Points

- Neurologic diseases are a major source of non-obstetric morbidity and mortality during pregnancy and the decision to operate should be primarily neurosurgical rather than obstetric.
- Anesthetic management during pregnancy must be designed to avoid fetal asphyxia, teratogenicity, and induction of preterm labor while being mindful of maternal physiologic changes during pregnancy.
- Rapid-sequence induction of anesthesia with succinylcholine is recommended along with administration of agents to attenuate the hypertensive response to laryngoscopy and tracheal intubation.
- No modern anesthetic agent has been shown to have teratogenic effects; inhalational, balanced, or total intravenous techniques can be used safely.
- Hyperventilation, osmotic diuresis, and deliberate hypotensive techniques should be used with caution and limitations, whereas moderate hypothermia is safe.

Abbreviations

ACLS	Acute cardiac life support
AVM	Arteriovenous malformation
ATLS	Acute trauma life support
CBF	Cerebral blood flow
CNS	Central nervous system
CSF	Cerebrospinal fluid
FHR	Fetal heart rate
GCS	Glasgow Coma Scale
ICP	Intracranial pressure
mGy	milliGray
SAH	Subarachnoid hemorrhage
TBI	Traumatic brain injury

Contents

- Intracranial Tumors
- Traumatic Brain Injury
- Surgical Timing and Delivery
- Anesthetic Management
- Postoperative Considerations
- Further Reading

Introduction

Neurological disease during pregnancy, although rare, represents a significant source of severe long-term morbidity and mortality. Pregnancy is a hypercoagulable state with altered hemodynamics and vascular wall changes that increase the risk of both ischemic stroke (4–10 per 100,000 deliveries) and cerebral venous thrombosis (1–2 per 10,000 deliveries). Although rare, both posterior reversible encephalopathy and reversible cerebral vasoconstriction syndrome can occur during pregnancy and post-partum. These rare conditions can occur in pre-eclamptics secondary to cerebrovascular hypertension, increased vascular permeability, and associated edema. Although other neurological disorders can arise during pregnancy, hemorrhagic stroke, intracranial tumors, and trauma are the most prominent among the non-obstetric causes of maternal mortality. Optimal management requires planning and treatment by a coordinated multidisciplinary team that considers the pathology of the neurological process, the physiological changes of pregnancy, fetal well-being, mode and timing of delivery, and appropriate risk/benefit patient counseling regarding care for both the mother and fetus.

Hemorrhagic Stroke

Intracerebral hemorrhage during pregnancy often follows a hypertensive crisis, with pre-eclamptic or eclamptic patients having a fourfold increase in the relative risk of stroke. The incidence of SAH from ruptured intracranial arterial aneurysms and AVMs is increased in the peripartum period with a rate of 3–7 per 100,000 deliveries and accounts for 5%–12% of all pregnancy related in-hospital mortality.

Management should be based on neurosurgical rather than obstetric considerations. ICP monitoring should be considered in patients with GCS < 8, blood pressure goals determined in consultation with a neurologist and obstetrician, and any coagulopathy reversed. Besides administration of magnesium for pre-eclamptic or eclamptic patients, seizure prophylaxis is not recommended unless convulsive movements are seen or seizure activity noted on the electroencephalogram (EEG).

Since morbidity and mortality associated with aneurysmal bleeding is significant, timely definitive treatment of ruptured aneurysms in the gravid patient is usually recommended at all stages of pregnancy. During temporary aneurysm clipping, EEG burst suppression can be safely achieved with propofol.

Vasospasm following SAH, with typical onset 4 to 10 days after initial hemorrhage, can be safely treated with nimodipine to prevent ischemic changes. Magnesium sulfate is ineffective and statins pose a teratogenic risk. Hypervolemia, hypertension, and hemodilution therapy for vasospasm prevention has limited evidence, and vasopressor induced hypertension is preferred instead by some clinicians. However, use of high dose vasopressors for extended periods during pregnancy can decrease utero-placental perfusion, risking fetal well-being, and increasing abruption risk. A multidisciplinary discussion for SAH pregnant patients should include not only treatment options, but also plans for vasospasm prevention, monitoring and optimal timing, and method of delivery.

It remains unclear if pregnancy increases the risk of hemorrhage from AVMs. Pregnant women with a non-ruptured AVM and those who are stable post-hemorrhage can safely reach term gestation with elective post-partum excision of the AVM. The decision to operate should be neurosurgical rather than obstetric.

Intracranial Tumors

Although the incidence of intracranial tumor does not increase during pregnancy, clinical symptoms can be exacerbated by hormonally induced acceleration of tumor growth, edema, blood vessel engorgement, and decreased immune system function. Neurological diagnosis is often challenging and frequently delayed during pregnancy by symptoms mistaken for normal pregnancy or a related illness such as preeclampsia (e.g., headache, nausea and vomiting, visual changes, and seizures). Early use of imaging is advocated for pregnant patients with neurological symptoms. MRI is preferred because it avoids fetal radiation exposure and has increased sensitivity. Surgical removal is preferred for most symptomatic and expanding intracranial tumors. Both adjuvant radiotherapy and chemotherapy during pregnancy have potential for harmful fetal effects. Complete tumor resection is associated with a favorable prognosis, and significant delays can cause progressive neurological deterioration. Decisions about resection timing should consider tumor type, location, and predicted course during pregnancy, with goals to balance optimum maternal outcome with fetal considerations.

Often neurosurgical intervention can be appropriately deferred until after delivery of a reasonably mature neonate. When resection is postponed until after delivery, the presence of an intracranial tumor in the peripartum period does not necessitate cesarean delivery. Although CSF pressure increases with uterine contractions and pushing, epidural analgesia, and instrument-assisted vaginal delivery can decrease the degree of ICP elevation. However, unintentional dural puncture in a woman with elevated ICP risks brain herniation.

Traumatic Brain Injury

In pregnant patients, TBI is commonly secondary to motor vehicle accidents and represents a significant cause of maternal morbidity and mortality. Acute management should follow ATLS guidelines, as appropriate resuscitation of the mother is also beneficial for the fetus. Immediate management is focused on prevention of additional brain injury from hypoxemia, hypercarbia, hypotension, or hyperthermia, and maintaining cerebral perfusion pressure with fluid resuscitation, vasopressors, and blood products if needed. Hyperventilation to a P_aCO_2 of 25–30 mmHg can transiently decrease ICP, but normal P_aCO_2 in pregnancy is 28–32 mmHg and values below 25 mmHg can significantly reduce blood flow to the fetus. Steroids are not recommended, but both mannitol and hypertonic saline can be used, despite potential adverse fetal effects.

Surgical Timing and Delivery

The neurological process, associated risk, maternal condition, and gestational age of the fetus all influence the surgical timing and delivery plan. When delivery is planned prior to neurosurgery, the mode of delivery and role of neuraxial anesthesia should be determined only after a multidisciplinary discussion of neurosurgical pathology and maternal condition to ensure all management details have been addressed.

Elective neurosurgery procedures should always be delayed until after pregnancy. Surgical procedures early in pregnancy carry the risk of spontaneous abortion, while procedures later in pregnancy are associated with premature labor and delivery. Non-urgent but essential operations are delayed until after the first trimester to minimize teratogenic effects on the fetus, but pregnant women should never be denied an indicated surgical procedure. For non-emergent maternal procedures involving a preterm fetus, maternal administration of steroids should be considered to improve fetal lung maturity in the event of an emergent delivery.

Use of FHR monitoring should be individualized in consultation with obstetricians. An external Doppler FHR monitor will usually detect FHR after the 16th week of gestation. For the pre-viable fetus, assessment of FHR before and after the procedure can be sufficient. However, even for a pre-viable fetus, FHR monitoring can be valuable before and after maternal positioning, where fetal bradycardia might signal an abnormality in maternal blood pressure, ventilation, uterine perfusion, or umbilical blood flow. Prompt maternal position change, treatment of maternal hypotension, hypoxia, or measures to improve cardiac output are essential for the fetus to have the best chance of surviving with an intact nervous system. If viable, persistent signs of non-reversible fetal distress should result in temporary suspension of the neurosurgical procedure while an emergent cesarean delivery is performed.

Planning should include the possibility of maternal arrest and emergent cesarean delivery. According to ACLS protocol, evacuation of the uterus should occur when a perfusing rhythm is not present after 4 minutes of resuscitation efforts. In addition, the procedure should be at an institution with neonatal teams, personnel to interpret the FHR, and an obstetrician readily available for possible cesarean delivery.

Anesthetic Management

Preoperative Assessment and Premedications

Perioperative management during pregnancy must meet the goals dictated by the neurosurgical intervention, optimizing cerebral perfusion, maintaining appropriate utero-placental blood flow, and avoiding fetal asphyxia. Physiological changes in almost every maternal organ system pose potential maternal and fetal challenges. Prior to the procedure, prophylactic medications should be administered to reduce gastric acidity and the risk of aspiration.

Monitoring

In most cases, invasive arterial pressure monitoring should be considered prior to induction to allow quick intervention for hemodynamic changes. Fetal and maternal temperatures are closely related, and maintenance of normothermia is associated with improved maternal and fetal outcomes.

Induction, Intubation, and Positioning

A rapid-sequence intravenous induction with endotracheal intubation should be performed to decrease aspiration risk. For patients in whom intubation can be difficult, an awake, fiberoptic intubation with topical local anesthesia to the airway is appropriate. To avoid a hypertensive response to laryngoscopy, placement of pins for head fixation or incision, administration of beta-blockers, opioids, and/or vasodilators is recommended. Positioning the patient in a left lateral tilt avoids aortocaval compression, and improves MAP and cardiac output.

Anesthetic Technique

No modern anesthetic agent or technique has been shown to have teratogenic effects. The anesthetic approach should be based on underlying morbidity and surgical procedure. All volatile agents decrease uterine tone and their concentrations should be reduced following a cesarean delivery to decrease risk of uterine atony.

Ventilation

The use of hyperventilation is limited in the pregnant patient. Pregnancy induces a compensated respiratory alkalosis resulting in a normal maternal $PaCO_2$ of 30–32 mm Hg, a pH of 7.42–7.44, and a HCO_3 of 20–21 mEq/L. Significant hyperventilation ($PaCO_2 <$ 25 mmHg) decreases umbilical blood flow, induces a leftward shift in the oxyhemoglobin dissociation curve, and decreases placental transfer of oxygen to the fetus and is not recommended. However, mild hyperventilation is probably safe. $PaCO_2$ values greater than 32 mmHg during pregnancy represent relative hypercapnia, which increases CBF and produces fetal respiratory acidosis. Excessive positive-pressure ventilation is avoided because it can increase intrathoracic pressure, decrease venous return, and reduce both cardiac output and uterine perfusion. Use of lower tidal volumes and slight head-up position helps reduce ICP.

Hyperosmolar Agents

Mannitol can adversely affect the fetus by inducing maternal dehydration, maternal hypotension, uterine hypoperfusion, and fetal injury. Mannitol crosses the placenta to a variable extent and can accumulate in the fetus, leading to fetal hyperosmolality, reduced lung fluid production, fetal dehydration with decreased blood volume and decreased urine production, and fetal hypernatremia. However, low doses of mannitol (0.25–0.5 g/kg) have been used during pregnancy without adverse fetal or maternal outcome. Furosemide crosses the placenta and may induce dose-dependent fetal diuresis partially mediated by increases in fetal vascular pressure, but has been administered in pregnancy without adverse effects. Cautious use in certain circumstances may provide an alternate to mannitol.

Vasopressor Agents

Vasopressors may be necessary during periods of intraoperative hypotension, or during arterial occlusion with use of temporary proximal clips. Phenylephrine and ephedrine in typical doses are not associated with adverse fetal effects. Although the safety and efficacy profile of norepinephrine in pregnancy is not complete, its use is associated with a greater maternal heart rate and cardiac output than phenylephrine and does not appear to adversely affect the fetus.

Nitroglycerin can be administered as a maternal intravenous antihypertensive agent without adverse fetal effects. Sodium nitroprusside can be used safely as an antihypertensive for short periods, but readily crosses the placenta and over time its metabolites can cause a reduction in fetal arterial perfusion pressure. Regardless of agent, risk of fetal distress and asphyxia increases with significant maternal hypotension. If controlled hypotension is necessary, blood pressure reduction should be limited in depth and duration, and FHR monitored.

Neurointerventional Procedures

Interventional radiology is often required for angiography, angioplasty, and coiling of aneurysms and AVMs. Risk of fetal abnormalities from ionizing radiation is dependent on both fetal age and cumulative exposure. Neurons are especially at risk during neuroblast proliferation and cortical migration (weeks 8 through 15). Although radiation is directed at the maternal cranium, abdominal shielding is essential to reduce fetal exposure. The minimal threshold for adverse CNS effects may be in the range of 60–310 mGy, and risk of fetal anomalies, growth restriction, or abortion have never been reported with radiation exposure of less than 50 mGy. For trauma assessment, diagnostic imaging should never be withheld, but consultation with a radiologist is beneficial when planning multiple imaging sequences, to minimize fetal exposure.

Postoperative Considerations

Appropriate postoperative analgesia should be provided using a multimodal approach, although anti-inflammatory medications are often avoided after intracranial procedures secondary to their antiplatelet and potential undesired fetal effects. Prophylactic tocolysis with agents such as nifedipine can be used to reduce the risk of premature labor. Tocodynamometric uterine contraction monitoring is often used postoperatively as reliance on abdominal pain for labor has poor sensitivity. The hypercoagulable state of pregnancy confers significant risk of thromboembolism, and non-pharmacological prevention methods should be used perioperatively (e.g., sequential compression devices, antithromboembolic stockings). Prophylactic heparin administration should follow a multidisciplinary risk/benefit discussion.

Further Reading

American College of Obstetricians Gynecologists' Committee on Obstetric Practice. Committee Opinion No. 656: Guidelines for diagnostic imaging during pregnancy and lactation. *Obstet Gynecol* 2016; **127**:e75–e80.

American College of Obstetricians and Gynecologists' Task Force on Hypertension in Pregnancy: Hypertension in pregnancy. Report of the American College of Obstetricians and Gynecologists' task force on hypertension in pregnancy. *Obstet Gynecol* 2013; **122**:1122–1131.

Bader, A.M.: Neurologic and neuromuscular disease. In: Chestnut D.H., Wong C.A., Tsen L. C., Ngan Kee W.D., Beilin Y., Mhyre J.M. (Eds.).

Chestnut's Obstetric Anesthesia: Principles and Practice, 5th ed. Philadelphia: Elsevier Inc; 2014: 15–38.

Bonfield, C.M., Engh, J.A.: Pregnancy and brain tumors. *Neurol Clin* 2012; **30**:937–946.

Chowdhury, T., Chowdhury, M., Schaller, B., et al: Perioperative considerations for neurosurgical procedures in the gravid patient. *Can J Anaesth* 2013; **60**:1139–1155.

Edlow, J.A., Caplan, L.R., O'Brien, K., et al: Diagnosis of acute neurological emergencies in pregnant and post-partum women. *Lancet Neurol* 2013; **12**:175–1788.

Flood, P., Rollins, M.D.: Anesthesia for Obstetrics. In: Miller, R.D., Cohen, N.H., Eriksson, L.I., Fleisher, L.A, Wiener-Kronish, J.

P., Young, W.L. (Eds.) Miller's Anesthesia, *8th ed.* Philadelphia: Elsevier Inc.; 2014.

Lipman, S., Cohen, S., Einav, S., et al: The Society for Obstetric Anesthesia and Perinatology consensus statement on the management of cardiac arrest in pregnancy. *Anesth Analg* 2014; **118**:1003–1016.

O'Neal, M.A.: Neurology of pregnancy: A case-oriented review. *Neurol Clin* 2016; **34**:717–731.

Pacheco, L., Howell, P., Sherwood, E.R.: Trauma and critical care. In: Chestnut, D.H., Wong, C.A., Tsen, L.C., Ngan Kee, W.D., Beilin, Y., Mhyre, J.M. (Eds.). *Chestnut's Obstetric Anesthesia: Principles and Practice, 5th ed.* Philadelphia: Elsevier Inc.; 2014:1219–1242.

Practice Guidelines for Obstetric Anesthesia: An updated report by the American Society of Anesthesiologists Task Force on Obstetric Anesthesia and the Society for Obstetric Anesthesia and Perinatology. *Anesthesiology* 2016; **124**:270–300.

Razmara, A., Bakhadirov, K., Batra, A., et al: Cerebrovascular complications of pregnancy and the postpartum period. *Curr Cardiol* 2014; **16**:532–537.

Verheecke, M., Halaska, M.J., Lok, C.A., et al: Pregnancy ETFCi: Primary brain tumours, meningiomas and brain metastases in pregnancy: Report on 27 cases and Review of Literature. *Eur J Cancer* 2014; **50**:1462–1471.

Chapter 53

Neuro-Rehabilitation

Fahim Anwar, Harry Mee, and Judith Allanson

Key Points

- Rehabilitation is a process of assessment, treatment, management, and ongoing evaluation of a patient to achieve their maximum potential for recovery.
- Early rehabilitation is essential in reducing physical, emotional, psychological, and psychiatric complications.
- Rehabilitation involves a multitude of disciplines as well as family members and carers, working together to improve the quality of life of the patient.
- The role of the rehabilitation physician includes leading a multidisciplinary team and combining medical skills in diagnosis and treatment of conditions causing complex disability.
- There is good evidence that early specialist rehabilitation for patients with complex needs is highly cost-effective.
- The UK-adapted functional independence measure and functional assessment measure are recognized as reliable scoring systems for independent functioning.
- The rehabilitation prescription is used to document the rehabilitation needs of patients with severe illness/injury and identify how they will be addressed. It should be initiated at an early stage and regularly reviewed.

Abbreviations

FAM	Functional assessment measure
FIM	Functional independence measure
ICF	The international classification of functioning, disability and health
ICU	Intensive care unit
NICE	National institute for health and clinical excellence
RP	Rehabilitation prescription
UKROC	UK rehabilitation outcomes collaborative

Contents

- Introduction
- The Multidisciplinary Team

- Role of the Rehabilitation Physician
- International Classification of Functioning Disability and Health
- Cost-Effectiveness
- Outcome Measures
- Rehabilitation Prescription
- Conclusion

Introduction

Rehabilitation is a process of assessment, treatment, management, and ongoing evaluation of the individual (and their family/carers) to achieve their maximum potential for physical, cognitive, social, and psychological function, participation in society and quality of life. Patients admitted to an ICU are prone to problems secondary to their length of stay, medications, interventions, and severity of their illness. These problems can be physical, emotional, psychological, or psychiatric in nature and may have long-lasting effects on a patient's quality of life following their discharge from the ICU (Figure 53.1). Early rehabilitation is essential in reducing these complications.

Rehabilitation should start as soon as an injury or a neurological event occurs. It usually involves the assessment, treatment, and management of an individual with repeated evaluation, and it continues throughout the patient's hospital stay as well as discharge to the community (Figure 53.2). Often the input is limited to assessment, giving advice, setting expectations, and organizing relatively simple interventions. A significant number of patients will have more complex needs requiring prolonged involvement from a multidisciplinary team with expertise in general rehabilitation. A smaller number will have highly complex needs, especially if there is neurological impairment, and require specialist rehabilitation.

The Multidisciplinary Team

Early rehabilitation involves a multitude of disciplines as well as family members and carers, working together to improve the quality of life of the patient. The multidisciplinary rehabilitation team consists of

- specialist physician in rehabilitation medicine (leader),
- physiotherapists (trained in managing patients on ventilators),
- occupational therapists,
- speech and language therapists (trained in tracheostomy management),

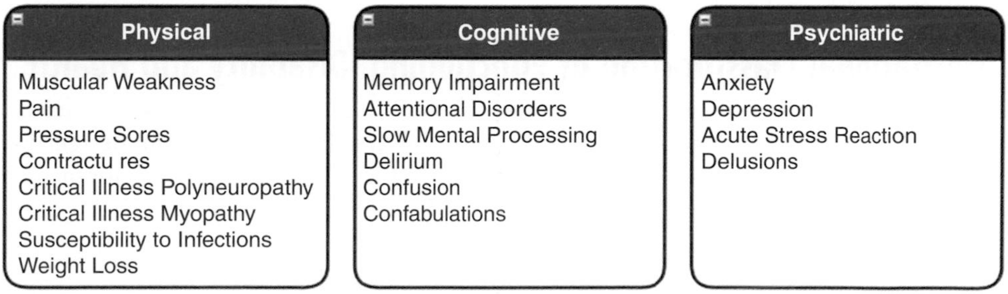

Physical
Muscular Weakness
Pain
Pressure Sores
Contractu res
Critical Illness Polyneuropathy
Critical Illness Myopathy
Susceptibility to Infections
Weight Loss
Cognitive
Memory Impairment
Attentional Disorders
Slow Mental Processing
Delirium
Confusion
Confabulations
Psychiatric
Anxiety
Depression
Acute Stress Reaction
Delusions

Figure 53.1 Consequence of prolonged intensive care stay

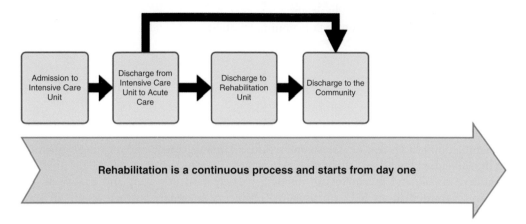

Figure 53.2 Process of rehabilitation

- clinical psychologists (trained in managing acute stress reactions),
- dieticians,
- pharmacists, and
- rehabilitation support worker/coordinators (role is to support families).

Maximizing physical, cognitive, social, and psychological function are some of the key areas the multidisciplinary team focus on during the process of rehabilitation, which often lasts years and undoubtedly goes beyond a patient's admission. The delivery of effective rehabilitation within the ICU environment can reduce the impact of subsequent physical and mental health impairment.

Role of the Rehabilitation Physician

In addition to leading a multidisciplinary team, the rehabilitation physician must be able to combine common medical skills in diagnosis, treatment, and general care of conditions causing complex disability. They must be knowledgeable about potential impairments and imposed restrictions in activity and participation a patient may acquire following a neurological illness and trauma.

The role of the rehabilitation physician is a vital one in the acute care pathway of a patient. This frequently involves advice on clinical matters as well as planning specialist services for patients with complex needs and networking to support local nonspecialist services. Some of the roles of the rehabilitation medicine physician in the acute care pathway are outlined in Figure 53.4.

International Classification of Functioning, Disability and Health

The International Classification of Functioning, Disability and Health (ICF) is a framework approved by the World Health Assembly in 2001, universally recognized and designed to allow a patient's health condition to be mapped alongside their medical and nonmedical needs within the rehabilitation process (Figure 53.3). The general principles of the classification are as follows:

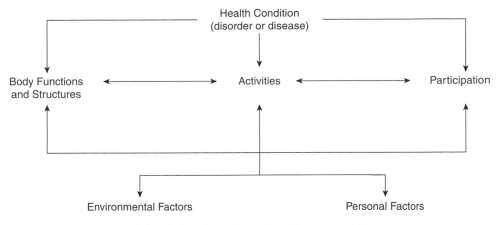

Figure 53.3 The International Classification of Functioning, Disability and Health (ICF) framework

Medical	Physical and Psychological	Other
•Advice regarding management of agitation, dysautonomia, pain, hypersalivation, autonomic dysreflexia, neurogenic bladder and bowel •Management of patients in post-traumatic amnesia, delirium and acute confusional state •Assessment and management of patients in prolonged disorder of consciousness •Advice about posture, tone and early mobility in the acute care setting •Advice regarding tracheostomy weaning •Advice regarding sleep disturbances	•Help the team with assessment of cognition and communication •Advice regarding prognosis and functional outcomes •Involved in decisions affecting the long-term rehabilitation •Assessment of long-term rehabilitation needs, sign positing and facilitating referrals to appropriate rehabilitation services •Assessments of mental capacity and best interest decisions •Prognostication •Advocacy role	•The development of a coordinated and resourced multidisciplinary team to ensure the delivery of rehabilitation during the acute care •Supporting the families •Improve communications within the MDT through regular team meetings, joint teaching and accurate sharing of patient information •Facilitating transition from intensive care to the general wards •Involving haedway and other charities in supporting families

Figure 53.4 Role of rehabilitation medicine physician in the acute setting

1. It is universally applicable to all patients and can be used without change by different clinicians.
2. The circumstances or disability of the patient does not alter the structure of the classification.
3. It has neutrality and environmental influences are captured within the model.

The model allows the clinician to individualize a patient's rehabilitation plan by separating different domains such as (1) body functions and structures, (2) activities, (3) participation, and (4) environmental factors. These domains are then interlinked with each other to aid a collaborative approach to a patient's rehabilitation needs.

Cost-Effectiveness

There is convincing evidence that early specialist rehabilitation for patients with complex needs is highly cost-effective. A recent study by Turner-Stokes (2016), looked at the cost-effectiveness of specialist inpatient rehabilitation for working-aged adults with complex neurological disabilities and found that the mean reduction in "care costs" was £760/week (~$900) in the high-dependency group, £408/week (~$500) in the medium-dependency, and £130/week (~$160) in the low-dependency group. The time taken to offset the cost of rehabilitation was 14.2 months in the high-dependency group, 22.3 months in the medium-dependency group, and 27.7 months in the low-dependency group. However, actual costs and savings will vary according to the health-care system.

Outcome Measures

A scoring system to measure disability was developed in the United States and subsequently adapted for the UK population. The FIM is used for measuring disability in a wide range of conditions and consists of 18 items each scored on seven levels, ranging from complete independence to total assistance required. The FIM can be scored alone or combined with the FAM which consists of 12 additional items addressing cognitive and psychological function, important in the assessment of brain-injured patients. The UK-adapted FIM and FAM are recognized as a reliable measure of independent functioning. Patients are scored on activities of daily living, physical ability, and cognitive/emotional rehabilitation, which is performed at varying intervals during their rehabilitation process with the results representing a quantitative measure of a patient's recovery.

In the United Kingdom, the Rehabilitation Outcomes Collaborative (UKROC) database collects all episodes for inpatient rehabilitation within specialist units. The dataset (apart from collecting FIM and FAM) consists of (1) a rehabilitation complexity scale, which measures the need for nursing and medical care along with therapy and equipment support; (2) a nursing dependency scale, measuring the need for skilled nursing; (3) a therapy dependency assessment, which measures the need for therapy interventions; and (4) a Barthel Index, which consists of ten items that measure a person's daily functioning, particularly the activities of daily living and mobility.

Rehabilitation Prescription

The RP may be used to document the rehabilitation needs of patients with severe illness/injury and identify how they will be addressed. Ideally, the RP should be initiated at an early stage, usually within 2 to 3 days of admission to the acute care service. It may be started by any suitably qualified member of staff, allied health professional or therapist, but is completed by the multidisciplinary team throughout the patient's journey. The prescription should be reviewed at regular intervals until the patient is discharged or transferred to a rehabilitation unit, when the RP is replaced by rehabilitation processes (goal setting, multidisciplinary reviews, etc.). In general, while RPs may vary between services, they have several different components as shown in Figure 53.5.

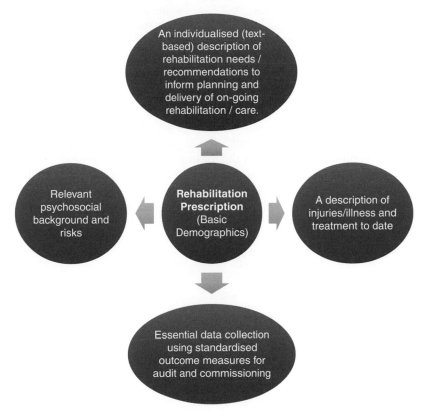

Figure 53.5 Components of the rehabilitation prescription

Conclusion

The importance of early rehabilitation in critical care has been recognized in the United Kingdom by the National Institute for Health and Clinical Excellence (NICE) Guidelines – "Rehabilitation after Critical Illness." These emphasize the importance of continuity of care throughout a patient's rehabilitation pathway and the need for clinicians coordinating a patient's rehabilitation, to have adequate competencies. Other key elements of the guidelines include regular reviews of rehabilitation goals; structured and appropriate therapy in a timely and safe manner; and liaising with appropriate primary, secondary, and tertiary services as applicable. These guidelines provide a reference for the transition from critical care to rehabilitation services. A well-coordinated and clinically led rehabilitation service, when started early in a patient's clinical pathway, can achieve good functional outcomes, improve quality of life and is cost-effective.

Further Reading

1. *Specialist Neuro-Rehabilitation Services: Providing for Patients with Complex Rehabilitation Needs*. London: British Society of Rehabilitation Medicine. 2010.

2. Needham D.M., Davidson J., Cohen H., et al. Improving long-term outcomes after discharge from intensive care unit: report from a stakeholders' conference. *Crit Care Med*. 2012; **40**:502–509.

3. Parker A., Sricharoenchai T., Needham D. M. Early rehabilitation in intensive care unit: preventing physical and mental health impairments. *Curr Phys Med Rehabil Reports* 2013; **1**(4): 307–314.

4. Turner-Stokes L., Paul S., Williams H. Efficiency of specialist rehabilitation in reducing dependency and costs of continuing care for adults with complex acquired brain injuries. *J Neurol Neurosurg Psychiatry* 2006; **77**:634–9.

5. Turner-Stokes L. Cost-efficiency of longer-stay rehabilitation programmes: can they provide value for money? *Brain injury* 2007; **21**:1015–21.

6. Turner-Stokes L., William H, Bill A., Bassett P., Sephton K. Cost-efficiency of specialist inpatient rehabilitation for working-aged adults with complex neurological disabilities: a multicentre cohort analysis of a national clinical data set. *BMJ Open* 2016; **6**: e010238.

7. Rehabilitation for patients in the acute care pathway following severe disabling illness or injury: BSRM core standards for specialist rehabilitation. Available from: www.bsrm.org.uk

8. Specialist Rehabilitation for Patients with Highly Complex Needs: D02 Service Specification. London 2013; Available from: www.endland.nhs.uk

9. Rehabilitation after Critical Illness: National Institute for Health and Clinical Excellence Clinical Guideline 83; March 2009. Available from: www.nice.org.uk

Chapter

54

Clinical Information Resources

Shymal Asher, Ricardo Andrade, and Keith J. Ruskin

Key Points

- Trusted, online medical resources such as PubMed and ClinicalKey provide access to high-quality, peer-reviewed information.
- A variety of web-based resources, such as BrainInfo and the Whole Brain Atlas can be used for background information for research and clinical care.
- Users are advised to verify information from non-reviewed websites with other trusted sources before using it for patient care.
- Accidental release of protected health information can result in large fines and loss of reputation.
- Computers that are used for patient care should be managed by an information technology professional.

Abbreviations

AANS   American Association of Neurological Surgeons
ATM   Automated teller machine
PIN   Personal identification number
SNACC   The Society of Neurosurgical Anesthesia and Critical Care

Contents

- Introduction
- PubMed
- Electronic Journals and Databases
- Privacy and Security
- Conclusions
- Further Reading

Learning Objectives

After reading this chapter, the learner will be able to:

- Use PubMed to quickly and efficiently find relevant articles in journals indexed by the National Library of Medicine.
- Use online journals and textbooks as references for research and at the point of care.

- Take appropriate precautions to prevent computers from being infected by malware and minimize the risk of protected health information being compromised.

Introduction

Clinical information from textbooks, specialty websites and latest journal articles is available to any clinician through the Internet. In addition, there has been a proliferation of smartphone applications allowing access to numerous medical resources. This chapter provides an update on clinical information resources, latest available applications for smartphones, and information security.

PubMed

PubMed (www.pubmed.gov) provides online searches of every journal indexed by the National Library of Medicine. The government of the United States provides this service free of charge. More than 24 million articles have been indexed in medical journals since the 1960s. If the article is available online, the reference will include a link to it. PubMed is free, and many hospitals and medical schools provide online access to the full text of journal articles through institutional subscriptions. Some health care institutions offer literature searches and online journals through Ovid (www.ovid.com) or ScienceDirect (www.sciencedirect.com). These fee-based services provide much of the information contained in PubMed, social sciences journals, and other medical resources. MEDLINE, the online version of Index Medicus, provides the information used by PubMed, Ovid, and other search engines. MEDLINE contains more than 25 million references, which may cause some searches to return thousands of articles, many of which may have nothing to do with the desired topic.

PubMed offers search tags that allow the context of a given keyword to be specified. Tags are enclosed in square brackets. For example, typing in Ruskin [au] will return any article in which Ruskin is an author. Adding English [la] to a search phrase will return only articles that are written in English. A search for malignant hyperthermia [majr] will return only articles in which malignant hyperthermia is a major topic. The tag [pt] refers to publication. Boolean operators are always capitalized and include 'AND,' 'OR,' and 'NOT.' A search for subarachnoid hemorrhage AND English [la] AND review [pt] will return review articles on subarachnoid hemorrhage that have been written in English. An easy-to-read tutorial is available on the website that will allow users who are using the system for the first time to conduct fast, productive literature searches in less than an hour. The tutorial offers tips on how to use the subject, author, publication type, and other information to limit results to just a few highly relevant articles. One quick way to create focused searches is to use the 'limits' tab on the PubMed home page, which offers useful check boxes to help narrow search results. PubMed Clinical Queries allows a busy clinician to do a highly focused literature search. Clinical Queries searches return articles pertaining to a specific clinical study category, and will also return systematic reviews and medical genetics citations. PubMed Health is designed for both clinicians and patients returning articles that focus on 'what works.'

Electronic Journals and Databases

Most medical journals and major textbooks offer web and print versions. Most publishers offer access to online journals for subscribers and charge nonsubscribers a fee for individual articles. Many anesthesia societies include a journal subscription in the membership fee. Anesthesiology (www.anesthesiology.org) and Anesthesia and Analgesia (www.anesthesia-analgesia.org) are available on the Internet to members of the American Society of Anesthesiologists (www.asahq.org) and International Anesthesia Research Society (www.iars.org). The Journal of Neurosurgical Anesthesiology (www.jnsa.com) is available to subscribers.

There are many specialty and disease-related societies with useful webpages. The Society of Neurosurgical Anesthesia & Critical Care (www.snacc.org) hosts a very useful bibliography that is regularly updated. It is organized by subject but is not searchable. There is also an outline of required knowledge in neuroanesthesia adapted from the American Board of Anesthesiologists guidelines. Washington University hosts a website devoted to cerebrovascular clinical trials that also details stroke scales and other useful links (www.strokecenter.org/trials). The tumor section of the AANS has a page with much useful information about brain tumors (www.tumorsection.org/patient/info.htm), and the AANS has some additional useful educational links (www.aans.org/education/).

ClinicalKey (www.clinicalkey.com) previously called MDConsult, is a fee-based service that offers access to textbooks, journal articles, and Clinics of North America. Some hospitals and most medical schools have purchased 'institutional subscriptions' that allow anesthesia providers, employees, and students to access journal articles and other resources. More information about how to gain access to institutional subscriptions is usually available from the medical library (Table 54.1 and Box 54.1).

Privacy and Security

Everyone should be concerned about the security of his or her computers and information. Unauthorized access to health information can have devastating consequences for physicians and their patients. Unintentional release of information about disease processes, medication use, or visits to health care providers can result in stigmatization, difficulty obtaining credit or employment, or disruption of family relationships. Most importantly, unintended release of information can result in a breach of trust between the patient and physician. In response to these concerns, the European Union, United States, Australia, Japan, and others have enacted stringent regulations that cover the sharing and protection of health information. Most of the requirements for storage and transmission of health care information in the United States are covered under the Health Insurance Portability and Accountability Act of 1996 (HIPAA) and the Health Information Technology for Economic and Clinical Health Act of 2009 (HITECH). In the United Kingdom, the relevant statute is the Data Protection Act 1998 and compliance is regulated and enforced by the Information Commissioner's Office. Any physician who uses a computer in a patient care setting should use precautions to maintain the security of patient information and ensure that it complies with institutional policies.

Attacks on personal computers in the form of viruses, keystroke loggers, and 'phishing' are a growing threat. Viruses are small programs attached to email messages or disguised as useful programs that once activated can destroy information or simply slow the computer down as they send copies of themselves to thousands of other computers. Viruses may also allow the computer to be remotely controlled, turning it to pornography websites, made to pose as a financial website to collect credit card information, relaying more phishing emails, and so forth. Keystroke loggers can be used to collect

Table 54.1 Internet Resources for Neurosurgical Anesthesiologists

Internet Resource	Website Address	Summary of Information Available
Braininfo	www.braininfo.org	Information about brain structures. Type the name of the structure for pictures and information
NeuronDB	http://senselab.med.yale.edu/neurondb/	Information about neurophysiology, including locations and types
Journal of Neurosurgical Anesthesiology	www.jnsa.com	A peer-reviewed journal devoted to neurosurgical anesthesiology
Society for Neurosurgical Anesthesia and Critical Care	www.snacc.org	US Neurosurgical Anesthesia Society
Whole Brain Atlas	www.med.harvard.edu/AANLIB/home.html	A neuroimaging primer with CT, MRI, and three-dimensional images of the brain
Stroke registry	www.strokecenter.org/trials	Inventory of ongoing cerebro-vascular trials and useful resources
American Association of Neurological Surgeons	www.aans.org/education/	Contains useful links, including a link to Neurosurgical Forum
Cochrane Reviews	www.cochrane.org	Free summaries of Cochrane Systematic Reviews; Evidence-Based Medicine (EBM) methods, definitions, etc.
Access Anesthesiology	http://accessanesthesiology.mhmedical.com/	McGraw-Hill Textbooks
Anesthesia and Analgesia Neuroanesthesia articles	www.anesthesia-analgesia.org/cgi/collection/neuroanesthesia	A collection of neuroanesthesia articles published in Anesthesia and Analgesia
Brain Trauma Foundation guidelines	http://braintrauma.org/	Guidelines with indications of the level of evidence for all aspects of head trauma management
Neurosciences search engine	www.neuroguide.com/	Extensive links to all aspects of the neurosciences

sensitive information such as credit card numbers, social security numbers, or login credentials for other websites. Unfortunately, the only sign that a computer may be infected is that the Internet connection seems much slower than it did before.

The most common method used by criminals to get credit card or bank account information is called phishing. This scam involves sending an email message that usually

---

BOX 54.1 Smartphone Applications for Medical Resources

Epocrates	A compendium of drug information, laboratory values, and calculators.
Dynamed	An evidence-based clinical reference tool for healthcare providers for use primarily at the point of care with clinically-organized summaries to answer most clinical questions in practice.
Read by QxMD	Provides a single place to keep up with new medical and scientific research and search PubMed.
Open Anesthesia	Sponsored by the International Anesthesia Research Society offering study resources for residents and anesthesiologists seeking CME through an encyclopedia and question banks.

---

alleges that the recipient's bank account has been corrupted and then directs the computer to a realistic webpage with a login screen. As soon as the ATM card number and PIN are entered, the criminals begin to withdraw money from the bank account or use personal information to steal the victim's identity. Needless to say, all suspicious messages should be deleted immediately and the financial institution contacted by telephone if fraud is suspected.

Fortunately, a few simple precautions, combined with common sense, can minimize the risk of information theft or damage. All access to websites, especially those of financial institutions, must be protected by a carefully chosen password, which should ideally consist of a series of letters, numerals, and punctuation marks. A good password is easy for its owner to remember but should be difficult for anyone else to guess. Passwords should never be given to anyone else, sent by email or posted on a webpage. Remote access to home computers that may not have the latest security updates should be allowed only when necessary. It can be difficult to remember many complex passwords, but a commercial password manager can securely store passwords and enable sharing between devices.

Hardware and software tools decrease the probability that a computer can be infected by a virus or be compromised by a hacker. Antivirus programs are an essential tool that should be installed on every computer. It is important to update the programs frequently because new viruses are released frequently, and 'zero-day' exploits (malware that takes advantage of a newly-discovered security problem) are increasingly common. Most of these programs also protect against known keystroke loggers and Trojan horses. Software or hardware firewalls prevent unauthorized programs from using an Internet connection and thus protect against spyware or adware. Router firmware should be updated regularly and old routers should be periodically replaced, as these devices may also have security issues.

Conclusions

A wealth of information is available to any clinician with access to a computer. Online literature searches and journal articles, continuing medical education, and clinical guidelines are just a few of the many resources available. The availability of many software and hardware tools along with a degree of common sense will help protect the security of patient information and minimize the risk of infection with a computer virus.

Further Reading

Saichaie, K., Benson, J., Kumar, A.B.: How we created a targeted teaching tool using blog architecture for anesthesia and critical care education–the A/e anesthesia exchange blog. *Med Teach* 2014 August; **36**(8):675–679.

Sharma, V., Chamos, C., Valencia, O., Meineri, M., Fletcher, S.N.: The impact of internet and simulation-based training on transoesophageal echocardiography learning in anaesthetic trainees: A prospective randomised study. *Anaesthesia* 2013 June; **68**(6):621–627.

Chu, L.F., Young, C.A., Zamora, A.K., et al: Self-reported information needs of anesthesia residency applicants and analysis of applicant-related web sites resources at 131 United States training programs. *Anesth Analg* 2011 February; **112**(2):430–439.

Liu, V., Musen, M.A., Chou, T.: Data breaches of protected health information in the United States. *JAMA* 2015 April 14; **313**(14):1471–1473.

Chapter

55

Case Scenarios

Claas Siegmueller and Oana Maties

Abbreviations

CPP	Cerebral perfusion pressure
CSF	Cerebrospinal fluid
CT	Computed tomography
DCI	Delayed cerebral ischemia
DCS	Direct cortical stimulation
ED	Emergency department
EVD	External ventricular drain
GBM	Glioblastoma multiforme
GCS	Glasgow Coma Scale
ICP	Intracranial pressure
MAP	Mean arterial pressure
MEP	Motor evoked potential
MILS	Manual in-line stabilization
MRI	Magnetic resonance imaging
PEEP	Positive end-expiratory pressure
SAH	Subarachnoid hemorrhage
SBP	Systolic blood pressure
SCI	Spinal cord injury
TBI	Traumatic brain injury

Contents

- Traumatic Brain Injury
  - Case Summary
  - Key Issues
    - Airway Management and Ventilation
    - Cerebral Perfusion Pressure Management
    - Blood Pressure Management
    - Intracranial Pressure Management
- Supratentorial Tumor
  - Case Summary
  - Key Issues
    - Preoperative Optimization
    - General Anesthesia for Motor Mapping
- Cervical Spine Injury
  - Case Summary
  - Key Issues
    - Steroid Therapy for Spinal Cord Injury
    - Anesthesia and Acute Spinal Cord Injury

Subarachnoid Hemorrhage

(See Chapters 16 and 35)

Case Summary

A 54- year-old female presented to the ED complaining of a severe headache, vomiting, and an episode of syncope that started suddenly 3 hours previously. She was alert, orientated, and without any neurological deficits. Past medical history included smoking and poorly controlled hypertension. A CT scan showed a SAH in the area of the anterior communicating artery. The patient was admitted to the intensive care unit for observation. An intra-arterial catheter was placed to help manage the blood pressure in the context of a suspected unsecured ruptured aneurysm. The patient had a cerebral angiogram performed the next day under general anesthesia which showed a ruptured 8 mm aneurysm on the left anterior communicating artery which was then treated by coil embolization.

Key Issues

Clinical Presentation and Treatment

SAH represents only 5% of all strokes but its mortality is high (around 40%). Risk factors for aneurysmal rupture include hypertension, smoking, alcohol use, and having a first degree relative with SAH. The initial management of patients focuses on airway protection if required, blood pressure treatment in order to avoid a rebleed and obtaining an urgent non-contrast CT. If the initial CT is negative but the clinical suspicion is high, a lumbar puncture is performed and a CSF sample is examined for xanthochromia. Aneurysms can be treated by surgical clipping or endovascular coiling, depending on their position and anatomical characteristics, as determined by angiography. There is good evidence to suggest that patients who had their aneurysms coiled have lower morbidity and disability but a slightly higher risk of rebleeding in both the short- and long-term future.

Endovascular treatment of the cerebral aneurysms is an expanding field and presents the anesthesiologist with challenges related to the environment (remote locations, ionizing radiation, and unfamiliar surroundings) and to managing the hemodynamic requirements related to the disease and treatment. Hypo and hypertension can both be detrimental to an unsecured aneurysm so the insertion of an intra-arterial catheter has become routine. Sedation is commonly used for diagnostic angiograms while general anesthesia is usually required for intervention as it provides better image quality. Good communication with the interventionalist and an understanding of the procedure are essential.

Neurological Complications

Rebleeding

The risk of rebleeding is higher in the first few days after hemorrhage, with 15% of patients affected in the first 24 hours. In patients who survive the first day, the risk of rebleeding decreases in a progressive fashion, with a cumulative risk of rebleeding of 40% in the first month without intervention. Strategies to prevent rebleeding include early intervention to secure the aneurysm and blood pressure management to ensure SBP <160 mmHg and/or MAP <110 mm Hg with unsecured aneurysms.

Hydrocephalus

Obstructive hydrocephalus has an incidence of 20%–30% in the first three days. It presents with a progressive deterioration of the level of consciousness over a few hours. In symptomatic patients, the management includes placement of an EVD. Sixty percent of these patients develop chronic hydrocephalus which requires placement of a shunt.

Delayed Cerebral Ischemia

Delayed cerebral ischemia (DCI) is defined as "the occurrence of focal neurological impairment (e.g., hemiparesis, aphasia, apraxia, hemianopia, or neglect), or a decrease of at least 2 points on the Glasgow Coma Scale (GCS – either on the total score or on one of its individual components) lasting for at least 1 hour, and cannot be attributed to other causes by means of appropriate studies." DCI occurs in 30% of SAH patients between days 3 and 14 and is the most significant cause of disability and mortality. Treatment includes, administering nimodipine (60 mg every four hours), maintaining euvolemia inducing hypertension, maintaining a hemoglobin concentration of 8–10 mg/dl and endovascular intervention with transluminal angioplasty and intra-arterial injection of arterial vasodilators.

Traumatic Brain Injury
(See Chapters 23, 33, and 34)

Case Summary

A 35-year-old male was brought to the ED following a motor vehicle accident. On admission his GCS was 7 (E2M3V2) and the pupils were noted to be unequal (R fixed at 3 mm and L reactive at 5 mm). The remaining physical examination was unremarkable. The patient was intubated with a rapid sequence induction using MILS, placed in a cervical collar, given 1 g/kg of mannitol 20% and transported urgently to the CT scan. The non-contrast CT showed a left 3.8 cm extradural hematoma with midline shift. The CT scan of the cervical spine revealed no bony abnormality. The patient was taken immediately to the operating room and a craniotomy was performed under general anesthesia to evacuate the hematoma. At the same time an EVD was placed. After the bone flap was replaced, the patient was transported intubated to the intensive care unit for further management.

Key Issues

Trauma patients often present with multiple injuries that need to be discovered during the initial examination and treated appropriately in order to maintain cardiovascular stability and oxygenation. While the primary injury to the brain tissue is very rarely reversible, the secondary injury can be minimized by interventions targeted at maintaining homeostasis.

Airway Management and Ventilation

Any patient with a GCS <8 or who is unable to protect their airway or maintain oxygen saturations >90% should have their airway secured by endotracheal intubation. Five percent of patients who have a severe TBI have also a cervical spine injury. Therefore, intubation is done with a rapid sequence induction and MILS in order to minimize the neck extension during laryngoscopy. The front part of the collar can be taken off during intubation to facilitate the placement of the laryngoscope blade. There is some evidence that videolaryngoscopes facilitate the intubation with less neck movement compared to traditional direct laryngoscopes. Succinylcholine is commonly used for muscle relaxation due to the optimal intubating conditions it provides, its short duration of action, and only a transient rise in ICP without proven long-term consequences. Ventilatory management of these patients targets normal oxygen saturations (PaO_2 > 60 mmHg) and normocarbia ($PaCO_2$, 35–40 mmHg) as both hypocarbia and hypercarbia can be detrimental. PEEP <10 cm H_2O will have minimal effect on the ICP and is used as part of the lung protective ventilation strategy and to improve oxygenation.

Cerebral Perfusion Pressure Management

CPP is managed by controlling MAP and ICP. The guidelines recommend CPP to be maintained between 50 and 70 mmHg. CPP over 70 mmHg in the absence of cerebral ischemia should be avoided due to high incidence of acute lung injury. The optimal CPP for any individual patient can be identified by multimodal neurological monitoring.

Blood Pressure Management

Systemic hypotension (SBP < 90 mmHg) is an independent predictor of poor outcome in brain injured patients. Intravenous isotonic crystalloids, inotropes, and vasopressors have to be titrated carefully in order to maintain adequate perfusion pressures, serum osmolarity, colloid oncotic pressure, and circulating blood volume. Systemic hypertension (SBP > 160 mmHg) can aggravate vasogenic brain edema and intracranial hypertension. As systemic hypertension may be a physiological response to reduced cerebral perfusion, lowering the blood pressure should be done cautiously, especially in the absence of ICP monitors.

Intracranial Pressure Management

Consensus guidelines recommend treatment of an ICP >20 mmHg. This is done by a combination of measures including: (1) head positioning to facilitate venous and CSF drainage, (2) hyperosmolar therapy including mannitol 0.25–1 g/kg intravenous bolus administration or hypertonic saline, (3) ventricular drainage if available, and (4) modest hyperventilation to achieve $PaCO_2$ of 30–35 mmHg. TBI patients have CBF in the ischemic range in the first 24 hours, so hyperventilation in this window may be detrimental. Resistant intracranial hypertension can be further managed with barbiturate therapy, further CSF drainage, moderate hypothermia (33°C–35°C) and decompressive craniectomy in selected cases.

Supratentorial Tumor

(See Chapters 11, 15, 20, 21, 49, and 50)

Case Summary

A 64-year-old woman with a past history of hypothyroidism was evaluated for progressively worsening headache with nausea and vomiting. CT and MRI revealed a 2.5 × 2.5 cm right periventricular mass arising from the right posterior parahippocampal gyrus having features consistent with a GBM. Imaging did not show hydrocephalus, midline shift, or other mass effect. No focal neurological signs were clinically detectable. Treatment with dexamethasone 3 mg three times a day was commenced. In addition, the patient received ondansetron 6 hourly, levetiracetam 500 mg twice daily for seizure prophylaxis and analgesics to treat her headache. Preoperatively, another MRI scan was performed with scalp fiducial markers to allow for calibration of a surgical navigation system. The plan was for surgery to involve intraoperative mapping of the motor cortex due to its proximity to the tumor.

After premedication with midazolam 2 mg, anesthesia was induced with propofol 2 mg/kg, lidocaine 1 mg/kg, two remifentanil boluses of 1 mcg/kg, and topical anesthesia of the larynx and trachea with lidocaine 4%. No muscle relaxants were used. Endotracheal intubation was performed. A radial intra-arterial catheter and a second intravenous cannula were placed in the right arm. The patient was positioned in a left semi-lateral position. The left arm and leg were covered in a clear sterile drape as to be visible to the surgical team during motor mapping. Maintenance of anesthesia was achieved with 65% nitrous oxide in oxygen, desflurane 0.3 MAC, and a remifentanil infusion of 0.2 mcg/kg/min. Phenylephrine 10–30 mcg/min infusion was administered as required to maintain a MAP >75 mmHg. The surgeon requested mannitol 1 g/kg and dexamethasone 10 mg to be given after induction and asked for hyperventilation to a target end-tidal carbon dioxide partial pressure of 35 mmHg.

During motor mapping the patient suffered a seizure which was not controlled by cold irrigation of the surgical field but abolished by a propofol bolus of 1 mg/kg. Following resection of the tumor nitrous oxide administration was stopped and desflurane increased to 0.9 MAC for surgical closure. After stopping the remifentanil infusion and administering repeated fentanyl 25 mcg boluses titrated to the patient's respiratory rate, extubation was performed "deep" to avoid coughing and straining during emergence.

Key Issues

Preoperative Optimization

Primary brain malignancies have no "typical" initial presentation and symptoms can range from a subtle headache to a new-onset seizure as a first sign. In addition, tumors can also cause focal neurological deficits depending on their location, for example, localized weakness and loss of sensation, visual field defects, or balance problems. ICP can be elevated, either due to a direct mass effect from the tumor, surrounding tissue edema or obstructive hydrocephalus.

Steroid therapy is often commenced at the time of diagnosis to provide some symptom relief by reducing peritumoral edema. For cases of obstructive hydrocephalus and markedly elevated ICP an EVD is sometimes placed before definitive surgery is attempted.

Seizure prophylaxis is empirically prescribed by many surgeons, although the evidence supporting this practice is weak. Phenytoin, once the traditional drug of choice for perioperative seizure prophylaxis, is now less frequently used in favor of levetiracetam which has a superior side-effect profile and reduced propensity for drug interactions.

General Anesthesia for Motor Mapping

Mapping of the motor cortex under general anesthesia typically involves eliciting MEPs through DCS with a hand-held probe by the surgeon. Motor responses on the contralateral side of the body are either observed clinically or measured with electrodes placed in relevant muscles.

Which general anesthetic technique is best for motor mapping is controversial. Volatile anesthetic agents cause a marked depression of MEPs, and should be avoided in concentrations >0.4 MAC. Nitrous oxide, propofol, or dexmedetomidine infusions can be used alternatively or as adjuncts for a balanced technique. Muscle relaxation is obviously not desirable. A single dose of an intermediately acting non-depolarizing muscle relaxant such as rocuronium for intubation is usually not problematic.

Depending on the electrical stimulation pattern used and duration of application, DCS can induce seizures in up to 9% of cases. The first step in treatment is immediate cold irrigation of the operative field by the surgeon. If unsuccessful, an intravenous bolus of either propofol or thiopental is given to abolish seizure activity.

Cervical Spine Injury

(See Chapters 24 and 25)

Case Summary

A 38-year-old male was admitted to ED after a fall while mountain-biking. He had been positioned on a spinal board and his neck immobilized with a hard collar at the scene. On arrival to the hospital the patient was alert and orientated, denying previous loss of consciousness. Examination of the airway and cardiovascular system was unremarkable. However, the patient was found to have diaphragmatic breathing, complete paralysis of both lower limbs, partial paralysis of the upper limbs, and absence of sensation below the C5 dermatome. During "log-rolling" a loss of anal sphincter tone and lower cervical spine midline tenderness were detected. The remainder of the primary and secondary survey examination were normal. CT of the spine showed anterior column injury with a C6 vertebral body fracture and spinal cord compression. The decision was made not to administer high-dose steroids. Within a few hours, the patient was transferred to the operating room for anterior decompression, cervical vertebrectomy, cage, and bone graft implant, along with plate spinal fusion. Following premedication with glycopyrrolate 0.2 mg iv, general anesthesia was induced with a rapid sequence induction and cricoid pressure using propofol 3 mg/kg, fentanyl 1.5 mg/kg, and suxamethonium 1.5 mg/kg. Intubation was performed with MILS of the cervical spine and videolaryngoscope assistance. An intra-arterial catheter was placed for invasive blood pressure monitoring. The patient remained hemodynamically stable during induction and surgery and was extubated uneventfully.

Key Issues

The main goal of management of patients with SCI is to prevent or limit secondary neurological injury while providing general organ support. The anesthesiologist's focus is on airway maintenance while immobilizing the spine and providing respiratory support as needed, particularly for high cervical injuries. These can lead to loss of intercostal function and more importantly, diaphragmatic function if the SCI affects C3 to C5, i.e., the phrenic nerve origin. In addition, hemodynamic instability, particularly during induction of general anesthesia in the acute spinal shock phase, can present a challenge.

Steroid Therapy for Spinal Cord Injury

High-dose steroids have been used to limit secondary injury in acute SCI for decades. A few large trials support their use in improving neurological outcome, but have been criticized for methodological flaws. Furthermore, it is not clear whether improved neurological outcome translates into better functional results for these patients. On the other hand, there is convincing evidence that steroid administration in the context of SCI is linked to a higher incidence of respiratory complications, in particular pneumonia, and more ventilator days. An increasing number of centers therefore do not routinely administer steroids to SCI patients.

Anesthesia and Acute Spinal Cord Injury

Recent evidence supports early decompression, less than 24 hours after trauma, to improve neurological outcome in SCI. Patients with a high thoracic or cervical SCI presenting to the operating room for early surgical intervention display varying degrees of a neurogenic "spinal shock" due to a loss of sympathetic innervation with preserved parasympathetic tone, causing vasovagal hypotension and brady-arrhythmias, mainly in the first 24 hours following injury. As these can be particularly problematic during induction of general anesthesia and intubation, premedication with glycopyrrolate or atropine is a useful preventative measure.

Administering suxamethonium to patients with SCI should be avoided between 72 hours and 9 months following injury. Loss of upper motor neuron innervation from an SCI effectively causes a spread of motor synaptic endplates over the whole muscle cell membrane, a situation in which depolarizing muscle relaxants can cause a large potassium efflux, and significant acute hyperkalemia.

Maintaining spine immobilization while managing the airway is crucial. During bag-mask ventilation and laryngoscopy, MILS is preferred over a rigid collar. MILS is more effective in limiting cervical movement and allows better mouth opening, which in turn facilitates laryngoscopy. Of the basic airway maneuvers, only jaw thrust does not inevitably extend the cervical spine. Head tilt and chin lifting must be avoided. Although direct laryngoscopy causes movement mostly in the atlanto-occipital joint, extension might also occur at lower vertebral levels, particularly if injured. There is conflicting evidence, depending on which device is used, whether videolaryngoscopy significantly reduces cervical spine movement compared to conventional laryngoscopy. Application of cricoid pressure in cervical SCI is also a controversial issue, and if used should be applied bi-manually, i.e., one hand applying cricoid pressure and the other supporting the cervical spine from the back to prevent accidental movement.

Index